DISABLED CHILDREN: CONTESTED CARING, 1850–1979

STUDIES FOR THE SOCIETY FOR THE SOCIAL HISTORY OF MEDICINE

Series Editors: *David Cantor*
Keir Waddington

TITLES IN THIS SERIES

www.pickeringchatto.com/sshm

DISABLED CHILDREN: CONTESTED CARING, 1850–1979

EDITED BY

Anne Borsay and Pamela Dale

PICKERING & CHATTO
2012

Published by Pickering & Chatto (Publishers) Limited
21 Bloomsbury Way, London WC1A 2TH

2252 Ridge Road, Brookfield, Vermont 05036-9704, USA

www.pickeringchatto.com

BRITISH LIBRARY CATALOGUING IN PUBLICATION DATA

Disabled children : contested caring, 1850–1979. – (Studies for the Society for
the Social History of Medicine)
1. Children with disabilities – Care – History – 19th century. 2. Children with
disabilities – Care – History – 20th century. 3. Children with disabilities – Services for – History – 19th century. 4. Children with disabilities – Services for
– History – 20th century.
I. Series II. Borsay, Anne. III. Dale, Pamela, 1975–
362.4'083'0903-dc23

ISBN-13: 9781848933613
e: 9781781440087

Typeset by Pickering & Chatto (Publishers) Limited
Printed and bound in the United Kingdom by the MPG Books group

CONTENTS

ACKNOWLEDGEMENTS

This volume began as a conference, entitled 'Children, Disability and Community Care from 1850 to the Present Day', held at Sketty Hall, Swansea, in October 2007. The event was co-organized by Anne Borsay and Pamela Dale with support from Swansea University School of Health Science. The University of Exeter Centre for Medical History generously supported the conference as part of a 2003–8 Wellcome Trust Strategic Award entitled 'Health, Heredity and the Environment, 1850–2000'. We would like to thank all our Swansea and Exeter colleagues, especially Professors Joseph Melling and Mark Jackson, for their assistance. Thanks are also due to the Society for the Social History of Medicine (SSHM) who did much of the publicity work and Claire Keyte (Centre Co-ordinator) who handled the administration. The conference presentations and discussions helped shape this volume at all stages of production and we are indebted to all the delegates for their thoughtful contributions. We would also like to thank David Cantor (SSHM Series Editor) and staff at Pickering and Chatto for all their assistance with the production of the volume.

ACKNOWLEDGEMENTS

NOTES ON CONTRIBUTORS

María José Báguena, MD and PhD, is a Senior Lecturer in the History of Science at the Institute of History of Medicine and Science López Piñero, University of Valencia. Her research focuses on the history of infectious diseases, public health and Valencian medicine.

Rosa Ballester, MD and PhD, is Professor of History of Science at the Miguel Hernández University in Alicante (Spain). She has done extensive research on the social history of paediatrics, public health and the history of poliomyelitis.

Anne Borsay is Professor of Healthcare and Medical Humanities in the College of Human and Health Sciences at Swansea University. She is currently writing a cultural history of disability in Britain between 1500 and 2000 which examines how disabled people are represented in literature and the visual arts.

Pamela Dale is an Honorary Research Fellow based in the Centre for Medical History, University of Exeter. She has published many journal and book articles exploring public health and learning disability topics.

Staffan Förhammar is Professor of History at The History Unit/Department for Studies of Social Change and Culture (ISAK), Linköping University, Linköping, Sweden. He is a pioneer in the study of disability history in the Swedish context.

Corinne Manning is a Research Fellow at Monash University, Victoria, Australia. Her work on the Kew Cottages History project has led to numerous publications and Corinne has also written about aspects of Aboriginal culture and Australian peacekeepers.

Mike Mantin is currently undertaking a PhD studentship at Swansea University on disability history in Wales. His thesis will focus on the Cambrian Institution for the Deaf and Dumb in Swansea.

Lee-Ann Monk is an Honorary Research Associate in the History Programme at La Trobe University, Australia. In 2005, she won an Australian Research Council (ARC) Post-doctoral Fellowship (Industry) to research the history of Kew Cottages, Australia's first purpose-built institution for people with learning disabilities. Lee-Ann is currently completing a book on the history of the Cottages.

Marie Clark Nelson is Professor of Social History at The History Unit/Department for Studies of Social Change and Culture (ISAK), Linköping University, Linköping, Sweden. Although her dissertation dealt with hunger crises in the Swedish context, her later work has dealt with the development of health legislation and the ways in which societies have responded to epidemics of infectious diseases.

José Martínez-Pérez, MD and PhD in Medicine, is a Senior Lecturer at the University of Castilla-La Mancha (Spain) in the History of Science Unit at the Faculty of Medicine where he is currently Dean. He has published many papers on the relationship between medicine and social exclusion, focusing on mental illness, hygiene and occupational safety. He is currently undertaking research on the history of disability in Spain.

María Isabel Porras, MD and PhD, is Senior Lecturer in History of Science in the Medical Faculty of Ciudad Real at the University of Castilla-La Mancha (Spain). Her main research fields are the history of diseases, the history of physical disabilities and social protection. She has published widely on the history of physical disabilities.

Amy Rebok Rosenthal received a PhD in history from Indiana University in 2010 and is Chair of the Department of History at Pacific Union College, located above the Napa Valley in Angwin, California. Her research interests include children in Victorian society and the history of medicine in nineteenth-century Britain.

Matthew Smith is a Lecturer and Wellcome Trust Research Fellow at the University of Strathclyde's Centre for the Social History of Health and Healthcare. His monograph, *An Alternative History of Hyperactivity: Food Additives and the Feingold Diet*, was published by Rutgers University Press in 2011.

Pat Starkey is an Honorary Research Fellow in the School of History at the University of Liverpool. Her principal research interests are in the history of charities and voluntary social work agencies working with families, women's history and the history of social work.

Steven Thompson is a lecturer in modern history in the Department of History and Welsh History at Aberystwyth University. His research has focused on various aspects of Welsh history and he has published work in the fields of medical, labour and sports history. His monograph, entitled *Unemployment, Poverty and Health in Interwar South Wales*, was published by the University of Wales Press in 2006.

Angela Turner received her PhD from the University of Strathclyde in 2010 for her work on the history of learning disability in Glasgow since 1945. This project was funded by the University of Strathclyde. Current areas of interest include the history of special education, social work, community care and voluntary organizations. Angela has worked at developing inclusive research methodologies using 'life story' approaches with people with learning disabilities.

Sue Wheatcroft completed her PhD thesis exploring the impact of the Second World War on disabled children at the University of Leicester in 2009. She is currently an Honorary Visiting Fellow at the University of Leicester. Sue has presented numerous conference papers on aspects of urban history, children living with learning disabilities, voluntary action and post-war planning.

INTRODUCTION:
DISABLED CHILDREN – CONTESTED CARING

Anne Borsay and Pamela Dale

The essays in this volume span many countries and different time periods, but they are united by a common set of approaches to childhood disability. These stem from seeing experiences as the outcome of personal circumstances and social structures, and offer an experiential critique of the dominant 'social model' originating in disability studies and developed within materialist histories of disability. The 'social model' tends to emphasize 'disabling' factors contributing to the exclusion of disabled people from the mainstream of society and contrasts with 'individual models of disability' that rely on notions of personal impairment. The intention of this volume is to develop a sense of contested caring. Rather than concentrate on the role of institutional factors contributing to disability the focus is on exploring how they shaped experiences of childhood disability in a variety of complex, unpredictable and sometimes contradictory ways. The book explores the varied, but distinctive, experiences of disabled children through their interaction with a range of specialist educational (Chapters 4 and 11) and medical services (Chapters 1, 2, 5, and 7–10). Provision for disabled children initially evolved in an institutional context (see Chapters 1–5, 7 and 9) and such segregated care often involved lengthy separations from families and communities. Over time the reach of these services was extended, and care was offered in new ways. Specialist provision could still be offered in residential institutions, but day-services were also important and the home, the school and the clinic became centres for diagnosing and treating various disabling conditions (Chapters 3, 6, 8 and 10–12). The imperative to provide such care meant that countries (and regions within them) that developed children's services could present themselves as modern and progressive (Chapter 9), while 'slow adopters' had to excuse and overcome their own 'backwardness' (Chapter 3). Most important for this volume, whether 'modern' or 'backward', these varied and changing institutional contexts helped to shape the often complicated experiences of disabled children.

This is not the first history of disability to explore the kinship and community support networks available to groups of people with special needs in different places at various times, or to combine such analysis with an assessment of the emergence of specialist provision. Nor is it the first to highlight the shared experiences of disabled people (across time and space) or to connect historical study with the identity politics associated with the modern disability rights movement. On the contrary, a growing historiography has highlighted the role of class, gender, race, type and severity of any disability as important determinants of a disabled person's life chances and experiences of care. What differentiates this volume is its focus on childhood. The book starts from the premise that the experiences of disabled children, now and in the past, are fundamentally different from those of disabled adults. It is further argued that the distinctive voice of the disabled child has been silenced by both the historical marginalization of disabled people and the focus of the disability rights movement on adult priorities. We argue that the social model is especially relevant to the experiences of adults of working age living with a physical or sensory disability. This helps explain why historical studies of disability issues have tended to overlook childhood experiences.

The voices and experiences of disabled children have been buried within the historical record, but they can be recovered by paying attention to what was distinctive about the services offered to disabled children and their families. This volume seeks to highlight why children were singled out by pioneering service providers, and how these organizations and facilities shaped experiences of childhood disability. It foregrounds the role of the state and a particular conceptualization of the respective roles of families and experts in raising the citizens of the future. A series of nineteenth- and twentieth-century reforms, in many western countries, tended to reconfigure the relationship between children and parents and between the family and the state. Children received additional protections, and greater investment, but this was accompanied by increasing surveillance over their development. As restrictions on child labour made children economically worthless, parents were encouraged to see their offspring as emotionally priceless in ways that complicated responses to childhood disability.[1] There were an increasing number of experts available to encourage and even coerce families into engaging with officially approved health and education services. The very operation of such services, and their bureaucratic and professionally determined boundaries, helped forge the identities – and shaped the experiences – of disabled children.[2]

Scholars from many disciplines have developed important insights into the historical experiences of disabled children, aided by a growing commitment to inclusive participant research.[3] Yet, paradoxically, the involvement of adult activists, and the promotion of the social model, tends to divert historical attention elsewhere for two main reasons. Firstly, although concern about the health of children, and the development of specialist medical and other care for sick and disabled children, is evident over many centuries,[4] the only really distinctive historiography concentrates on the development of special schools. It is the evaluation of this limited provision that has tended to marginalize the historical experiences of disabled children. This volume redresses this imbalance by exploring a wider range of institutional contexts for care while also building on insights from histories of the special schools where these adopt the conceptualization of sick and disabled children as children in need. This was an important spur to voluntary and statutory assistance. Yet hand-in-hand with an impulse to care often went a desire to control. Interest in the care/control paradox unites many strands of the historiography but reveals more about the intentions of service-providers than client responses. The purpose of this volume is to identify the shared experiences of disabled children, to distinguish them from those of both non-disabled children and disabled adults, and to examine the debates through which their care and control were contested.

The second reason for overlooking disabled children is a tendency, within the social model, for the promotion of independence to inadvertently foster the historical neglect of groups reliant on support services managed by third parties. Jan Walmsley has raised this concern in relation to provision for adults with learning disabilities, but disabled children are also vulnerable.[5] The marginalization of the history of disabled children, which struggles to escape the care/control paradox, is not easily corrected with reference to the social model. Therefore, while many have found it theoretically robust, and personally and professionally empowering, the promotion of the social model, unaligned with a careful appreciation of the historical development of children's services, may be unhelpful in shaping current and future provision.

The Social Model and Services for Disabled Children

This volume argues that one of the ways to overcome the limitations of the social model is to recognize that the delivery of children's services, now and in the past, is complicated by factors that are perhaps less relevant to the experiences of disabled adults. Compared to the oft-mentioned neglect of the elderly and chronic sick (viewed as economically unproductive), children were historically targeted for interventions that were meant to promote their independence. Thus a child with a hearing or visual impairment unremarkable in an older person was increasingly classified as having special needs and brought within the ambit of targeted medical and educational provision. Disabled children, now and in the past, therefore arguably had to navigate their way through a larger array of services than disabled adults. This journey was complicated by other issues. A variety of experts historically claimed jurisdiction over the disabled child. This inevitably created conflict over the best methods of care and questions about accessing and financing this. Care was contested within as well as between groups offering health and education services. There was also potential for conflict between service providers and service users, since the child's right to either have or refuse medical treatment/ specialist educational services was contingent upon a number of factors that changed over time. An important determinant of the care historically offered to disabled children was the triangular relationship between service-providers, their parents and themselves. Each was fraught with difficulties, resulting in conflicts that shaped the experiences of many disabled children.

Modern public policy documents rightly stress that service users are *The Same as You*,[6] but historically specialist provision for disabled children was shaped by notions of difference. Research also suggests that parents tended to parent their disabled children differently. For example, parents are typically very boisterous when handling blind infants apparently with the hope of eliciting the anticipated welcoming smile spontaneously given by sighted babies.[7] These emotionally charged experiences now, and particularly in the past, are not easily captured by the social model. There are two further departures from the social model that need to be considered when evaluating the historic experiences of disabled children. Both relate to the dependence of the child on carers (usually adults who do not define themselves as living with a disability) who may be isolated from (and even rejecting of) groups representing the rights of disabled people. Parents (and other carers) may prefer to stress the individuality of their child and/or the common humanity of all children rather than a distinct and separate identity that celebrates difference. Disabled children (or more realistically carers making decisions for them in early life) are also likely to either seek or be forced to accept a medical model of care (especially during the initial diagnosis and stabilization phase) that still focuses on individual pathology and the disabled body/mind rather than social barriers to inclusion.[8]

While professionals can downplay the historic difficulties of inclusion,[9] parents were and are often acutely conscious of problems with other children at home and at school.[10] Changing expert opinion has also been problematic. Parents have been especially worried about their mid-twentieth-century designation by experts as a 'disabled family', and have also explicitly rejected scientific work that had identified 'the neurotic or rejecting mother' behind every atypical child.[11] These concerns, and an explicit need to protect others, introduce a certain negativity into (auto)biographical work that otherwise celebrates either the personal achievements of a person living with a disability or the dedication of their carers.[12] In one of the first parent-authored books about raising an autistic child in the USA, Clara Claiborne Park mentions the interactions between E and her siblings but more attention is given to the way the other children were protected from any negative consequences stemming from either E's behaviour or the parents' understandable preoccupation with E's care.[13] A similar set of issues appear in contributions from British parents. Interestingly recent work tends to echo much earlier books, although the role/attitudes of professionals and the availability of paid domestic help does show significant periodicity.[14]

Each of the books written by parents tells the unique history of their family and its response to raising a disabled child but many common themes emerge. Yet, it is difficult to avoid the conclusion that it is the more affluent and articulate parents who have historically found opportunities to record their experiences. In the same way organizations seeking to elicit donations and/or state support traditionally published the life-stories of their most successful former clients with little regard to their true representativeness. A not-untypical example appears in Chapter 7 where Staffan Förhammar and Marie Nelson discuss the much-publicized case of Petter Bernhard Savela who overcame poverty, illegitimacy, abuse and ill-health with the assistance of the Apelviken institution before making his fortune in real estate. This type of selection, providing at best a snapshot of events, tends to further isolate the child receiving care from their wider family environment. Yet services designed to prevent, identify and even treat various disabling conditions in the home have been amongst the most maligned in contemporary and historical accounts. The health-visiting activities described by Pamela Dale (Chapter 8) were clearly often viewed as intrusive by families and also, significantly, failed to attract support from sections of the medical community.

The health visiting profession is often described as an uncertain one,[15] but doubts about the care (and control) needs of disabled children infused the responses of state agencies, philanthropists, citizens and parents across the whole period covered by this volume. Indeed the proliferation of services, and fears that other countries were doing more and progressing further in developing their human resources, was as much a feature of Cold War politics as the earlier, and better known, boost twentieth-century conflicts gave to health and welfare reform. Even where the immediate physical needs of disabled children were apparently met there was increasing anxiety about their intellectual and emotional development and mental health issues (see Chapters 10–12). The gradual expansion of children's services could provide more resources for the disabled child, but all too often the preference for specialist and targeted services only contributed to the marginalization of disabled children and adults. Paradoxically the recent policy commitment for inclusion can also work to the detriment of people with special needs as there is pressure to open up specialist resources, often acquired at great difficulty in the past through dedicated fund-raising, to general access.[16]

These issues and debates, and different perspectives on them, help explain the 'subjectivity and contingency of historical accounts' noted by Felicity Armstrong in her survey of research and literature relating to the history of the education of disabled children.[17] It can be argued that scholars interested in the experiences of disabled children face unique difficulties. Thus while the focus on experiences has been aided by the search for new source material (including oral histories), multiple and discordant voices have often emerged from such materials leaving partial, fragmentary and confused accounts. The history of disabled children is beset by difficulties surrounding both memory and the ownership of narratives belonging to families and communities as well as individuals. These problems, perhaps inherent in studies of all socially marginal groups, have received most discussion in relation to the history of insanity, but even in this field the historiography benefits from active participation by those who define themselves as either living with or recovering from mental health issues.[18] By contrast, in the case of disabled children the situation is more complicated because children are unable to independently critique the historiography, determine research goals or even collaborate with investigators. Parents and parent groups may wish to speak for children, but their interest in the history of services is shaped by competition for the right to make decisions about their future configuration and individual placements within them.[19] Implicit within these discussions is often a rejection of earlier care practices and the assumptions that underpinned them in a way that prohibits developing an understanding of either past experiences or historic opportunities for participation, negotiation and resistance.

Recovering the voices of disabled children is all the more difficult because capturing them was not the main purpose of surviving records. Indeed official documents often silenced the child by denying the legitimacy of their experiences and prioritizing the opinions of professionals, and to a lesser extent parents. This theme is explored by Lee-Ann Monk and Corinne Manning with reference to the Kew Cottages in Australia (Chapter 5), and is also documented by Amy Rebok Rosenthal in Chapter 2, dealing with an English asylum. Educationalists were perhaps keener to tell children's stories, especially as an aid to fundraising, but also placed limits on what children could say for themselves and had predetermined ideas about the prospects of their pupils. Mike Mantin (Chapter 4) shows how desired outcomes for deaf pupils were determined by ideas about class and gender as well abilities and disabilities. The disappointments, isolation and stigma experienced by these children often have to be inferred from silences in the records. Psychological trauma arising from separation from home and parents, as well living with a serious disabling condition, also tends to be understated in documents created by residential services for physically disabled children. However, the records do at least hint at some of the physical and emotional pain experienced by child patients at the House of Charity (Chapter 1) and Apelviken in Sweden (Chapter 9). Similar hints of the suffering of disabled children who had not gained access to specialist medical services can be found in work on the coalfield communities (Chapter 3) and health visitors (Chapter 8), although these narratives were designed to advocate for better provision not relate individual experiences.

The chapters of this book are organized chronologically. As we move towards the present day it might be assumed that parents and professionals, responding to the evolving disability rights movement, offered disabled children more opportunities to speak for themselves and determine their own care. Where documentary and other sources become more child-centric over time it is certainly easier for scholars to recover both the voice and experiences of the child but this process was neither automatic nor straightforward. Although it is erroneous to assume that children in the distant past were totally silenced it is also inaccurate to suggest that later generations of professionals (and parents) consistently sought to empower children. Attention to the rights of children and parents involved recognition of tension between the two and also risked conflicting with professional interests. Arguably children were only empowered when and where professionals committed to this agenda. This orientation also served to encourage the collection of oral testimony and retrospective accounts from service-users. The rich potential of these initiatives is shown by Angela Turner's evaluation of special education in Glasgow (Chapter 11). Yet, this chapter demonstrates it is often painful and difficult to tell these personal stories; when they challenge powerful state bureaucracies it may even be dangerous. This theme is developed further in relation to the Spanish polio survivors (Chapter 9), whose experiences have only come to light as a result of political change in that country. Here recent activism associated with maintaining and improving services for survivors in the present day has facilitated efforts to understand the past through discussions that highlight personal, family and community experiences of disability.

The importance of these factors is highlighted by Chapter 10 where Sue Wheatcroft explores child guidance services for 'hard to place' evacuees. While there is a growing historiography (drawing on oral testimony and written records) about child evacuees this group is conspicuous by its absence. We argue that this is because there is no survivor network in place to help this group identify itself and no independent way of tracing its former members, many of whom had only a brief encounter with facilities that quickly disappeared. Vulnerable people need help to tell their stories from contemporary actors as well as current scholars and activists. Here the attitude of professionals appears to have been unhelpful. In its pioneer days the child guidance movement was inward looking and expert-led so the voice of the child is often absent. Similar problems of relating expert debates to actual experiences apply to the chapters looking at advice literature and hyperactivity (Chapters 6 and 12). In both cases professional concerns were heavily mediated by the way parents responded to the advice and modified their own practices. Very young children typically retain limited personal memories of this period of their lives. Although some parents do recount their experiences it is not entirely clear how their parenting styles were influenced by either the child's disability or their own or other people's response to it. In the case of hyperactivity, the willingness of parents to talk about their child's problems and their efforts to overcome them have dominated the debates. Work by Matthew Smith and others is only just starting to probe their children's responses. In these accounts, it is noticeable that some of these now adult children are supportive of their parent's faith in various experts, but others reject not just the recommended treatments but the idea that they had a disability. It is difficult to assess how influential the advice literature was without a defined set of service users, for example patients admitted to a specific institution. However, it is probable that people who were unusually accepting or rejecting of the advice offered are prominent amongst those coming forward to share their experiences. And, these are likely to be presented as personal biographies and family sagas that will tend to downplay wider social, economic and political issues. The family is obviously central to the experience of growing up, but for the disabled child the role of the state (and/or wider community support networks) also needs to be kept in focus.

The State and the Disabled Child

This volume explores the experiences of disabled children with particular emphasis on the contested nature of their care. Discussions about the contested delivery of publicly-funded care and the development of state services, usually under expert direction, foreground these issues. While individuals may or may not have viewed themselves as a disabled child, expert opinion in our study period offered strict, though changing, definitions of childhood and disability and allocated people to services deemed appropriate for them. The very existence of such provision did much to define what disability was (as definitions expanded from conditions easily recognized by lay people to those requiring expert diagnosis) and how different conditions should be managed.[20] Growing interest in both children and disability issues was an international phenomenon that dated from the mid-nineteenth century. In this volume, Pat Starkey (Chapter 1) locates pioneering initiatives to support disabled children within a network of charitable activities and highlights the importance of religious beliefs and royal patronage in creating and sustaining services. In the United Kingdom, and elsewhere, medical innovators and/or educationalists combined with philanthropists to develop new provision for various groups of disabled children. At other times these pioneering projects developed under the aegis of the local and national state, sometimes as part of national projects that celebrated and furthered the role of the state (Chapters 7 and 9 dealing with tuberculosis care in Sweden and polio services in Spain). Conflict within and between states also provided an important impetus for service-development, although a focus on children as the future of the nation encouraged a certain ambiguity towards disabled children. Such children were simultaneously viewed as potential future citizens and also a likely source of deviance and dependency. These issues are explored in an important collection of essays edited by Roger Cooter, but his focus on childhood tends to neglect the experiences of different groups of disabled children.[21] By the mid-twentieth century, Matthew Smith (Chapter 12) argues that 'disabilities' were not conceived in terms of recognizing an individual's special needs but were instead defined by an inability to contribute to the goals of the state.

Throughout this volume the case studies reveal that the expansion of state services for disabled children was a contested process. Here it is essential to recognize that the much-discussed maternalist policies adopted by many nation states in the first decades of the twentieth-century did not start from the position of a blank canvas. Parents, and others, had an established concern with child health although changing expert opinion increasingly politicized debates about child rearing.[22] Increased state support for and surveillance over families went hand in hand with anxieties about the financial commitment involved. This encouraged discussion about the most appropriate balance of providers in a mixed economy of care. There was also a concern to enforce rather than undermine family responsibilities while promoting the future economic independence of the disabled child by providing specialist training that the family might well not be able to afford. All these themes are discussed by Steven Thompson (Chapter 3), who draws attention to the often neglected point that provision, both in terms of the scope of services and their underlying ideologies, varied as much within as between different countries.

Childhood disability was an issue for all social groups. Yet the organization of state services meant that the poorest were singled out for official intervention. In the past it was too readily assumed that socially marginal groups had a disproportionate number of inherent defects. Anxiety about the implications of this for the future of national economies, social and political institutions, and gene pools fed unattractive eugenic arguments while also providing a spur to service development.[23] Nowadays there is greater recognition that disabling conditions are both the cause (through loss of family income and additional expenses incurred to meet special needs) and consequence (as people in poor districts are exposed to worse environmental conditions, have greater vulnerability to life-changing accidents, are more likely to suffer nutritional deprivation, and have less access to preventative healthcare and treatment services) of poverty,[24] but this can still lead to suspicion of clients of health and welfare services (whose case records and the negative comments therein are accessible to researchers).[25]

This source-base paradoxically may lead historians to neglect the experiences of other disabled children whose parents made private arrangements for their care.[26] Since the role of experts has been identified as a problem in the care of all disabled children it seems possible that wealthier children suffered disproportionately from more frequent contacts with a wider range of professionals. This might encourage parents to either pursue overly aggressive treatment options and the often vain search for a cure,[27] or send the child away to a private institution.[28] Health surveillance and the identification/treatment of conditions that the child might not experience as disabling but surrounding adults had a problem with were also likely to be earlier (and more intense) experiences for the more affluent family.[29] The quest for the perfect child in the twentieth century increasingly required interventions by medical experts (including the recent involvement of geneticists), often with mixed results for the child.[30] Wealthier children were not necessarily healthier children, or less prone to congenital or acquired disabilities.[31] An important collection of essays edited by Mark Jackson makes it clear that although there was persistent concern on both sides of the Atlantic about the threats to health posed by the material (and moral) environment of slum dwellings there were periods in the twentieth century when the hazards of the middle-class home received even greater scrutiny.[32]

It remains true, however, that the majority of children living with disabling conditions fell into the ambit of state-supported services and were assessed as being dependent as well as disabled in some way. The problematic association of dependence with deviancy cannot be overlooked when evaluating services and children's involvement with them but it is important not to forget the difference small services could make to deprived children's lives. In the United Kingdom, the Edwardian School Medical Service first noticed that many needy children were unable to read because of poor eyesight. The provision of spectacles helped, although there were many obstacles to developing other schemes to address more complex problems.[33] Since poorer people were more reliant on state aid their experiences were determined by the way this was delivered. In England the workhouse was reviled by many working-class communities but historians continue to emphasize its importance as an embryonic social service, especially for the elderly and infirm.[34] Children were also an important client group for the Poor Law authorities but by the late nineteenth century statutory and voluntary effort encouraged their redirection towards specialist services which emphasized education and training. These concerns embraced children with special needs, and residential schools emerged from the end of the eighteenth century to cater for blind and deaf pupils. Over time, other groups were identified and offered distinctive provision. Assessment of the aims, methods and achievements of this special schooling shows much continuity over time and commonality between countries although many published histories celebrate particular institutions and pay only limited attention to wider developments in health and welfare policies.[35] A more thoughtful account, that notes the contested nature of many developments in the fields of deaf education, can be found in Mike Mantin's work on the oralism debate (Chapter 4). He reveals conflict between the key actors and the continuing importance such educational policies have for understanding Deaf/deaf culture.

While the appropriateness of special education can be debated, it was for many years quite a marginal but somewhat exclusive activity underpinned by strict entry criteria for pupils and the social status of patrons, board members and donors. Although some services were configured to meet regional as well as local need there was no sense of coordination, and such provision as there was must have been easy to avoid if unacceptable to parents until the last decades of the nineteenth century. It was the introduction of compulsory schooling, itself part of a reassessment of the state's duties to and rights over its future citizens, which did more than anything else to reveal the number of children with special needs.[36] Subsequent legislation encouraged recourse to existing and new facilities but the principles of voluntarism were increasingly replaced by official medical assessments and bureaucratic arrangements for the correct disposal of cases. Here it is hard to escape the dualisms identified by Harry Hendrick at the heart of increasing concern about child welfare from the 1870s. These included children as victims and threats, children's bodies and minds and the management of the normal and abnormal.[37]

Understanding the Past, Looking to the Future

Tension between the rights of adults and the needs of children has become an important theme in recent work exploring changing meanings of welfare. Harry Hendrick attributes many modern anxieties about the nature of childhood and the status of children in western societies to cultures of adult individualism and economic uncertainties that took root in the 1970s. He views feminism as a particularly insidious influence on policies and practices that affected children without necessarily being child-friendly.[38] This analysis however has little to say about children with special needs, although journalists have recently used the abusive care of disabled children as the ultimate examples of selfish parenting.[39] Likewise, disability research has embraced many feminist perspectives, but its focus on adult experiences and opportunities for self-expression and self-determination says little about children living with a disability or the special needs of the children, disabled or not, growing up in a household where one or more of the other children or adults has a disabling condition. There is also concern that there may be discrimination even within the disability movement, with people living with learning difficulties (traditionally viewed as child-like regardless of age) apparently the main victims of this.[40]

The rhetoric of independence and social inclusion, derived from the social model, is strong, but the way this might apply to children living with disabling conditions in the past, present or future is still underexplored and it seems possible that specialist services (even additional support provided to facilitate access to mainstream provision) designed to promote such goals may unintentionally frustrate them, especially in medical and educational settings.[41] The legacy of past services, together with assessment of their ideological roots and institutional cultures, is also clearly important here. However, with the explicit scholarly rejection of any whiggish notion of linear progress in the provision of disability services any sense of change and continuity over time may be lost in analysis of power-relations embodied in professional practices and/or particular institutional settings. Children's historic experiences of coping with ill-health and disability in a variety of settings and contexts thereby risk being lost,[42] even as more attention is given to oral history projects and life-story work.[43] The special needs of disabled children can too easily become marginalized within wider debates about both children and disability.[44]

This was a historical problem but is particularly acute today given present anxieties about children in the social investment state (where scarce public resources are targeted to address future labour-force requirements) and concern about the financial burden of caring for an ageing population.[45] The global economic downturn following the banking crisis in 2008 has also raised significant questions about the ability of either the statutory or voluntary sector to sustain let alone develop the existing level of services in many countries. The full impact of these events is as yet unknown but it is not unrealistic to suggest a similar loss of confidence to that seen at the end of the long boom in the western economies in the early 1970s. This was associated with a decline of support for collectivist principles, reduced funding growth, restricted entitlements for service-users, and significant new pressures on staff that fed into a developing literature on stress and burnout.[46] It is no coincidence that the 1970s and 1980s saw the promotion of 'inclusivity' alongside the closure of large-scale, long-stay institutions.[47] This positively asserted the normalization agenda and brought many benefits but it was also associated with the withdrawal of specialist support, the inappropriate use of facilities poorly adapted for those with special needs and a heavy reliance on family carers.[48]

It seems unlikely that families will be able to do more indefinitely.[49] Indeed recent developments have tended to encourage expectations that disabled young adults will leave home at the same time as their peers to access opportunities for education, work, independent living and new relationships.[50] New barriers to independence are likely to be resisted and resented by service-users and carers. Such arrangements are also likely to dismay professionals whose commitment to client empowerment through improved person-centred support services now risks becoming rhetorical cover for removing access to valued facilities. Client dissatisfaction and staff morale problems seem inevitable in the current climate of cuts.

Other emerging problems also threaten to redirect resources away from disabled children and their families in a situation where vulnerable groups will have to compete for reduced resources. Recently, new charities have drawn public attention to the needs of injured veterans of armed conflict to a degree that has arguably not been seen in the United Kingdom for many decades.[51] At the same time adult victims of road accidents, industrial injuries and various diseases have pursued distinctive campaigns to get their specialist needs recognized.[52] While many disabled children now achieve adulthood, prompting concern about managing the transition from child to adolescent and adult services, it is correct to say that increasing proportions of adults with disabling conditions (including but not limited to age-related infirmities) have no experience of childhood disability. This is a significant challenge for those seeking to assert the special needs of the disabled child and compete for support from tax revenues, philanthropic endeavour and charitable donations. These problems are being compounded by evidence of increased adult mistrust of, and disengagement from, the world of the child.[53]

1 CLUB FEET AND CHARITY: CHILDREN AT THE HOUSE OF CHARITY, SOHO, 1848–1914

Pat Starkey

Introduction

Charitable activity grew rapidly in Britain from the late eighteenth century and disabled people were caught up in this expansion. Blindness and deafness were popular causes because these sensory impairments denied access to the word of God and hence appealed to Christian sympathies. Support for physical disabilities was slower to arrive, gathering pace after the 1870 Education Act revealed how many 'crippled' children did not receive schooling. Therefore, the House of Charity for Distressed Persons, founded in Soho in 1846, was unusual in caring for physically disabled children. This was not part of its original plan. The House was largely the achievement of a group of Anglo-Catholic laymen, known as the Engagement, whose members agreed to perform regular acts of charity.[1] Their aim was twofold; to provide temporary shelter for suitably selected or recommended persons in London, and to give an opportunity for association with charitable activity to those too busy to get directly involved themselves.[2] Its involvement in the provision of temporary accommodation for children with disabilities came about almost by accident. Although contrary to the founders' original intentions, it was probably a necessary response to the urgent need to keep its beds full, both to ensure a regular income from those benefactors who pledged to pay for the care of individual inmates, and to satisfy the spiritual needs of those of its supporters for whom the financial support of the House of Charity was a religious exercise, as well as a response to pressure from its supporters for a place of refuge for children receiving treatment in the capital. This chapter will suggest that this broadening of the activities of the House also intersected with a growth in charitable foundations that supported advances in paediatric medicine and surgery and the foundation of specialist hospitals in London.

Why Children?

In 1846 the founders had assumed that recipients of the care funded by their beneficence would be adults or families, fallen on hard times through no fault of their own, who needed short-term assistance until they could get back on their feet. They were the deserving, not the casual, poor. As it happened, the supply of that sort of person dried up fairly quickly, probably because the general economic situation improved during the 1850s and fewer people were in need of assistance. Driven by the need to continue to give its donors a locus for their charitable giving, the House began to diversify its activities. For example, it lowered its standards for admission and took in increasing numbers of men and women who failed to meet the original criteria. It also made arrangements with several London hospitals to provide convalescent beds and in the mid-1870s it even entered a short-lived, and not very satisfactory, arrangement with the Charity Organization Society (COS) whereby COS clients were admitted to the House.[3] Between 1848 and 1914 more than 240 unaccompanied children and persons aged eighteen or younger were admitted to the House of Charity.

The staff at the House were not unfamiliar with children. From its earliest days, it had followed a policy of admitting families with children. Additionally, more than a hundred unaccompanied children were taken in as emergencies at the instigation of Catherine Gladstone during the cholera epidemic of 1866.[4] Most of these had been orphaned by the effects of the disease which seriously affected parts of East London and they stayed for a very short time, until they could be placed with family members or sent to orphanages. The reception of those children was formally agreed at a meeting of the Council, but there is no record of any decision to admit those other children found in the House who were suffering from a variety of medical conditions, most of which could be classified as disabling or potentially disabling. As well as helping to meet the House of Charity's need to keep its beds full, their presence in central London also allowed emerging medical specialties patients on whom to practise their new skills and reflected an increasing interest in the welfare of the handicapped child.[5] It is also evidence of a tension between philanthropy and medical expediency: hospital governors needed to avoid their beds being occupied for long periods of time by patients who were more or less convalescent and frequently wished, therefore, to concentrate on treating acute cases, so as to maintain any income dependent on charitable giving. But many medical procedures necessitated long periods of bed-rest and supervision and patients needed somewhere to stay within easy reach of the hospital so that they could attend the outpatients department at regular intervals.[6] By accepting children for whom this was the case, the House of Charity enabled other charitable foundations, the voluntary hospitals, to maximize their contribution. This is explicit in the sad case of Ellen

Meagher, aged eight, who had congenitally dislocated hips. In April 1869, after twelve weeks in St Bartholomew's Hospital, Rochester, she was discharged in spite of the fact that she was deemed to need six months' further care. The reason given was that because the hospital was 'so small and the urgent cases so numerous' the house surgeon was unable to allow her to stay. Although the House of Charity admitted her, presumably with the intention of looking after her for six months, she did not return to Rochester because she died of scarletina, a disease that quite frequently was contracted in hospitals, three weeks later.[7]

Children Admitted to the House

If the children admitted to the House are divided into groups according to their diagnosis, by far the greatest number (thirty-six) is represented by those, like Ellen, who suffered with orthopaedic problems. Some are given very vague descriptions in the case books, for example 'no use of legs' or 'lameness' or 'cripple', but the conditions affecting some of the others are described more specifically. A number of children were admitted with recognized diagnoses like club feet or curvature of the spine, and a couple were reported to be suffering the after-effects of infantile paralysis (poliomyelitis). Other distinct groups were those with ophthalmic problems (twenty-two children); eleven were admitted with epilepsy or mental health problems, which tended to be grouped together; and a further group, not really a group at all, had chest diseases or dental problems. This chapter will concentrate primarily on the orthopaedic cases, although reference will also be made to children with other conditions.

Rapidly improving techniques for dealing with common orthopaedic conditions meant that increasing numbers of children and young people were treated at general hospitals in London. For example, among those admitted to the House of Charity was Hannah Larter, a thirteen-year-old from Suffolk with a spinal curvature. She was an outpatient at Guy's Hospital where her spinal support was fitted and maintained. Her stay in the House of Charity lasted from January to May 1878, because, as the case book records, 'her parents were too poor to pay for the journey back and forward to London and too ignorant to understand the necessity for her attending hospital, even if money were available'. Encased in her spinal support, she went 'to Guys from time to time when a new splint was required'.[8] Another child at the House of Charity who was treated at a general hospital was Mary Fuzzle, who was twelve years old and a patient at St George's Hospital in May 1889 with 'contraction of the muscles in the leg'.[9] Mary had been admitted to his own ward at the hospital as a personal favour by one Dr Ewart, but sadly nothing could be done for Mary 'but to leave well alone'. She was discharged home after three weeks in the House. In Mary's case, 'home' was almost certainly the Anglican convent of St John Baptist in Clewer, near Windsor. Close links were maintained with that institution, whose sisters managed the housekeeping services in the House as well as running a home for 'fallen women' nearby.[10] In the extensive grounds of their mother house at Clewer, in addition to a House of Mercy for penitent women, were both an orphanage and a convalescent hospital, which meant that both homeless children and those with complaints necessitating care and nursing over a long period could be sent there.[11] Children in the care of the Clewer sisters were sent to stay at the House while they received treatment in London, and the journey in reverse was taken by children needing convalescence or longer-term care. One such was nine-year-old David Hall whose lower body was paralysed and who was admitted to the House of Charity in October 1872 while his mother gave birth. After a few days he had to be sent to Clewer because he needed more care than the staff at the House of Charity could provide.[12]

Children Suffering from Orthopaedic Conditions: Club Foot

Although general hospitals continued to provide orthopaedic treatment for patients like Hannah and Mary, increasingly such children were to be found in those specialist institutions that had their origins in the first half of the nineteenth century. The Infirmary for the Correction of Club Foot and Other Contractions, for example, was founded in Bloomsbury in 1838. It quickly changed its name to the Orthopaedic Institution, and by 1855 it had seen 6,000 patients including 1,600 who had deformities resulting from rickets. The Orthopaedic Institution had also treated 500 patients with foot deformities and 450 for spinal problems. It became known as the Royal Orthopaedic Hospital in 1845.[13] Some sufferers would have been admitted as inpatients, while others would have attended outpatients clinics. Many, perhaps most, would have had the initial stage of their treatment performed while they were resident in the hospital and then have attended for aftercare as outpatients. Not all of them would have been children, of course, but it must be assumed that because childish deformities were deemed to be more susceptible to treatment than those afflicting adults, the average age in such hospitals would have been quite low. In fact, as Roger Cooter has argued, because orthopaedic hospitals catered very largely for children they became quasi-children's hospitals,[14] and their services were increasingly in demand. The growing numbers of patients presenting for treatment at the Royal Orthopaedic Hospital prompted its governors to consider the need to extend their building as well as to make plans for a completely new orthopaedic hospital.[15] Its waiting list of more than 300 'crippled poor' at the Royal led to the foundation of the City Orthopaedic Hospital in Hatton Garden for 'the gratuitous surgical treatment of poor persons of every nation afflicted with club foot, contractions or distortions of the limbs, curvature of the spine or other bodily deformities' in 1851.[16] A third institution, the National Orthopaedic Hospital was founded in 1864.[17] These figures are very remarkable: in little more than a generation a medical specialty whose origins, though long and honourable, lay more with the mechanics of bone-setting and therefore with trauma than with responses to deformity, whether congenital, pathologically acquired or idiopathic, now found itself expressed in specialist hospitals in the capital as well as with practice in general ones.[18]

Such voluntary hospitals employed various means to fund their work. Beds at the Royal Orthopaedic Hospital were allocated according to the incomes of the patients. Some were expected to pay, but others could benefit from the hospital's charitable income, very largely derived from gifts from generous benefactors; its designation as 'Royal' witnesses to one such benefaction by the Prince Consort who became a patron in 1842, with a gift of twenty-five guineas. In 1846 the Queen also became a patron and contributed £50; and in 1850 she gave 250 guineas in order to obtain for the Prince of Wales (then aged ten) the right always to have one patient under treatment.[19] In addition to such benefactions, which gave the donor rights of nomination to beds, governors of the institution were permitted to recommend one inpatient and two outpatients annually. This privilege cost one guinea for one year, five guineas for ten years and ten guineas for life. Would-be patients were interviewed by a committee whose responsibility it was to enquire into their finances and decide whether they could be treated by the charity, or whether they were deemed to be able to pay, or have paid for them, the sum of £10. The City Orthopaedic Hospital, whose first president was Lord Shaftesbury, operated a scheme that purported to dispense with interviews and letters of recommendation and to provide free treatment with no strings attached. It raised funds, though not always with notable success, at annual festival dinners, at special sermons by eminent ecclesiastics in smart churches, and by encouraging subscriptions. In 1852, at its first festival dinner, it was reported that there were 799 patients on its books. [20]

We do not know which hospital treated eleven-year-old Emily Cooper, who was admitted to the House of Charity in October 1855, and neither do we know whether she was one whose family finances had been assessed sympathetically by a committee or whether a governor had exercised his right to nominate her, but we do know that a 'ticket for the orthopaedic hospital' had been procured for her. We also know that she had been admitted to the House 'because she has not the means of remaining in London to attend the hospital'.[21] Her stay in the House of Charity would also have been paid for by some sort of benefaction: a supporter or associate of the House would have had to recommend her as a worthy recipient of their hospitality and to have paid for her keep there. It would not be surprising if the person who paid for her stay in the hospital also paid for her stay in the House. The council and associates of the House tended to be upper-middle-class and aristocratic men who supported numerous charities. The ability to utilize the services of those with complementary functions would have been an efficient and elegant way to reassure the benefactor that his money was being carefully spent. In addition, it is clear that local parish clergy throughout the country exploited the links between members of the national Anglo-Catholic network in order to access beds for their parishioners. Those from outside the capital, and possibly those from its outskirts, would have needed temporary accommodation to recuperate after medical or surgical intervention and more easily attend outpatient clinics. One such was ten-year-old Sophia Meech, from Puddletown in Dorset. She spent four nights in the House of Charity before being admitted to what is described as the 'Spinal Hospital' in August 1861.[22] Another was Claud Brown, aged nine, from Southsea, whose spinal curvature required a support and who spent two months at the House between November 1890 and January 1891.[23] It must be assumed that parents or more likely someone else in their home area made arrangements for the children to stay in the House before they made the journey to London, although case notes rarely mention such details.

If we consider the conditions for which treatment was considered feasible, amongst those admitted to the House of Charity club feet and curvature of the spine feature largely. Surgical treatment for club foot had originated in France and Germany, with varying degrees of success, in the last decades of the eighteenth century. In England it dates from the early 1830s. Until then, it had been considered untreatable, left to the mercies of the bonesetters or treated by various forms of splinting.[24] In 1834, a London doctor, William John Little, himself afflicted with an acquired form of the deformity, went to Berlin to learn the surgical technique from a successful German practitioner, Johannes Muller, and two years later Louis Stromeyer of Hamburg performed an operation to realign Little's foot.[25] According to his own account, Little's surgery was performed while he sat on a comfortable sofa and, of course, without anaesthetic. So successful was it, that Little introduced the operation, which involved dividing the Achilles tendon, to this country and within the next decade other surgeons in England as well as the United States were employing the technique, sometimes dividing either the tibialis anticus or the tibialis posticus and also the flexor tendon of the big toe in addition.[26] The instrument used was a slender, round-ended knife (a tenotome) that was passed so as to divide the tendon from within outwards. It appears that the wound was then dressed and splinted so as to prevent the extremities of the muscle from reuniting.[27]

Surgery became such a popular form of treatment that in 1857 Little himself complained of its overuse, arguing that splinting should not be abandoned and that in slight cases non-operative treatment gave better results.[28] Not all children were subjected to surgery. Some were given more conservative treatment. But most had some sort of splinting and even those for whom surgery was thought appropriate were required to wear special boots after surgery in order that correct alignment of the foot was maintained. Annie Turner, aged four, had a boot fitted, and so did Caroline Webster, from Torrington in North Devon. There is no mention of surgical intervention for either of them.[29] But Henry Radbourne, who was aged twelve and from Banbury, was a patient at Kings College Hospital in October 1879. He had surgery to one of his legs and returned in December to have a boot fitted. Henry was obviously from a very poor family. He spent some time in the House, where he was given some warm clothing, before being sent to the Sisters of St John Baptist at Clewer, where he convalesced in St Andrew's Hospital before he finally went home to Banbury once the boot was made to fit satisfactorily.[30]

We know nothing more about Henry's progress. The notes do not say whether his foot functioned normally or whether, as was the case for many such children, the operation succeeded in only in a partial correction of the deformity. A similar question arises in the case of Emily Cooper who went home 'quite better' in December 1855. Annie Turner was 'too young and sickly' to stay at the House while her club foot was treated in June 1868, and she was discharged two days later to a Mrs Chapman in Frith Street.[31] We have no idea who Mrs Chapman was, but there is nothing in the case book to suggest that she was related to Annie or anything to tell us who made the arrangements or paid for her care. As there is no reference to parents or other family members, it must be assumed that Annie had been admitted from one of the many orphanages with which the House authorities maintained links.

Although surgery would have been performed without anaesthetic in the early part of the century, it is likely that the procedures to correct club foot in children would in most cases have been under nitrous oxide or chloroform by the 1850s. An apothecary was appointed to the Royal Orthopaedic Hospital in 1869, and one of his duties was to administer chloroform, a practice in the hospital that dates at least to 1862.[32] Manipulations were performed under chloroform there by 1873, and by the end of the century an anaesthetist was appointed because of the large number of major operations that were being performed.[33] More than 6,000 anaesthetics were administered in 1896 at the London Hospital.[34] But this may not have been general practice. As Cholmeley has pointed out, there was no anaesthetist or resident medical officer at the City Orthopaedic Hospital until 1894 and no reference is made to an operating room.[35] That could, of course, suggest that all treatment there was conservative rather than surgical, or that operations continued to be performed, like William Little's own, from a comfortable sofa.

Children Suffering from Spinal Deformities and other Orthopaedic Conditions

Curvature of the spine, what today would probably be diagnosed as an idiopathic, adolescent scoliosis affecting the lumbar region, was another condition which was treated both at general hospitals and at London's new orthopaedic ones. Many patients presenting with spinal deformities would, of course, have had tubercular lesions of some kind, but the condition treated by mechanical apparatus, described by an American surgeon, J. D. Brown, as 'frames of iron' was more likely to have been an idiopathic one. Its perceived increase in the early nineteenth century and its greater incidence amongst women was, however, according to Brown, the result of poorly constructed seats in schools or the wearing of stays. He argued that one encouraged bad posture and the other allowed the muscles to weaken.[36] His form of treatment consisted of braces, exercises and a 'spinal spring support', but he also applied leeches and blistering, though the rationale for those methods is unclear.[37] British surgeons were also active in the treatment of this condition. Charles Verral, for example, who moved from Seaford in Sussex to London in 1850, specialized in spinal problems and founded the Society for the Treatment at their Own Homes of Poor Persons Afflicted with Diseases of the Spine, Chest, Hip etc which later became the National Orthopaedic Hospital.[38]

Anne Stroud, who was eleven yeas old when she was admitted in July 1870, was among those suffering from the condition who spent some time in the House of Charity. All her expenses at the Spinal Hospital were paid by someone called Miss Thompson although we are not given details about the treatment given. And Mary Jane Thrush, a ten-year-old, spent three days in the House, while she waited to be examined at the orthopaedic hospital. She was sent home for a further wait, this time for a vacancy in the hospital.[39] It has to be assumed that Annie Bronham's scoliosis was less severe, though it is at least possible that it was believed to be untreatable. She spent a week in the House, attending the hospital as an outpatient, before being discharged home.[40]

The shortage of hospital beds and suitably trained practitioners meant that only a minority of children were able to access treatment. However great the unpleasantness of nineteenth-century orthopaedic treatment, whether or not it involved surgery, there can be little doubt that those children submitted to it were the fortunate ones. As Cooter has argued, most children with bony deformities would have been labelled as 'crippled' and have received merely custodial care and many were destined to remain in workhouses along with others, like the blind or insane, whose value as workers was negligible. That was certainly not true of those who stayed in House; they had been admitted specifically so that treatment could be found for them. Nevertheless, a child or young adult unable to be self-supporting, and with no prospect of ever being productive, could be an intolerable burden on domestic finances, sometimes making the difference between family survival or destitution. Even though children admitted to the House did have access to medical care, some still found themselves sent to the workhouse once treatment was finished. In 1855, George Whitmore, who was fifteen, was unable to continue his work at Price's candle factory because of 'his disordered state of health and lameness'. Although he went to Margate for several months, almost certainly to the convalescent home with which the House had links, supported by the factory, and although his condition improved, he was unable to accept his employer's offer of further work 'because [in] his state of health it would be cruelty to do so'. Because of his family's financial difficulties, the casebook notes that 'there was nowhere for him to go but the Union in the end'.[41] And in May 1863, Richard Grizzell, an eleven-year-old with a fractured thigh, was discharged to St George's Workhouse.[42]

Children with Epilepsy and Mental Health Problems

Orthopaedics was only one of the many medical specialisms making rapid advances in the middle years of the century. Neurology was another. Attempts to understand the 'falling sickness' (epilepsy) advanced as a result of work in London and Paris. Acknowledgement of its particular character meant that in county asylums in England, the confinement of epileptics in wards separate from those housing other patients became the established procedure around 1859, but as with orthopaedics specialist institutions began to appear. For example, the National Hospital for the Paralysed and Epileptic in Queen Square, now the Institute of Neurology and part of University College Hospital, opened in 1859. Owsei Temkin sees its foundation as part of the process whereby people with epilepsy began to be distinguished from patients with mental illnesses, although the aetiology of the disease the hospital set out to treat was by no means understood.[43] At least one theory posited a link between epilepsy and 'idiocy', arguing that the former was a condition which developed in childhood, 'where the mind has never been fully developed but is afterwards destroyed by successive attacks and we have the idiot whose course is generally cut short in early life or where some considerable amount of intelligence has been developed but is afterwards destroyed by successive convulsive attacks'.[44] At the same time, experimental forms of treatment, some pretty heroic, to replace automatic incarceration began to be discussed in the medical literature. These included surgery, the performance of tracheotomy, and medication with silver nitrate or bromide of potassium, all of which carried considerable risk but give an indication of the perceived intractability of the condition and the anxiety of physicians to pursue any course which might alleviate the worst symptoms.[45] It was not until John

Hughlings Jackson did his seminal work on the pathology and aetiology of epilepsy in the 1860s, that a more accurate definition began to appear; this was
refined in 1873 to the broad definition that 'epilepsy is the name for occasional
sudden, excessive, rapid and local discharges of grey matter'.[46]

Given the uncertainty about the diagnosis of epilepsy in the mid-nineteenth
century, it is interesting to note the number of times that the term is used
unquestioningly to describe the difficulties experienced by some of the children
admitted to the House of Charity. None of them appears to have been submitted to any of the more adventurous treatments. John Holland, who was aged
eighteen, was admitted so that he could be an outpatient at the Middlesex Hospital. The case book notes suggest that at first he appeared to benefit from a
course of mesmeric influence (a form of hypnotism) but that this had very little long-term effect on what are described as his 'very awful and very frequent
fits'.[47] We are told neither the length of his stay nor where he went at the end of
it, but we do know that another inmate subject to frequent fits, sixteen-year-
old Jane Price, stayed for a month, although 'she was not liked in the House'.[48]
Caroline Read, on the other hand, who was thirteen, was left at the House from
February 1859 until the following August when her fits apparently subsided.[49]
Another brief entry tells us about George Schooling, aged eleven when he was
admitted in April 1862. He is described as 'idiot and epileptic' and was quickly
discharged, where we do not know, because 'he was too helpless and annoying
to the inmates'.[50] No information is given about any treatment that either he or
Caroline might have received; perhaps their stay in the House was simply in
order to provide temporary accommodation while some permanent shelter was
found. But George Darwood, admitted in January 1867 when he was twelve
years old, was sent to the House specifically in the hope that some medical care
could be found for him. Normally a resident of the orphanage in the grounds
of the Gladstone family home at Hawarden, he was expected to stay in London
'until he could go to the epileptic hospital', but he was discharged on 22 April to
Woodford Hall.[51] There appears to have been no mental hospital of that name
and the fact that John Wren, aged ten, who had to have his leg amputated after
an accident, was also admitted there suggests that this was either a convalescent
home or, conceivably, an orphanage. As John was eventually sent to a Boys'
Home in Regents Park, that suggests a more temporary function for Woodford
Hall.[52] We are not told whether George was eventually admitted to the 'epileptic
hospital', but the note on Robert Middleton, another twelve-year-old from the
orphanage at Hawarden, says that it was very difficult to access beds there, which
might explain why George was sent to Woodford Hall instead.[53]

Experience of Care in the House of Charity

To what extent can we uncover the experience of the children admitted to the House of Charity? Our knowledge of their personalities, their conditions and their treatment is conveyed in the words of others, whose medical knowledge was very limited and whose notes on their young charges are often brief. As a result we can claim only to have some slight insight into how the children were seen and described by the staff at the House. Moreover, the questions that would enable us to discover more about the day-to-day detail of the life of children in the House are more or less unanswerable. For example, how were the journeys of children like Hannah Larter, who had to attend the hospital outpatients clinic for examination or treatment, accomplished? Sadly, the case notes give no clue. Presumably someone pushed them in wheelchairs or spinal carriages, but we are not told who that was or who provided the necessary equipment. It is possible that the House had equipment of its own, although there is no record of any decision to purchase it. Who supervised and assisted the children with basic washing and toileting? Were they all able to feed themselves? And who helped Timothy O'Keefe, who was blind, to find his way round the House during the six weeks that he stayed there?[54] What sort of support was in place for the two poor blind girls from the Blind School in Avenue Road, Regents Park who were sent to the House for their school holidays, incidentally demonstrating that although most children were admitted for medical reasons some just had nowhere else to go.[55]

It has to be assumed that the Sisters of St John Baptist, in their role as managers of the household, took responsibility for organizing the care of the children. Moreover, as other residents, particularly the women, were expected to help with basic household tasks, it is likely that some of them assisted. Even those with some disability were given jobs to do and it may be that ambulant children were also given tasks. Bessie Frost, a thirteen-year- old from Torquay, who was deaf and stayed in the House while attending the Middlesex Hospital, was recorded as being 'useful in the House as far as her deafness would allow', but we are not told whether her usefulness extended to helping with the other children.[56]

The psychological welfare of children and the maintenance of contact with their families, something that has assumed great importance since the work of John Bowlby in the years following the Second World War (see Chapters 6 and 10), was not a preoccupation of the staff of the House of Charity. We have no idea whether or how often parents were able to visit, neither are we told how the children travelled home once their period of treatment was over. Some, as we have seen, came from as far afield as Devon. In 1921, Elsie White, who was twelve and a victim of the 'infantile paralysis' that she had contracted when she was three, was sent home to Hungerford on the train, the arrangements for her travel having been made by the lady almoner at St Thomas' Hospital.[57] In the absence of any information about discharge arrangements in the period before 1914, we can only guess that perhaps train tickets were purchased for other children. The case notes record the poverty of many of the families whose children spent some weeks in Soho, so it is very unlikely that they would have been able to travel to visit or to collect their progeny.

In spite of the limitations of the records, and even though the numbers accommodated are small, it is possible to ask whether the reception and treatment of disabled children at the House of Charity gives any indication of differing attitudes towards particular conditions. For example, the notes on the children reveal a much greater sympathy for the plight of those subjected to surgery or to immobility in corrective appliances than those with conditions that manifested themselves in behaviour that was difficult to handle. We have already noted that George Schooling was 'helpless and annoying to the inmates', and others who excited distaste or disapproval included Emma Ricketts, whose diagnosis was given as 'imbecility' and who was described as 'stupid and obstinate'.[58] None of the children with other conditions attracts comments quite like that, although Dinah Wood, who was admitted for 'rest and food' in April 1854 is described as a 'poor fool of consumptive habit'.[59]

In addition, the children's destinations after discharge throw some light on their families' acceptance of their conditions and their ability to cope with them at home. Of the thirty-six children with orthopaedic complaints at least eighteen were admitted from their family homes and fifteen were eventually discharged there, even if it was necessary for them to convalesce in nearby orphanages or convalescent homes until they were properly fit. And some of those children had severe disabilities, necessitating considerable care. We are told, for example, about four-year-old Richard Humford, whose 'back had grown ... so as to endanger his life by contraction of the neck' as a result of a fall. He was admitted to the House in June 1866 and finally discharged home in August 'after correct good food'. For some reason the casebook record is incomplete, noting that that his mother 'would not allow him to be put in a cripples home where he would have been ...'.[60] How was the sentence supposed to end? Was it going to express disapproval of Mrs Humford's decision and to suggest that the child should be institutionalized, or was it going to hint that he would be better off at home because he might not have received good care in the 'cripples home'? That it was thought necessary to record that he had been carefully fed while in the House suggests that Richard's family was not well-off, and that looking after him at home might well have put a strain on the family economy, especially if his care prevented his mother from working. It is possible to argue, though, that Mrs Humford's determination to look after her child, gives a clear indication that he was valued, in spite of the attendant difficulties. Claud Brown was also clearly valued by his family. He was admitted to the House with a congenital curvature of the spine, which was deteriorating, and he sent to London so that a spinal support could be fitted. He was discharged home to Southsea in January 1891 after two months' stay, during which time he had obviously endeared himself to the staff. The casebook notes that he was 'very patient amid much suffering' and that he had 'a beautiful voice and great love of music'.[61] It is possible that Richard and Claud illustrate Cooter's argument that the nineteenth century witnessed changes in views both about childhood and about the value of the physically disabled child. The growth of services for 'crippled' children, he has claimed, 'illuminated a context in which socio-economic, ideological, political, technical and professional factors were increasingly intertwined and interdependent' and reflected an increasing interest in the welfare of the handicapped child. Evidence for this can be detected in the numbers of charities that were founded for the care of 'crippled' children – over forty of them in Britain between 1870 and 1914, including the wonderfully named Crutch and Kindness League and the Guild of the Brave Poor Things.[62] And the presence in the House of children from orphanages demonstrates that even those children without families were deemed to be worthy of treatment. But Cooter's argument that compulsory education from 1890 meant that all children were removed from the workplace and became economically unproductive, thereby providing a sort of level playing field for children with disabilities, does not address the fact that the latter group threatened to remain unproductive and a long-term strain on family finances. If they survived, both Richard Humford and Claud Brown would have cost a lot to keep, feed and care for and would probably have been incapable of making any sort of financial contribution to the household.

If the experience of physically disabled children can be said to have improved by the end of the century, the records of the House of Charity suggest that children afflicted with epilepsy or mental health difficulties were less likely to benefit from greater understanding. Of the eleven children suffering mental health problems, four were admitted from orphanages or institutions described as 'schools'. None was definitely admitted from home, although in some cases no note has been made of where they came from. And none appears to have been discharged to his or her home. Although Temkin argues that from the first half of the nineteenth century major trends in neurological medicine were characterized by enthusiasm for 'pathological anatomy, clinical observation and an appreciation of statistical data', neurological disease appeared, and was, more intractable and disturbing than those conditions which affected the skeleton and whose largely mechanical malfunctions were more easily understood.[63] That epilepsy was singled out as a distinct and definable disability is evidence of some hope and greater understanding, but its association with what was known as 'imbecility' or 'idiocy' still left a legacy of anxiety in the minds of families and carers, something that was to continue well into the twentieth century. And the anxiety occasioned in those who observed children suffering severe seizures, while understanding little of what had caused them, cannot be underestimated.

Conclusion

Examination of the cases of those children admitted to the House of Charity either for convalescence after treatment or while they attended outpatients clinics demonstrates ways in which networks of charities helped to make treatment available or possible. Practitioners of emerging medical and surgical specialities needed to be able to employ and perfect their new skills, but hospitals could not afford to have very long-stay patients occupying beds which could more usefully and profitably be used for new patients. They needed to concentrate on treating only acute cases, or those in an acute stage of treatment, so as to ensure a regular income dependent on charitable giving.[64] But many procedures took weeks or months to complete and patients needed to be able to stay somewhere within easy reach of the hospital so that they could attend outpatient clinics at regular intervals. Accommodation at the House of Charity, well placed as it was within relatively easy reach of the major hospitals, helped both the hospitals and the House to keep their beds full. But the House could accommodate only a handful of children; it did not have appropriate staff and its primary purpose was to offer temporary shelter to adults and families. There must have been many other such refuges in the capital, like the House of Charity, offering beds to children in addition to pursuing their original aims. J. A. Cholmeley has argued that patients at the Royal Orthopaedic Hospital had travelled there from every county in England and Wales, from Scotland, Ireland and from the Channel Islands. His comments about orthopaedics must also apply to neurology and ophthalmology and the other medical specialities beginning to establish themselves in the second half of the nineteenth century. Those from outside the capital, and possibly those from its outskirts, who wished to avail themselves of specialist care would have needed temporary accommodation so that they could more easily attend clinics or so that they had somewhere to recuperate after medical or surgical intervention. Whatever the limitations of what it had to offer, the House of Charity made it possible for a small number of children to receive treatment.

2 INSANITY, FAMILY AND COMMUNITY IN LATE-VICTORIAN BRITAIN

Amy Rebok Rosenthal

Introduction

In the era known to modern scholars of British history as 'the age of improvement', Victorians sought to better identify, categorize and manage those individuals who were unable to conform to society's expectations. At this time disabled children living with physical and sensory impairments, and/or what we would now understand to be learning difficulties and/or mental health problems, came under increasing scrutiny. Although histories of childhood and disability issues have tended to neglect mental health, insane children arguably represented a particular problem for Victorian society. This was because contemporary actors believed their disabilities compromised their ability to function within their own families and within the larger community. With children seen as the nation's future, questions relating to the care and control of young people stood precariously between the family and the state. An insane child was not only likely to cause family anguish but also to create concern, even fear, within the local community. One writer described such children as 'a plague on the neighbourhood'.[1] Such thinking tended to encourage official intrusion into the private, domestic world of the family to protect the public and/or defend insane people from neglect or abuse.

While many aspects of the care of disabled Victorian children are unrecorded and elude historians, the committal of insane children to lunatic asylums created voluminous paperwork. Surviving records provide a rare opportunity to look more closely at the experiences of these young people before, during and after official confinement. A further window into the lives of insane children and their families is provided by the writings of leading British alienists. These sources suggest that contemporary actors were even more disturbed by cases of childhood insanity than they were worried about insane adults. This was because insane young people contradicted fundamental Victorian ideas about children and childhood. Investigations into the care of insane children also reinforced commonly-held beliefs about the family and class relations. Since family members, local people and officials all played active roles in the process of confinement there was inevitably an element of contested caring in decisions about the care/control of the insane child that did not apply to other groups of disabled children. If insane young people were treated differently than other groups of disabled children it remains to be seen whether or not their experiences can be distinguished from those of insane adults. This chapter provides an opportunity to evaluate the potential of applying modern historiographical trends in the history of asylums to the experiences of children with mental health problems and/or disabilities. Insane children and youths were diagnosed in similar ways to adults. They were also treated using the same methods as adults and they were confined in institutions shared by adults. Yet it is incorrect to simply assume that the commitment of young people to lunatic asylums was driven by the same factors that provided the catalyst for the admission of insane adults. To date, the historiography has concentrated almost exclusively on the adult experience.[2] A number of scholars have drawn attention to the active agency of close kin who were prepared to use institutional care for unproductive insane adults as part of a family economic survival strategy.[3] The focus on cases of childhood and youth insanity in this chapter reveals more significant roles for the public authorities and also, a perhaps unexpected, reliance on testimony from neighbours. One voice that is rarely heard is that of the insane child; instead we learn about them through their reported interactions with family members, local people and various 'experts' concerned with the management of the insane poor. For, although mental disorder was not class specific, it was the poorer sections of society who used the public asylums whose records are so attractive to historians.[4] There is plenty of detail about individual cases but the experiences of insane children have to be distilled from records created for quite different purposes. Even the opinions attributed to their relatives and neighbours have to be recovered second-hand from committal papers and other medical notes.

This chapter reviews a number of debates about insane children in the Victorian period and then goes on to explore contemporary ideas about links between poverty and morbid heredity. Such thinking, it will be shown, did much to undermine the notion of a private, domestic world represented by home and family. It is therefore no coincidence that insane young people were amongst the first group of children to be targeted by legislation that envisaged not only state protection for vulnerable individuals but conferred on state officials the right to remove such persons from their homes. In the final section of the chapter a number of individual cases are explored to examine the experiences of insane children and their families.

Debates over Insane Children

Theoretical discussions about childhood insanity involved a number of interested parties. Medical men, for example, debated the question of not only *if* a child could be insane, but at what point in the experience of childhood insanity could be present. Practitioners focused on the distinction between the sane and insane mind. Scottish physician William Ireland noted: 'Sanity is generally regarded as a natural and healthy growth of a man's character, and insanity as something diseased or abnormal'.[5] A mind clouded by insanity, then, clearly deviated from the normal characteristics of childhood espoused in contemporary discourse by corrupting the natural innocence of children and by manipulating their natural tendencies. Practitioners also sought to identify the stage at which the mental capacities of children were such that they could be insane. Renowned practitioner Henry Maudsley considered the question, 'How soon can a child go mad?', and thought, 'obviously not before it has got some mind to go wrong, and then only in proportion to the quantity and quality of mind which it has'.[6] During the second half of the nineteenth century, practitioners identified that insanity (though not conditions we would now understand as learning disabilities) was rare if not unknown in very young children. Symptoms emerged as children developed, with age of onset typically seen as eleven to fifteen years.[7] It was older children and adolescents who accounted for the vast majority of child admissions to the county asylums.

The Victorian classification system of mental disorders used by medical practitioners and asylum personnel covered a plethora of conditions. Terms such as 'idiot', 'imbecile' or 'feebleminded' were in common usage amongst members of the medical profession and the public. Insanity, on the other hand, was a term used to describe disorders signifying mental illness in which the healthy mind deviated from normal activities and patterns, as often evidenced by behaviour considered socially unacceptable. The medical community and the public used both 'insanity' and 'lunacy' to refer to these individuals. If any distinction is to be made, evidence suggests that the medical practitioners may have favoured the term 'insanity', whereas 'lunacy' was preferred in legal contexts. Historians have argued that identification of lunatics in the Victorian period conformed more to legal definitions of insanity than to medical diagnoses, thereby justifying the grouping together of children suffering from both developmental disabilities and various forms of insanity.[8] Yet, in the theoretical context of Victorian medicine, the separation of these disorders and levels of deficiency had seemed fairly straightforward. Theorists also made a distinction between conditions stemming from a perceived lack of morality and those caused by other psychological disturbances.[9] Each condition had specific characteristics and degrees associated with it, and medical practitioners were generally clear on the definitions of each.

In reality, however, this apparent separation was, more often than not, a mirage, with mental disorders manifesting themselves in a variety of competing and contradictory diagnoses. For example, the behavioural characteristics of groups of children categorized as 'idiots', 'imbeciles' or 'feebleminded' could just as easily be discerned among children diagnosed as insane.

While medical men addressed the problems of diagnosis and treatment from a technical perspective, their work engaged with a number of contemporary discourses about insane youngsters. These revolved around debates about the place of children in Victorian society and the dynamic relationship between the family, insanity and the wider community. Inherently, insane children presented a paradox to the Victorians: How could childish innocence take on the demented characteristics of insanity? This question was particularly perplexing for British society, which had, by the nineteenth century, a very defined, albeit ideal, sense of childhood. For Hugh Cunningham, this was a middle-class ideal, which perpetuated 'the view that childhood was not only a separate stage in life, but the best of those stages'.[10] No longer were children conceptualized as small adults whose value was often established according to their usefulness to the family. Rather, children were valuable because they represented a purer form of humanity.[11] As such they were expected to conform to the accepted, or at least perceived, values of the community.

Class, Poverty and Heredity

Insanity in the young was a legitimate issue for nineteenth-century society and one which was difficult to separate from other community concerns. Embedded in public and professional discussions of mental illness were, for example, arguments about class, poverty, disease and degeneracy which were already having an impact on changing approaches to child welfare.[12] If, as James Walvin maintains, the Victorian image of children emphasized the innocence of a child and the distancing of children from the real world of adults this was not an ideal that was achievable for many if not most working-class families.[13] This situation perplexed reformers like Florence Davenport Hill, known for her work in prison and Poor Law reform. She noted:

> It is painful to set aside our ideal of a childhood of innocence and bright playfulness and to realise that there are among us thousands of children familiar with shocking vice, to whose tiny mouths disgusting words and even blasphemy come naturally and who, seemingly incapable of shame, pride themselves on their knowledge of evil.[14]

Other contemporary actors also drew connections between poverty and an apparent predisposition towards immorality, criminality and insanity. Henry

Maudsley, for example, suggested that socio-economic status directly impacted the development of children with intellectual deficiencies. He argued:

> Unequal to the social ways and regular work of their fellows they drift apart into idle brooding and sauntering, and, when they belong to the lowest classes, gravitate vagrantly into workhouse or gaol. From time to time one of this class commits arson, rape or even homicide.[15]

In the Edwardian period these concerns crystallized around the question of mental deficiency, but a close association between insanity and deficiency was a legacy from earlier Victorian discourses.[16] In 1870 the *British Medical Journal* suggested:

> It is only fair to conclude that, with an increased number of such persons [pauper lunatics] at liberty, drawn from a less safe class, we should have a much richer harvest of murders, acts of violence, and legal transgressions, committed by lunatics.[17]

This was seemingly a long way from the idealized innocence of childhood, but an essential component of child welfare concerns at this time was the connection between class, poverty and morbid heredity. A bond which, at least in the minds of many Victorian doctors and social commentators, predestined children to suffer the sins of their parents; thereby placing much of the blame for both character flaws and unacceptable behaviours on family genetics as well as environmental factors. Nowhere was this problem more marked than in the transmission of hereditary insanity. Although this was potentially a problem for all social classes it was the poorest that attracted most condemnation. Medical men generally believed that undesirable parents begot undesirable children. 'Seeing that bad mental organization is just as much a manufactured article as a bad machine', concluded Maudsley, 'it is not a little pathetic to see parents amazed and aghast in the face of such a product of them and their stocks'.[18] Maudsley doubted that such individuals could be treated or educated, speculating that only by 'touch[ing] the bottom of misery ... may here and there teach one of them self-control enough to enable him to get a living in the low social conditions to which his nature gravitates and in which alone it is at home'.[19]

Continental practitioner M. Brierre de Boismont affirmed the important connection between heredity and mental disorders, suggesting that eccentric, excitable or nervous parents were destined to pass these traits to their offspring, as the 'defects of his [the child's] sad heritage'.[20] He claimed, 'the majority of children born of such parents were uneven in temper, irritable, coarse, dishonest, sad, difficult to manage, obeying no rule'.[21] As a result of these concerns, practitioners and asylum personnel gave particular attention to the parents of patients, taking thorough medical histories to determine the role heredity might have played. The age of the parents at conception, any blood relationship between the parents and the habits of parents were all seen as key prognosticators of the mental health of their offspring.[22] 'The intemperate parent', suggested James Crichton-Browne (Superintendent of the West Riding Asylum in Wakefield), 'will transmit to his children a heritage of disease, and will inflict upon them ills innumerable'.[23] Such sentiments fed into wider public discourses about insane children and youths.

Home as Contested Space

An emerging consensus of opinion that viewed childhood as a, if not the, most important phase of life encouraged a public debate that both emphasized the importance of character formation and connected such concerns to wider anxieties about class, poverty and morbid heredity. Yet if the debate was a public one, most of its concerns centred on the private world of the home and family which children were raised within. Cunningham suggests that as the nuclear family retreated into the private sphere of the home, 'the community and the extended family lost their role as arbiters of moral issues'.[24] While the family enjoyed this privacy and autonomy, public pressure remained high for families to produce good, decent, and productive children. Popular publications placed the responsibility for child-rearing squarely on the shoulders of parents, emphasizing their essential role in determining the success or failure of their children in both childhood and adulthood. In 1869 *Bow Bells* magazine opined:

> Under the most favourable circumstances some children grow up to excellence, and, under the most virtuous influences, sometimes break down and become worthless. But such cases are clearly exceptions. They do not invalidate the general truth, that a child will go as he is trained.[25]

Parents were instructed to be persistent in training their children, as any lapse in oversight might leave a child teetering on the brink of delinquency. The article concluded:

> No parent can safely laugh at petty vices in his child, and neglect them with the easy plea that he will outgrow them. Some will outgrow these evils without parental care, but more, by far, will be overgrown by them.[26]

The sheer volume of advice to parents might suggest a popular perception that many parents, even those striving towards the ideals established by the Victorian community, were failing to train their children properly. This led to concern that parents themselves were insufficiently prepared for competent child rearing. 'To shape the character of a child aright', maintained the author of 'Early Training', 'is a task which perhaps only those who have themselves been wisely disciplined in youth are thoroughly competent to perform'.[27]

As faith in the ability of parents to guide children safely to adulthood waned, the privacy and autonomy of the family began to fracture, with politicians, reformers and philanthropists turning their attention to children as the future of the nation. 'Most people are convinced that the strength of England lies in her family life', suggested *Longman's Magazine* in 1895, 'and the keenest-sighted patriots are bending their energies to its maintenance and elevation'.[28] As British legislation codified the experience of childhood through the imposition of education requirements, labour laws and Poor Law Acts, families faced increasing pressure from the state and voluntary organizations to conform to new standards of parenting. From every direction parents were urged to make the 'right' decisions regarding the physical and mental upbringing of their children.

Harry Hendrick suggests that the changing relationship between the family and the state was influenced at least in part by the emerging image of nineteenth-century children as 'economically worthless' but 'emotionally priceless'.[29] Victorian children were becoming both the vehicle for the transmission of social ideals and an investment in the future of the family and the nation.[30] As a result, some reformers advocated increased governmental regulation of the private sphere. Florence Davenport Hill, who was especially concerned with the plight of pauper children, urged state intervention.[31] In *Children of the State*, Hill wrote:

> But though the action of the state has been much restricted by the growth of individual responsibility and the enlarging of individual liberty, she [the state] has yet to regulate many social conditions, and must interfere when private duties are neglected which ought to be performed without prompting.

She continued:

> ... If these [children] should be left without natural protectors, she has to assume parental authority over them; and if they should be also destitute, she must provide for them maintenance and education until she deems them old enough to fend for themselves.[32]

This increasing concern with children and childhood, suggests Cunningham, led to '[t]he identification of childhood as an area for state policy [which] was accompanied and to some extent caused by a declining confidence in the family'.[33] As a result, he continues, 'it was certainly no longer assumed that the rearing of children could be left to families with the state or voluntary organizations picking up the casualties'.[34] Such thinking perhaps went furthest in the case of insane children. Writing about admissions to Devon County Asylum, Joseph Melling, Richard Adair and Bill Forsythe note:

> It is possible to see a distinctive shift in policy principles away from the concept of the child as the property of the family to an assumption that the young person was under the guardianship of the state.[35]

Even when an insane person (child or adult) was kept at home the family could no longer be expected to be left alone. Indeed, '[I]f lunatics are kept at home', warned the *British Medical Journal* in 1866, 'one of the characteristics of the home which Englishmen prize – its privacy – must be surrendered'.[36] Since parents were often blamed for the behaviour of their children, children whose behaviour was suspect could no longer be entrusted solely to the care of such parents. Florence Davenport Hill, for example, recommended that there were 'children over whom, although their parents are living, the State must, for their good and for that of the community, exercise an absolute authority'.[37]

While the initial concern of reformers was apparently to protect children from 'vicious' parents, an increasing number of children were perceived to be at risk and targeted for state intervention.[38] This could take the extreme form of enforced removal from home. Given the significant attention given to child welfare issues in the late nineteenth century, it was no coincidence that medical practitioners often agreed with lay reformers that the sanctity of the family must be breached for the good of the child and society. Walvin suggests that changing public opinion regarding children and childhood paved the way for greater state involvement within the private sphere of the family and home. He argues that the family was so important in the eyes of the state that officials were willing, at times, to go 'to great efforts to create an artificial one' and to impose 'the social ideal to which deprived children ought, it was felt, to be exposed and directed'.[39]

One of the most contentious aspects of the new child welfare policies was the ability of the state to remove a child from its home. It seems no coincidence that some of the earliest legislation facilitating such policies applied to insane children, though it is also noteworthy that the succession of Lunacy Acts that were used by the public authorities to institutionalize such children were oddly silent on the whole question of the existence, let alone management, of the insane child. Melling and colleagues note:

> [T]he lunacy legislation of 1808, 1845, 1853 and even 1890, did not establish any clear age limits for the certification of the lunatic nor was specific provision made for the insane child.[40]

At first sight, the idealized image of the Victorian child seems incompatible with contemporary efforts to confine and thereby control lunatics. Yet the disturbing presence of the insane child or youth represented a danger that was readily apparent to lay as well as medical experts; and if the establishment of shared social values was the ideal that eminent Victorians hoped to achieve, the establishment of community security was the reality that they expected to attain. Public opinion was also favourable to this goal. While theory was often central to professional discussions of childhood insanity, for most people, the issue of security in the form of personal safety and protection of property seems to have been the primary concern. Indeed',[t]he easiest way to justify their [young lunatics] admission to the asylum was to emphasize the danger they posed to those around them'.[41]

The desire to confine insane children and youths also reflected a growing emphasis on custodial, rather than curative, institutions.[42] By the late nineteenth century, the problem of insanity had become an issue of public safety. Popular opinion viewed confinement as the best method of achieving the separation of lunatics from the general populace and as the only means of obtaining a potential cure.[43] This applied as much, if not more so, to mentally disordered children as insane adults. Such thinking found its ultimate expression in the 1913 Mental Deficiency Act but had long-informed child admissions to Victorian asylums.

Patients and their Families

Important as the care/control rhetoric was, and necessary as it is to understand how this interacted with a wider set of concerns about children and childhood, it is also vital to examine the lived experiences of insane children/youths and their families. This section draws on evidence from the County of Kent where the opening of a new lunatic asylum in 1875 coincided with what, in retrospect, can be seen as something of a turning point in the delivery of institutional care.[44] The original Kent County Asylum, located at Barming Heath near Maidstone, had opened in 1833 but by the 1870s was struggling to accommodate a rising inmate population.[45] As a result, a committee was formed to procure the location for a second institution at Chartham, near Canterbury.[46] Work on what became an extensive complex of brick buildings began in 1873, under the direction of architects John Giles and Albert Edward Gough.[47] The East Kent Lunatic Asylum (hereafter EKLA) opened its doors in 1875, although construction continued into 1876, with final costs amounting to over £200,000.[48] From the beginning, county officials and asylum staff strove to provide patients with more than medical treatment. The institution's farm, laundry, sewing rooms and artisan workshops provided inmates with employment. They also had access to amusements on the grounds, and patients were taken on occasional outings.[49]

The first children and youths admitted to the EKLA were transfers from the Barming Heath facility in April 1875. Over the next twenty-five years more than 300 young people were committed to the institution. Their admission to the EKLA followed strict procedures outlined by the 1845 County Asylums Act,[50] and the 1853 Lunatics Amendment Act.[51] Local Justices of the Peace were ultimately responsible for admission to and release from county asylums, but it was Poor Law officers who were responsible for much of the process.[52] Poor Law medical officers were required to undertake a quarterly review of all pauper lunatics not confined to an asylum, establishing the state of their mental health and, after 1853, issuing the medical certificates needed for admission to county institutions, substantiating the mental condition of the individual under examination.[53] Poor Law relieving officers handled the admission process, interviewing families and, at times, delivering the insane to the asylum.[54] Finally, the Justice of the Peace issued an Order for the Reception of a Private/Pauper Patient, a 'legal certificate transferring, from the guardian to the superintendent of the institution, the care of a person certified as insane'.[55]

Officially, nineteenth-century Poor Law authorities considered children to be those under the age of sixteen. It was these children for whom parents were responsible and, when lacking appropriate parental care, for whom the state took responsibility. Yet the definition of children established by Poor Law authorities does not accurately define what the term child meant to Victorians.[56] Evidence from patient records, published case studies and medical discourse greatly expands this notion of the child in both reference and identification. Many of the children and youths admitted to the EKLA, for example, lived at home and their families continued to be an important part of the commitment process. A not untypical case involved fourteen-year-old William G. who arrived at the doors of the EKLA during the evening of 3 July 1879. His father James G., a labourer from the town of Sheerness, Kent, in his middle fifties, testified to the boy's 'violent demeanour'.[57] Admission records also stated that the boy was observed 'gesticulating and talking with imaginary people'.[58] James indicated that his son's behaviour had gone on for more than two months, finally compelling him to seek the assistance of the asylum. Armed with an order to commit the youth signed by Edward James Athawes, a magistrate whose name was often found on admissions to the asylum and a medical certificate that was signed by another local practitioner, James G. made a thirty-mile trip to the EKLA, where he committed his eldest son to an institution for the insane.

Asylum officials recorded the cause of William's mania as 'fever fright', attributing the malady to a recent fever. Although excitable and restless upon admission, his condition gradually improved. On 10 November 1879, medical staff noted he 'has wonderfully improved in mental state and bodily health'.[59] This improvement was attributed at least in part to the use of cod-liver oil, a common remedy introduced in British medical practice in the late 1840s for 'wasting' ailments connected to diseases such as consumption and phthisis. William experienced a setback in December, however, prompting asylum personnel to comment: '[He] is getting very troublesome & saucy frequently interferes with other patients'.[60] By March of 1880, he was on the mend again, leading to his discharge on 13 April.

The inability of parents to control their children was a common theme among the admissions to the EKLA. Fifteen-year-old Ann E.'s mother Julia told officials that she had 'no control over her daughter'.[61] The girl was first brought to the attention of surgeon John Greasley after she was observed 'constantly following her [a lady] about'.[62] Admitted to the Canterbury hospital for five weeks, her behaviour improved. Upon discharge, however, Ann's condition worsened and she was admitted to the EKLA on 8 May 1883 as suicidal. Asylum officials reported that: 'She repeatedly complains to her mother of having something on her mind and must do something to herself'.[63] Melling and colleagues noted similar cases being admitted to the Devon County Asylum and concluded:

> [t]he threat posed by the lunatic child and adolescent to the safety, good order and respectability of the household and the wider community by 'unmanageable behaviour' was a vivid thread [in admission records].[64]

Such was the case of Edward P., a sixteen-year-old transfer patient from the Surrey County Asylum in Tooting admitted to the EKLA on 27 March 1882. Testimony from the medical certificate read:

> He has a wild look, is fond of messing with dirt, and does unaccountable things, a dead rat was found concealed in his bed. He is very passionate and violent so that his sisters are in fear of his committing [some] act of violence.[65]

EKLA admissions records confirmed a history of mania, identifying two previous bouts of insanity, the first of which occurred at the age of thirteen, during which it appears that Edward was admitted to Bethlem Royal Hospital. When admitted to the EKLA, his mother, the sole guardian of her ten children in 1881, was afraid her eldest son would 'commit some act of violence unless he is again removed from this house'.[66]

Propensity for violence outside the home was also of utmost concern. James F. was eighteen when he was admitted to the East Kent Lunatic Asylum for mania in March 1882. Testimony recorded on the Medical Certificate included the comments of neighbours and acquaintances, giving evidence of his disturbing behaviours:

> Mr. G. P. tells me that [James F.] came into his garden in a very excited condition and began dancing about and declared himself to be 'Jumbo', and that he talked in a very extravagant and exaggerated manner as to his abilities. Mr. Edward P [?] tells me that [James F.] has been jumping over fences & shouting out to the passing trains and calling 'Jumbo' out loud. Says all he does is by electricity.[67]

While these public displays were certainly odd, his actions also included more disturbing behaviours which posed a danger to himself and to the community. 'Mr. John C. tells me that JE [James F.] had in his possession a bottle of ... acid', the testimony continued, 'and that he had intended to commit suicide with it'.[68] Asylum personnel also noted that the youth had exposed himself to a local girl.[69] Admissions records indicated a family history of epilepsy and characterized his mother as 'addicted to drink', suggesting in the mind of mental-health professionals a predisposition to mental disorder.[70]

Lunatic children and youths like James F. behaved in ways that threatened life and personal possessions, and offended notions of public decency in regard to behaviours expected of young people of both sexes. Fourteen-year-old Matilda B., for example, was admitted to the EKLA in 1887 for '[p]eriodical attacks in which she throws herself about and exhibits violence to those in charge of her and while in these attacks [she] requires much restraint'.[71] At times these attacks were destructive: '[She] wander[s] aimlessly through the streets at night[,] damaging the furniture in her house [and] rushes out into the streets in her nightgown'.[72] The fact that the girl was repeatedly found in the neighbourhood at night seems to have been particularly disturbing (to her family as well as officials), undoubtedly casting further doubt on her mental (and perhaps her moral) state.

In the formal environment of the asylum, the evolving dynamics between asylum staff and the patients' families are intriguing. By the end of the nineteenth century, parents appear to have played less of a role in admissions to the EKLA. In the 1890s, admissions records became more streamlined and less 'personal', with testimony limited to brief statements from the medical certificate and medical histories abbreviated to a mere three or four lines. Family references could still be found in asylum records, but they were fewer in number. The records for Kate S., for example, limited the inclusion of family information to a reference to Kate's father as 'a drunkard' and her mother as having 'left him and gone to America'.[73] The sole familial reference in Emily S.'s admission record was to her father under the category 'relatives'.[74] We know even less about the experience of young patients after their discharge from the asylum. While a few were readmitted to the asylum over the years and some can be traced through the national census, most faded from the public eye.

Conclusion

Although neither histories of childhood nor disability issues have had much to say about the identification and management of the insane child this chapter has revealed that contemporary actors (from the most prominent alienist to the most humble neighbour offering witness testimony) were acutely aware of the serious conceptual and management problems these cases represented. Not only did the existence of insane children confound the emerging consensus that children should be childlike and innocent but their actions presented a very real threat to the welfare of individuals and society. Some of these hazards, such as the threat of national decline as the population degenerated, were perhaps better appreciated by concerned social commentators, but the immediate danger to people and property was obvious and the likely costs of care (in domestic as well as institutional settings) all too readily understood by relatives and local tax-payers.

The discourse surrounding public and medical concerns regarding the mental health of children and youths perched precariously at the intersection of two of the most pressing issues facing late-Victorian society. Victorians could accept the notion of the loss of sanity in adults and could rationalize the development of their often disturbing behaviour by applying commonly-held perceptions of class, gender, heredity and morality issues. It was much more difficult to explain insanity in children. In one arena, medical professionals and asylum personnel sought to better understand the nature of mental disorders and to devise more effective means of identifying and treating their patients. Simultaneously, changing approaches to children's welfare tended to increase the role of the state and undermine the authority of the family. Meanwhile, practitioners, lawmakers and conscientious citizens consistently lobbied for improvements and reforms in the operation and management of the asylums. Significant to both discussions of the treatment of mental disorders in the home and the management of the insane in county asylums were nineteenth-century assumptions about childhood. The idea of children as future members of the state and part of the nation itself, can be seen threading its way through the discourse surrounding insane children, providing medical men with the justification for penetrating the private realm of the home and the authority to usurp parental control for the good of the community and the state, establishing the legitimacy of both their diagnoses and their recommended methods of treatment. Evidence suggests, however, that at least some parents protested against increasing public interference when it came to matters of the family. The anonymous author of *The Cry of the Parents*, for example, criticized the increasing public emphasis on parental education and training advice, comparing such interference to 'the probe of the surgeon, necessary in disease but not in health'.[75]

By the late-Victorian period, then, childhood had become a very significant period of experience and children had become important individuals whose very beings were seen by some as embodying the hopes, dreams and values of an entire society. Given this idealized image of Victorian childhood, it is not surprising that British society found it so hard to deal with insane young people. These individuals were often seen as damaged products inclined toward disruption and disorder, the exact opposite of how many Victorians wanted to imagine childhood. It is not surprising that mental disorders in children emerged as a significant concern at this time. Indeed, the care and control of children with mental disorders were widely discussed in the late nineteenth century by philanthropists, medical practitioners and concerned citizens. In many ways, the question of institutionalization united both social reformers and medical practitioners and contributed to the changing dynamics in the relationship between the family, insanity and the Victorian state as part of a growing emphasis on 'preventative medicine, that is, a medical commitment to the solution of social problems primarily (but not entirely) through environmental reform, parental education, and the medical inspection and treatment of children'.[76]

3 THE MIXED ECONOMY OF WELFARE AND THE CARE OF SICK AND DISABLED CHILDREN IN THE SOUTH WALES COALFIELD, *c.* 1850–1950

Steven Thompson

Introduction

Historians of welfare have utilized the idea of a mixed economy of care to explain the various combinations of welfare providers in different contexts in the past.[1] They have used the concept as a means to better convey the balance and interaction of public and private forms of provision in any consideration of the welfare system and as a means to examine the provision of welfare in its totality; for a later period, the phrase very usefully reminds us of the variety of providers overlooked by use of the term 'welfare state'. In contrast to discrete studies of particular institutions or organizations, the concept changes the focus from a particular initiative to give more attention to the precise ways in which communities made provision for particular groups of the population or for distinct social 'problems', the conditions under which they did so, and the differential impact made by provision from different providers.

Despite criticisms of the *étatist* orientation of earlier accounts of welfare provision and the corresponding neglect of other, non-state providers, advocates of an approach that utilizes the mixed economy of welfare as a conceptual tool nevertheless adopt the state as the unit of analysis. Reminders that the mixed economy varied in space only seem to recognize that it did so *between* states and neglect to observe that it also varied *within* states. To date, very little attention has been paid to the regional or local particularities of the mixed economy of care.[2] And yet, a local or regional approach can allow us to better appreciate the varied and indeed contested nature of welfare provision in different parts of Britain and can complicate our understanding of this useful concept. It seems reasonable to assume that the precise mix of providers varied greatly between cities, industrial districts and rural areas or, to take a particular example, between Cardiff, Clydach Vale and Cilycwm. The particular social, industrial and political characteristics of the South Wales Coalfield, for example, resulted in a distinctive mixed economy of care that set it apart from other regions of Britain and, indeed, other industrial areas. Industrial south Wales, with its hazardous occupations, characterized, at least in the twentieth century, by a single, powerful and militant trade union and hostile, laissez-faire employers, lacking a significant middle class or wealthy local authorities, produced a distinctive mixed economy of welfare provision where working-class, mutualist provision was far more significant than in other areas of Britain and was, in many ways, more important than that provision made by other welfare providers within south Wales.[3]

But what did this mixed economy of care look like when viewed from the perspective of sick and disabled children? What were the consequences of the social, political and cultural characteristics of south Wales for the provision of medical, health and welfare services for the region's children? Did the mixed economy of child welfare and care differ from that which provided care more generally? Where exactly did disabled children sit within this particular mixed economy of care? How did their claim on the resources of coalfield communities compare with those of other children or the population more generally? Did any expansion of specialist services work to the benefit or detriment of disabled children and their families? Was provision designed to include or exclude? A chronological approach to these questions provides a broad perspective that allows the significant changes in modern British welfare provision to be observed more clearly. The focus on the South Wales Coalfield *c.* 1850–1950 captures both its breakneck industrialization and urbanization followed by economic depression and depopulation. This later period was when greater attention came to be placed on the health and well-being of children by the community. In this context, emphasis on frustrated aspirations, and obstacles to service development, usefully contrast with both celebratory accounts, that can easily overstate the contribution of specific institutions and prominent individuals, and pessimistic surveys that seek to highlight the deliberate neglect and marginalization of disabled people.

Mid-Nineteenth Century

Child welfare in south Wales in the mid-nineteenth century was, more so than in other parts of Britain, limited in scope and character. The care of sick and disabled children may have been particularly neglected in these circumstances. Workers' medical schemes in the iron-making communities at the heads of the valleys of Monmouthshire and Glamorgan, in contrast to schemes elsewhere, included medical attendance for wives and children.[4] In those same communities, certain employers made educational provision for the children of their workers,[5] but, for the most part, philanthropic activity was barely present in most valley communities at this time. The *Morning Chronicle* correspondent, for example, noted that Merthyr Tydfil, the largest town in the coalfield with a population of almost 50,000 people in 1851, possessed no almhouses, endowed charities or hospitals at mid-century despite the massive fortunes that had been accumulated in the town.[6] The South Wales Coalfield as a whole possessed none of the voluntary hospitals seen in other parts of Britain at this time. The small institutions founded in the southern coastal towns, such as at Swansea and, later, Cardiff and Newport, were only utilized by male workers whose employers or friendly societies had subscribed the necessary amounts to gain tickets of admission. Just about the only welfare provision made for children in such communities was through the residual and punitive Poor Law.

Poor Law facilities for the care of sick paupers in south Wales were meagre and inadequate. Merthyr Tydfil Union did not open a workhouse until 1853 but most unions in the region built workhouses within a relatively short space of time after the Act of 1834, despite popular opposition, and provided means within these workhouses to disaggregate paupers into various categories. These workhouses were, nevertheless, too small for the populations they were intended to support and did not have sufficient specialist provision for different groups of the population. Some had children's wards but these were small and inadequate; when infectious disease epidemics broke out amongst the children of the Merthyr workhouse, for example, the only space available for them was in the attics of the building.[7] In such circumstances, sick and disabled children too often ended up in the general rooms or wards of the workhouses.[8]

Given this paucity of provision, it is perhaps not surprising, therefore, that a Select Committee report published in the 1840s found that Poor Law authorities in Glamorgan spent less per head of population on medical relief than any other union in England and Wales with the exception of one other union.[9] This was primarily due to cultural attitudes to poverty and sickness. There was undoubtedly popular and official opposition in Wales towards the new Poor Law system that was seen as a cruel, alien imposition that clashed with Welsh values. Families preferred to care for sick or injured relatives at home and were loath to see them enter institutions.[10] During the cholera epidemic of 1866, for example, the Dowlais workmen passed a series of resolutions which included the demand that sick men, women and children should be treated in their homes, if possible, rather than be admitted to the Poor Law infirmary.[11] Correspondingly, Welsh Poor Law authorities preferred to give outdoor relief rather than build large, expensive institutions.[12] Care for children was bound up in this medical and political economy of provision. Little provision was made, and services tended not to meet the particular needs of disabled children. For the most part, the family continued to be their primary source of support and care.

Late-Nineteenth Century

Despite the development of the iron industry in the late eighteenth and early nineteenth centuries, and despite the existence of coal-mining during the same period, partly to serve the various metallurgical industries in the region, it was the rapid development of the export coal industry in the second half of the nineteenth century, and in the last few decades of the century in particular, that brought about the most significant urbanization and industrialization of the south Wales valleys. This resulted in a massive increase in population: the population of Monmouthshire and Glamorgan doubled from about 600,000 in 1871 to almost 1.2 million by 1901.[13] With the increase in population, and the unhealthy nature of these 'frontier' towns, the need for medical, health and welfare services increased. While it would be difficult to argue that welfare and medical provision kept pace with these developments, certain improvements did take place at this time. Children, with and without disabling conditions, were sometimes the intended beneficiaries but at other times were not.

For example, and perhaps rather unexpectedly, voluntary efforts resulted in a children's hospital being founded in Merthyr Tydfil in 1877. A sum of money was left over from a children's meal fund that had been established during an industrial dispute in the town. It was used as the nucleus of a fund to establish the Cefn and Merthyr Children's Hospital. The hospital, in a converted house, had accommodation for twelve patients and preference was given to orthopaedic cases, perhaps because such cases offered the best possibility of finite and effective treatment and suited the particular skills of surgeons in an industrial district such as Merthyr where orthopaedic injuries were so common. By the time of the hospital's second annual report in 1879, Dr Dyke, the honorary surgeon, expressed the hope that the hospital could be expanded to take in 'some of the slighter cases of disease amongst children' also but it seems that the hospital admitted mainly orthopaedic cases for the duration of its short existence.[14]

This Children's Hospital at Merthyr was the only such specialist hospital in south Wales until the twentieth century. More common were small cottage hospitals, founded in the years that followed, that possessed children's wards. The Aberdare Cottage Hospital, founded by the Marquis of Bute in 1881 and maintained by him in the years that followed, possessed a ward for women and children that contained four beds.[15] Such provision hardly constituted specialized or even adequate care for sick and disabled children and it is clear that the poverty of south Wales was reflected in this totally inadequate provision. In their annual reports to the Local Government Board, the Poor Law inspectors for south Wales often noted the absence of the better-off classes from coalfield communities and the consequent lack of charitable activity; similarly, critics of employers in south Wales pointed out their failure to invest adequately in social provision for the communities in which their works were situated.[16] Even within this limited provision, children came after breadwinners as the focus of welfare and medical initiatives.

And yet there was one area in coalfield communities where child welfare was prioritized and did indeed motivate voluntary effort, and this was in the wake of the mining disasters that devastated too many pit villages. In such instances, communities assumed responsibility for the children of miners killed and disaster funds not only provided a weekly sum of money to mothers or guardians as maintenance, but also made extra provision for the children in the event of sickness and disability. Colliery disaster funds paid monthly sums to local doctors, for example, to provide medical attendance for the children and also made additional payments to the guardians of disabled or sickly children where the additional income was required.[17] Extraordinary payments were made by the disaster funds to allow children to travel to hospitals to obtain surgical and medical assistance; examples include children being provided with the funds to attend Bristol Eye Hospital and the Cheshire Epileptic Asylum.[18] In other instances there were attempts to secure the long-term support and future economic productivity of mentally and physically disabled children. Disaster funds paid for such children to become apprenticed as dressmakers, shoemakers and in other occupations.[19] The funds continued to support disabled children after they reached the age of thirteen and were due to come off the funds.[20] In the case of an 'imbecile' boy relieved by the Park Slip Colliery Explosion Fund, the committee of the Fund made repeated attempts to persuade his mother to have him committed to the Western Counties Idiot Asylum at Starcross but she continuously refused and he continued to be cared for in the home.[21] This suggests perhaps the opposition that might have existed among many families towards sending their children to far-flung institutions that would have been very difficult for working-class families to visit. It also reminds us of the importance of the family as a source of care but also that where institutions were utilized, it tended to be those far removed from the coalfield communities in which these children lived. Such examples also demonstrate the increased complexity of the mixed economy of care by this time: the disaster funds, voluntarily raised, facilitated access to other charitable and philanthropic resources, in these instances institutions, for members of the community.

Nevertheless, colliery disasters were exceptional in the emotions and social relations they occasioned and the absence of philanthropic provision was the defining feature of most coalfield communities. This relative lack of voluntary philanthropic or paternalistic activity in the South Wales Coalfield was also reflected in the absence of provision for children with disabilities. Coalfield communities were forced to rely on institutions for blind and deaf and dumb children found in the larger, coastal towns to the south of the coalfield or in towns in close proximity to the coalfield, such as Bristol. Such towns possessed more varied social structures, were sufficiently affluent to make provision, and drew their patients from a much larger geographical area than their immediate vicinities. These institutions did take in some children from the coalfield but, as was noted in 1889, there were still large numbers of such children in the region who received no such specialized education or medical care whatsoever and who continued to be cared for by their families or the Poor Law.[22] Those children who gained entry into these institutions did so through Poor Law admission or, later on, through referral by educational authorities. In the mid-1870s, for example, the Pontardawe Board of Guardians sent child paupers to the Cambrian Institution for the Deaf and Dumb and the Institution for the Blind, both at Swansea for care and instruction.[23] Similarly, Neath Poor Law Guardians drew upon the services of the Bristol Blind Institution and the Blind, and Deaf and Dumb institutions at Swansea in the latter decades of the century.[24] The usual practice was for the Guardians to pay the cost of the fees and maintenance of those pauper children sent to such institutions. In addition, board deaf schools were founded by the local education authorities in Pontypridd and the Rhondda valley in the 1890s, but still most coalfield communities relied on the provision made in towns such as Swansea, Cardiff, Newport and Bristol.[25]

Poor Law Guardians in south Wales, therefore, were still some distance behind other unions in England in the provision of specialist services for children and the poor. Most unions built relatively small workhouses, and only very slowly were separate infirmaries added. Part of the reason for this later development in south Wales can be attributed to enduring Welsh attitudes to the Poor Law: again and again it was noted that Guardians in Wales preferred to give outrelief, and that indoor-relief was the exception rather than the rule.[26] The Poor Law Inspector for Wales estimated that out-relief accounted for almost 90 per cent of all relief given by Poor Law Guardians in south Wales in 1891.[27] Specialist provision in the form of industrial schools for pauper children and cottage homes for orphans was gradually made but specialist provision for children with disabilities was almost non-existent in the coalfield, either inside or outside the Poor Law system. The Poor Law Inspector for Wales claimed in 1900 that most unions had their share of 'imbeciles of a harmless and inoffensive type' who continued to be housed in workhouses. He insisted that while some would have benefited from specialized care in asylums, such asylums were too over-crowded to permit their transfer and that the majority of them were, in any case, 'happier' in workhouses than they would be elsewhere.[28]

Some use was made of institutions outside the region: efforts were made in the early 1880s to send a handful of children to the Royal National Asylum for Idiots at Earlswood, Surrey but these *ad hoc* efforts stood outside the Poor Law as citizens in Cardiff and Swansea attempted to raise enough money through philanthropic means to pay for the maintenance of children in this institution.[29] By the end of the century, it was found that Earlswood only contained a small number of children from Wales despite it being the only one of the five English voluntary idiot institutions that admitted children from the country.[30] Calls for the establishment of a similar Welsh institution, or even a modest local facility, did not come to fruition.[31] The vast majority of children we would now understand to have learning disabilities, therefore, remained within Poor Law accommodation or else were cared for by their families.

Twentieth Century

Developments in the twentieth century greatly changed the context within which provision for children was made and transformed the mixed economy of care. In some contemporary publications this was termed the new 'Children's Era'.[32] It placed greater emphasis on the value of infants and children to the community, and encouraged service development. Far greater provision was made, particularly by district councils and local educational authorities, but also by a number of other providers that emerged in the decades after the turn of the century. The emergence of these providers, and the many, various ways in which they interacted with each other, brought about an increasingly complex mixed economy of care. In addition, the particular political context of south Wales influenced the extent and nature of provision, with a far more extensive representation of working-class interests in local authorities in south Wales in comparison to other parts of Britain;[33] 'Labour women' were particularly vocal advocates of child welfare reforms.[34] Continued improvements were made to Poor Law services, partly as a result of central pressures but also due to the influence of larger numbers of female and working-class Guardians from the mid-1890s onwards.[35] The vast majority of children were housed separately from the main workhouse in Welsh Unions by the end of the Edwardian period in separate blocks or even in cottage homes on separate sites. Many unions appointed female officers as infant life protection officers following the Children Act of 1908 and such officers visited the homes of women who received relief to ensure their children were well cared for.[36] Sick and disabled children were likely to have received particularly close attention as part of these schemes.

The early twentieth century also witnessed some new developments in voluntary sector provision for physically disabled children in the region. Poor Cripples Aid societies were founded in Cardiff and Newport in imitation of similar organizations elsewhere and worked in various ways to assist individuals, mostly children but adults also, with disabilities. Payments of money were occasionally made but, in most cases, assistance to disabled individuals came in the form of surgical appliances and equipment such as crutches, artificial limbs, surgical splints, spinal jackets and orthopaedic boots.[37] The societies also arranged for children with disabilities to undergo surgical treatment at a range of hospitals throughout Britain, either through paying regular subscriptions, making donations, or paying the cost of the treatment in relation to those institutions. In the absence of specialist services in south Wales, the societies sent disabled children to institutions such as the Bristol Royal Hospital for Sick Children and Women, the Bristol Orthopaedic Hospital, the Victoria Hospital for Children, Chelsea, the Alexandra Hospital for Children with Hip Disease, Luton, the Lord Mayor Treloar Cripples Hospital and College at Alton, and the Royal National Orthopaedic Hospital, London. In the same way, the societies arranged entry into various convalescent homes and training colleges for the disabled throughout south Wales and the southern half of England. That these societies were forced to send children outside the region, and sometimes quite considerable distances, for specialist orthopaedic care and convalescence demonstrates once again the paucity of provision in the region relative to other parts of Britain, but the location of these charities in Cardiff and Newport also points to the inequalities in charitable resources *within* the region as the larger towns on the coast, with their larger, more varied economies, were better able to sustain such voluntary initiatives than the poorer communities of the coalfield. The Cardiff Poor Cripples Aid Society, for example, did aid some individuals from the mining valleys but, for the most part, it was the disabled people of the towns themselves that benefited most from the activities of the societies.[38]

Furthermore, the work of these charities provides a fascinating insight into the workings of the mixed economy of care. As shown, the Cardiff Society arranged for disabled children to access specialist orthopaedic surgical and convalescent care provided by other charities.[39] It usually bore the cost of entry or maintenance but there were a large number of cases in which the families of the children or indeed Poor Law authorities paid part or indeed all of the cost.[40] Where the Society did not incur any costs, it would seem that the Society's contacts and experience were utilized by parents or public bodies. This co-operation between a voluntary organization and public authorities was even more marked in 1927 when Dr Ralph Picken, Medical Officer of Health for Cardiff, requested the assistance of the Society. He met with the secretary of the Society in October 1927 and explained that the money he had been allocated for orthopaedic work on children of school age to March 1928 had already been overspent and requested that the Society should assist urgent cases among such children while he devoted what resources he possessed to children below school age. The Society agreed to this, despite its slender resources, and assisted as many cases as possible in the following months, though it did write to the County Borough Council a little later asking that it increase its funding to this type of work so that such a burden did not fall on the Society year after year.[41] The Society also had an arrangement with the Glamorgan County Council whereby the Council subscribed to the Society and sent it cases, although, as a result of economic pressures, this changed in 1931 when the Council decided to pay the Society on a case-by-case basis.[42]

Despite such voluntary initiatives, public bodies continued to be the most important providers of child welfare services. In this regard, the most important innovation in child welfare in these early decades of the twentieth century was the introduction of school medical inspection and school medical services. One socialist from south Wales welcomed the advent of school medical inspection as the dawn of socialism, but inspection itself was not enough.[43] Perhaps inevitably, a school medical service was developed within a short space of time. Some school clinics were established in the late Edwardian period: a clinic for the treatment of eye, ear and skin diseases was opened at Abertillery in 1910. In this case, the initiative was partly justified along the lines that such problems were not met by club practice in the area, that there was an absence of hospitals, dispensaries and nursing associations in the locality, and that the Poor Law system did not meet such need.[44] Despite its pride in having established the first school clinic in Wales, the Abertillery education authority was nevertheless frustrated by financial considerations in its attempts to further develop its school medical service in the decades that followed, and the service was soon surpassed by those offered by other authorities. The clinic treated eye diseases and defective eyesight, ear complaints and skin diseases but did not treat minor ailments or tonsils and adenoids.[45] Some minor improvements came in the next few years but the school medical officer could do little but recommend suggested improvements and enhancements to the service in his annual reports through the 1920s and 1930s. Recommendations that an assistant school medical officer be appointed, that new premises for the clinic be erected, that the dental clinic be extended and that a full-time dentist be appointed, that the x-ray treatment of ringworm be initiated, that remedial exercises for children be offered, that an open-air school be built, that school baths be made available, and that classes for 'dull' and 'backward' children be started, were made annually throughout the late 1920s and early 1930s but to little avail.[46]

This pattern of initial development followed by frustration in the interwar period was replicated in the other local educational authority areas in the coalfield. Monmouthshire County educational authority made good progress in the few years after the introduction of school medical inspection as staff were appointed, an eye clinic and a clinic for minor ailments were established, open-

air classrooms were erected at a number of its schools, and, in 1920, the school
medical service was coordinated with the maternity and child welfare department. Further clinics were added so that by 1922 there was a network of nine
clinics and one travelling clinic for the rural areas of the county. Attention in
Britain came to be focused on the orthopaedic care and treatment of children
with 'crippling defects' in the 1920s but the county was unable to make much
provision, despite plans in 1924 to build an Orthopaedic Hospital School at
Caerleon, and instead secured twenty-four beds at the Royal National Orthopaedic Hospital at London in 1924 for use by its children.[47] Prior to this, the
education authority had contracted with different hospitals in various ways to
procure surgical treatment: in 1914, for example, the authority paid £25 to the
National Orthopaedic Hospital for treatment for a child suffering curvature
of the spine, while an annual subscription of £10 to the Royal Gwent Hospital
allowed thirteen children to receive treatment, mainly surgical, for minor ailments.[48] Subsequent to this, however, and in light of the authority's failure to
develop its own comprehensive scheme, the medical officer could do no more
than extol the virtues of the facilities available to Monmouthshire children
at the Orthopaedic Hospital.[49] An orthopaedic consultant was appointed in
1932 and clinics were held on a few days each month at which children were
inspected for admission to the National Hospital or for the provision of orthopaedic appliances. Nevertheless, such provision did not come close to meeting
the considerable need that existed in the county as the number of children with
orthopaedic 'defects' numbered in the hundreds each year.[50]

Financial difficulties in the interwar period prevented the establishment
of an Orthopaedic Hospital School in the county, but they also limited other
areas of provision. While nine open-air classrooms had been opened by 1920,
for example, this number had fallen to three by 1934 as the classrooms were
put back into general use when the authorities were unable to provide enough
accommodation for the school population; Rocyn Jones lamented the inability
of the county to maintain and extend this important work for 'delicate' children.[51] He might have had in mind the successful open-air school opened at
Aberdare in 1914. The school had classes for mentally and physically disabled
children where a regime of suitable meals and dietary supplements, open-air
treatment, prescribed rest periods, medical attention, corrective exercises, and
educational instruction from specially trained teachers, was instituted and from
which many children, at least those with physical disabilities, were returned to
their former schools after a period of time. Those children described as 'mentally
defective' were engaged in practical work that was intended to prepare them for
their future working lives: girls were trained in various domestic skills and subsequently entered domestic service, while boys were given more practical tasks to
do around the school – many went on to do surface work at the local collieries.[52]

The financial limitations faced by local authorities in interwar south Wales are most starkly revealed in the case of the Rhondda Local Education Authority. By the early 1920s, its service was limited to dental and ophthalmic treatment while minor defects were treated by medical practitioners in the district since, as the school medical officer argued, most of the population was registered for medical attendance in the colliery medical schemes that, in south Wales at least, included dependent wives and children.[53] By the interwar period, however, he was forced to admit that many of the defects identified by school medical inspection were not treated because many ailments required specialist knowledge, skill or appliances and occasionally hospital care; medical practitioners too often did not possess these things, gave most of their time to the adult male patients in their practices, and did not have access to hospital facilities due to the paucity of provision in the district.[54] There was much variation in the treatment of tonsils and adenoids for many of the same reasons.[55] Differences in orthopaedic work were even starker, since local doctors were even less likely to have had sufficient experience to develop the necessary skills.[56] In the absence of orthopaedic provision, the Authority could do no more than arrange for admission of some of the worst cases to the Prince of Wales Hospital at Cardiff and, as was commented, 'in view of the … financial distress in the district, even this form of assistance has been limited to the narrowest possible extent'.[57]

Enhancements to Rhondda's limited school medical service came only very slowly in this period and were often initiated or assisted by organizations from the voluntary sphere. In the 1920s, for example, the Carnegie Trust made a grant of £100,000 to the Ministry of Health, to be shared between four district councils in different parts of Britain, for the establishment of infant welfare clinics. One of these clinics was situated in the Rhondda valleys.[58] It was completed in 1927, but, the clinic was not equipped and furnished until the end of the decade due to the inability of the local authority to afford the expense.[59] The medical department was only able to pay these costs as a result of funding from the Coalfields Distress Fund and the clinic was subsequently used for school medical service and orthopaedic purposes in addition to child welfare work.[60] The council itself was only able to make improvements in the late 1930s. New clinics were opened at Ferndale and Ynyswen, and another at Ystrad was rebuilt and opened.[61] A scheme for the treatment of minor ailments and an extended scheme of orthopaedic care were initiated at these clinics in 1938. An agreement was also struck with local hospitals and the former Poor Law institution at Llwynypia, now under the control of Glamorgan County Council, for the surgical treatment of chronic tonsillitis and adenoids.[62] Pleas by the school medical officer for the treatment of diseases of the ear and nose, for the supervision and treatment of rheumatic cases, and for open-air schools to care for delicate or convalescing children amounted to nothing.[63] It is noteworthy, however, that even these undelivered schemes helped establish a medical framework for care and tended to encourage the eventual development of specialist, and segregated, institutional facilities for sick and disabled children. This ultimately brought mixed benefits for disabled children.

This story of failure and retrenchment in the interwar period is most marked in relation to another of the responsibilities of the school medical service: physically and mentally 'defective' children. The story of provision in this area is one of almost complete failure. Various Poor Law unions in Glamorgan held a meeting in 1899 to discuss the possibility of a joint colony with the county council for epileptics and a school for 'idiot' and 'feeble-minded' children. Such an institution, it was claimed, could not be provided by the Guardians, even in combination, and needed to be organized with the county council for non-pauper children as well as those children under the care of the Poor Law. It was noted that if such plans came to fruition and led to the establishment of the two planned institutions for the whole of Wales and Monmouthshire, they would meet a want that had long existed and finally bring Wales up to the level of other parts of the United Kingdom.[64] Nevertheless, a joint scheme was still being debated when war broke out in 1914.[65] The smaller educational authorities resorted to making their own provision, albeit it on a small, inadequate scale: Barry, Mountain Ash and Pontypridd made school provision for forty, twenty and forty mentally defective children respectively.[66] No significant provision was made in Glamorgan in the interwar period,[67] but a small day-school for fifty 'educable' mentally defective children was opened by the Rhondda authority in 1932. The school medical officer noted that there were roughly 350 such children in the area and that seven or eight times as much accommodation was actually needed.[68]

Similarly in Monmouthshire, the educational authority initiated discussions with Ebbw Vale and Abertillery authorities in 1909, and invited Newport County Borough to join the discussions in the following year, over the joint provision of a school for mentally and physically 'defective' children.[69] A site at Caerleon was chosen and plans were further developed in the next few years to increase the size of the proposed institution and to include some form of accommodation for blind and deaf children; subsequent amendments included some form of open-air school on the same site.[70] These plans were eventually abandoned in 1932 in favour of an alternative plan for a Colony for Mental Defectives by the County Mental Deficiency Committee constituted under the 1913 legislation.[71] This similarly failed to materialize. Throughout this period, therefore, despite these various negotiations, plans and efforts, the vast majority of the hundreds of mentally and physically defective children classified as such each year continued to be educated in public elementary schools or else remained at home.

While financial pressures placed limitations on local authorities, these early decades of the twentieth century nevertheless witnessed the emergence of new providers in the welfare mix. One of these new providers was the labour movement, though the extent of its provision was limited. Pit lodges had supported local causes in the nineteenth century but the formation of the South Wales Miners' Federation in 1898, with its commitment to play an important social and cultural role in the lives of all the people of the communities in which its lodges were situated, gave a new fillip to efforts within the labour movement in the region to help and support children. Lodge committees undertook collections of money to aid individual children obtain specialist care and treatment. They also supported voluntary organizations such as specialist schools for disabled children or organizations such as Barnardo's Homes.[72] Most lodges subscribed to the Porthcawl Rest Convalescent Home on the south Wales coast and provided tickets not only for members and their wives, but also to allow the children of members to enjoy a stay at this institution to recuperate after illness or an operation.[73]

Nevertheless, despite these examples of provision and instances of awareness of the problems of child welfare, the labour movement was dominated by a conception of welfare needs that prioritized the protection of the earning capacity of male workers as the best means of ensuring the welfare of different members of the family and indeed the community as a whole. The South Wales Miners' Federation, for example, might have claimed that it aimed to defend the interests of all the people in which its lodges were situated, and might have been more generous in the distribution of aid and support than its rules allowed, but it nevertheless looked first to defend wages or supplement incomes and made little specialist provision for other members of the community.[74] The broad character of the Federation's social and welfare provision for its members far surpassed anything it provided for the 'dependent' wives and children of its members and, instead, it contented itself with the nomination and support of candidates in Poor Law, district, and county council elections, where, it was believed, the interests of women and children were best served. The particular needs of disabled children remained far in the background of this labourist conception of welfare.

Conclusion

An examination of the mixed economy of child welfare provision in south Wales, more so than studies of welfare and medical services more generally, demonstrates in more dramatic and clear terms the distinctiveness of south Wales. Here it is the paucity of provision for children, especially sick and disabled children, that is striking. The social structure of coalfield communities did not allow for any meaningful philanthropic activity and the particular character of coal employers in the region meant that industrial paternalism was largely absent. In addition, Welsh Poor Law authorities were less inclined to build large, expensive institutions and preferred to give out-relief. All these factors were responsible for creating a distinctive mixed economy of care and left it trailing behind just about every other region of Britain in the extent of provision made. This shortfall was even more marked in relation to provision for disabled children as attention was focused more on the nutritional and health status of the general school population rather than the specific and expensive needs of small sections of the child population. In the early decades of the twentieth century, local authorities attempted to make good the historic shortfall in provision. There were some notable successes, for example an expanding number of maternity and child welfare clinics, but services were not transformed and did not become comprehensive. This was partly as a result of the economic depression but primarily because of the relative poverty of coalfield communities.

To some extent, the inequalities relative to other regions of Britain were lessened as Labour-dominated local authorities put 'public welfare before private interest',[75] but regional inequalities remained nevertheless. Both the report of the consultative council on medical and allied services that was published in 1920, and the hospital survey published by the Nuffield Trust in 1945, demonstrated the paucity of provision of health services in south Wales that was even more marked in the provision made for children, especially for disabled children.[76] They demonstrated that south Wales was perhaps the most poorly provided for region in the whole of Britain. In addition, however, the mixed economy of *child* welfare provision differed from the mixed economy of care as a whole. The mixed economy of care in industrial south Wales, primarily intended to meet the needs of working men, was dominated by provision within the labour movement and, by the twentieth century, the South Wales Miners' Federation. The mixed economy of child welfare was clearly far less indebted to the labour movement. It was the state, particularly local authorities, that provided the vast majority of child welfare services, through the Poor Law, the educational system, and the maternity and child welfare service.

While the distinctive character of the mixed economy of care in the South Wales Coalfield resulted in a relatively low level of provision, it was nevertheless the case that, as provision increased, so the complexity of the mixed economy intensified. Different providers had interacted in different ways and in varying degrees in the early decades of industrialization as Poor Law unions drew upon the few specialized forms of child welfare provision made available in the voluntary sphere, usually in the seaport towns to the south of the coalfield or, more usually, across the border. But with the development of provision by a series of different providers, so the interactions between them increased, particularly in the twentieth century as the increased responsibility of local government combined with the entry of national voluntary organizations into coalfield communities due to the interwar depression; these organizations were themselves more willing to countenance working with local authorities perhaps as a result of their increasing marginalization by an increasingly interventionist state. Such complexity was not limited to south Wales, of course, but such complexities registered themselves in different ways in different parts of the British Isles.

4 THE QUESTION OF ORALISM AND THE EXPERIENCES OF DEAF CHILDREN, 1880–1914

Mike Mantin

Introduction

In 1880, the delegates of the International Congress on the Education of the Deaf in Milan met to discuss the direction of deaf education. Their attention was focused specifically on the role of articulation and speech, in contrast to the prevalent sign-language-based manual teaching methods. Of its 164 attendees, 139 represented the Italian and French clergy, five people each comprised the British and American delegations and only two were deaf.[1] On 11 September, the delegates voted 160 votes to four, for the 'incontestable superiority of speech over signs, for restoring deaf mutes to social life and giving them greater superiority in language'.[2] With hardly a single deaf voice, the Congress began the process of removing sign language from the education of deaf children across the world. A year later, British headmasters gathered at the Conference of Head Masters of Institutions and of Other Workers for the Education of the Deaf and Dumb in London. They discussed the 'pure oral' system advocated in Milan, which would teach articulation and lip-reading rather than signs. Richard Elliott, headmaster of the Old Kent Road and Margate schools, presented the opening paper, musing on the Congress's recommendation of the abandonment of signs:

> If I believed that the Congress at Milan had settled the question, I should have said change your system – I do not believe it has done so, so far as the English language is concerned, but it has brought forward prominently the claims of the system it advocates, and therefore, I say, try it – but try it without sacrificing the interests of any child in the enlightenment it seeks at your hands.[3]

Elliott's cautious optimism for the system epitomized the long, varied and often contradictory debate which Britain experienced in the years after 1880, neither wholeheartedly embracing oralism nor fighting the ideologies of normalization and language suppression that had been shaped at Milan.

The practice and legacy of what is now largely termed 'oralism' has become the most controversial and passionately-argued topic of modern deaf history, though some early histories of special education discussed it uncritically. For example, Kenneth Hodgson's *The Deaf and their Problems* (1953) presented deaf history from a distinctly medical perspective, the history of oralism fitting into a narrative of progress against the 'problem' of losing hearing.[4] Similarly, D. G. Pritchard found the earliest deaf schools' abandonment of oralism 'deeply to be regretted'.[5] More recently, however, a new strand of deaf history has emerged which studies deaf culture as a separate and richly varied entity, one which could be subject to oppression from the hearing majority.[6] For example, Paddy Ladd emotively asks:

> What could we have been had not sign language and Deaf teachers been removed from Deaf education after the Milan Congress of 1880, a date as pregnant with meaning for us as 1492 is for Native Americans.[7]

Ladd's juxtaposition of oralism's effect on deaf people with the colonization of Native American people's land demonstrates the strength of feeling about oralism. Historians have attacked oral teachers' dismissal and suppression of any kind of deaf community and its language, as well as the general failure of the system to achieve its main goal – enabling deaf children to write and speak English.[8] Moreover, historians are beginning to address the need for deaf voices in their own history. Cathy Kudlick notes the shift towards seeing deaf people as 'active agents of their own fate', standing up for their position as a 'legitimate linguistic minority'.[9] Studies such as Robert Buchanan's *Illusions of Equality* show a picture of organizational and personal resistance to the threat oralism posed to American deaf people's communities.[10] 'This record of sustained resistance through shared linguistic and cultural identification,' he argues, 'is remarkable, if not unique, in American history'.[11]

These contests over language were fought not just in the United States, but worldwide. This chapter aims to supplement existing studies and criticisms of oralism and its historical effects by focusing specifically on Britain. It will reveal a deeply fought contest for the identities and lives of deaf children which, from a national perspective, did not simply lead to an instant shift from manualism (the use of sign in the classroom) to oralism. The chapter will then focus on the Cambrian Institution for the Deaf and Dumb, the first and largest deaf institution in Wales. Its records – most significantly a collection of letters sent by its deaf principal Benjamin Payne – reveal an open but questioning, and frequently contradictory, attitude to the value and ideology of oralism. It will be argued that, in order to understand the complexity of the situation, the historian needs to consider the experiences of pupils and the deaf communities to which they belonged, alongside the far more widely documented opinions of educators and philanthropists. Payne's letters provide clues to the effects on the individual children's lives, while deaf newspapers reveal deaf resistance to oralism's destructive effects on the community. Though these deaf voices are hard to find, and in some cases require careful reading of institutional sources, they help to reveal the damaging effects of oralism and, crucially, resistance from the deaf people whose lives it affected.

Oralism in Britain

Whilst Milan marked a watershed for the replacement of sign language with oralism, Britain's pre-1880 deaf education was less homogenous than the extremes experienced by France and Germany. Despite some voices of opposition, the majority of French deaf students, beginning with those at the Abbé Charles-Michel de l'Épée's school in Paris in 1760, had used French Sign Language (FSL). This was until a dramatic shift to oralism as a consequence of Milan. FSL was banned in many schools from 1880 until the 1990s.[12] Conversely, Germany had mostly been using the pure oral system since Samuel Heinicke had founded its first deaf school in Leipzig in 1778, favouring the articulation-focused teaching method he had developed.[13] As several historians have pointed out, Britain's deaf schools had been mixing manual and oral methods long before 1880 and did not rely on one fixed interpretation of how deaf children should be educated.[14] Thomas Braidwood, whose Academy for the Deaf and Dumb in Edinburgh was the first school for the deaf in Britain, used what Jackson has called 'a form of total communication', which taught both speech and sign.[15] His early methods were primarily oralist and involved using mouth instruments to teach children sounds of words, moving to more manual-focused teaching later in his career.[16] Many of the emerging British deaf schools (which until the 1820s remained dominated by Braidwood and his family) used either the 'combined system' of sign and speech or occasionally, in the case of the Swiss headmaster Louis du Puget at the General Institution for the Instruction of Deaf and Dumb Children at Birmingham, manualism in the French tradition.[17]

The Milan Congress raised the profile of oralism in the UK, though the pure oral method had been spreading since the 1850s. This had started on a small scale through figures such as Susannah Hull in London and Gerrit van Asch in Manchester, and culminated in the founding in 1871 of the Association for the Oral Instruction of the Deaf and Dumb in Fitzroy Square, London.[18] Likewise, from 1879 the London School Board (LSB) introduced the pure oral system into their experimental Day Schools.[19] The LSB was one of few school boards to deal specifically with deaf children. It shunned the traditional institutional approach in favour of day schools, which most leaders of institutions considered insufficient to provide deaf children with a full education. Reverend William Stainer – appointed first as a teacher and later as Superintendent of Schools and Classes for the Deaf and Dumb Children of the Metropolis – presented this idea in a paper on 'The Advantages of Small Numbers in Day Schools over Large Numbers in Institutions' at the Headmasters' Conference of 1877.[20] He noted that a number of school boards (such as Sheffield) sought to emulate the LSB. However, the resulting discussion at the conference suggests his ideas received a less than enthusiastic response from the institutions' headmasters.[21] The institutions and school boards which *did* adopt the oral method also varied greatly in their execution. A letter to the *British Medical Journal* in 1884 praised the LSB but criticized institutions whose oral classes were ruined, according to the author, by 'the habitual practice of signs, and the manual alphabet in the daily teaching of its pupils'.[22]

Yet for all its unusualness, the LSB's adoption of oralism was indicative of increasingly receptive British attitudes towards the method. In the wake of Milan, oralism became a major facet of British deaf education. Oralism received widespread recognition as a valid educational practice and this encouraged rejection of sign language. Indeed, Stainer himself made what Pritchard calls 'a very sudden conversion' to pure oralism, having previously advocated the combined system.[23] The Royal Commission on the Blind, the Deaf and Dumb acted as an outlet and introduction for some of the key strategies and ideologies behind oralism. Initiated in 1885 by Lord Egerton to recommend state action for blind education, it began reporting on deaf education the following year. The Report emerged in 1889 as a forum for debate on oralism. It reprinted an American debate between Edward Miner Gallaudet and Alexander Graham Bell. Gallaudet, like his father Thomas Hopkins Gallaudet, helped give signs a major role in American deaf education, while Bell's work in deaf education focused largely on speech and articulation.[24]

The American interviews provided a backdrop to the Commissioners' own debates. Although the three panellists varied in their educational backgrounds, their conclusions came down firmly on the side of oralism. While shunning a total ban of signs, as in France, the adoption of the oral system in certain schools was presented as 'a step in the right direction'.[25] Perhaps more telling were the explanations offered as to why signs were to be sidelined:

> We have observed how the use of signs creates a tendency to live apart as a class rather than to mix with the world, and upon the consequent intermarriage of the deaf, which in Germany and Switzerland does not occur to the same extent under the oral system.[26]

The supposed dangers of deaf people marrying or cutting themselves off from hearing society were flagged throughout the report. The Commissioners printed research from a paper given by Dr David Buxton at the Medical Society at Liverpool. He argued that congenital deafness in children was seven times more likely if both parents were deaf, rather than just one.[27] Oralism was proposed by the Commissioners as the best solution to the supposed problem of deaf people failing to integrate into wider society. 'The use of articulate language and the power of lip-reading accurately', they argued, 'are the greatest alleviation to their isolated position'.[28] The reasoning behind the Royal Commission's findings demonstrates the importance of finding the underlying motivations behind oral education, and their effect on (and destruction of) deaf communities. Much research has already been done on the wider social motivations of oralism. Douglas Baynton has explored the 'linguistic Darwinism' at the heart of the theory. It was argued, even by Darwin himself, that contemporary sign language was 'used by the deaf and dumb and by savages', and was linked to the gestures used by humans before they mastered spoken language.[29] Oralism would therefore give teachers the responsibility and ability to instil spoken language in deaf people, returning them to hearing society and thus human evolution.

It was this evolutionary slant and normalizing ideology which made oralism more than compatible with the emerging eugenics movement. Alexander Graham Bell's warnings against 'the formation of a deaf variety of the human race' (this despite his wife's deafness) chimed perfectly with the eugenicists voicing their fears of the decline of the race and the reproduction of the 'unfit'.[30] Likewise, the Royal Commissioners' argument that schools should keep careful statistics (recording pupils' age of deafness, existence of deaf relatives, amount of hearing and physical condition) mirrored the meticulous race science methodology of Francis Galton and Karl Pearson.[31] The use of oralism was also deeply class-based and exclusionary. Oral methods were more expensive than manual and required smaller class sizes, and few claimed that all deaf children could be taught speech. It was, however, accessible to the 'parlour pupils', the private pupils taught exclusively by headmasters for an increased fee, which helped create a deep linguistic class divide.[32]

It is likely that this social engineering was actively encouraged. An interview with William van Praagh, the director of the Training College for Teachers of the Normal School of the Association for the Oral Instruction of the Deaf and Dumb, certainly suggests this. Asked why 'orally-taught deaf, after leaving school, seldom, if ever interest themselves in the welfare of their less fortunate brothers and sisters', he responded:

> Your remarks are perfectly correct. The deaf, taught to speak, feels his superiority, and the more advanced he is in speech and lip-reading the more he feels inclined to ignore his affliction and mix with the hearing. The pure oralist ought to encourage this feeling.[33]

Oralism's ability to divide and destroy deaf communities appears to have been actively encouraged by oralists hostile towards the very idea of a deaf community.

Yet for all its influence and power, Britain experienced a debate on oralism, not a full-scale revolution.[34] The headmasters' conference of 1881 revealed a receptive but uncertain community of deaf headmasters, willing to try the oral method but expressing doubts about its effectiveness and concern about the costs of introducing more expensive teaching methods into institutions precariously funded by donations.[35] Oralism tended to spread in England, but the combined system retained a firm hold on Scottish deaf education. Iain Hutchison rightly points out this may partly be explained by differences in the economic backgrounds of Scottish and English pupils.[36] Yet the place of oralism in British deaf education remained contested, even with social and economic factors taken into account.

The Cambrian Institution for the Deaf and Dumb

The Cambrian Institution for the Deaf and Dumb was Wales's primary deaf institution, and its records play out a contest between sign language and oral education.[37] The school used the combined method of teaching, but its minute books, letters and annual reports play out a discussion of oralist methodology and the social manipulation associated with it. Founded in Aberystwyth in 1847 with accommodation for twelve children, the Cambrian Institution moved to Swansea three years later, finding Swansea's transport links advantageous.[38] From the outset it showed ambitions of teaching deaf children to speak. A report in the *Welshman* in 1847 detailed the public meeting to establish the school, which included a customary display and examination of deaf children (the subjects here being a sixteen-year-old pupil at the Yorkshire Institution and a former pupil of the London Asylum).[39] After answering a question fingerspelled to him by headmaster Charles Rhind, one of the children pronounced vowels while placing his fingers on Rhind's throat to 'feel the muscles that were in operation in the pronunciation of articulate words'. The reporter noted the audience's fascination at 'this wonderful display of man's conquests over the difficulties and defects of nature'.[40] The normalizing processes of oralism – casting deafness as a 'defect' which must be corrected – were clearly aspired to from the very beginning.

Yet it was not until the tenure of principal Benjamin Payne (1876–1914) that the oralism contest was truly played out. Payne was one of few deaf headmasters in Britain, having lost his hearing through scarlet fever at ten years old.[41] Deeply involved in the debates occurring amongst deaf headmasters, he was a regular figure at the Headmasters' Conferences and at times acted as its only deaf representative. At the 1877 conference, he used this position as a man who 'for more than eighteen years had been most intimately associated with the deaf and dumb' to highlight the specific requirements of the deaf community. He defended the 'immense moral influence' that manualist teachers possessed over their students. The report of the conference details this personal attack on oralism:

> ... the pantomimist [sign language teacher] did not bid a final good-bye to his pupil at the schoolroom door, but followed him into his walk in life ... Did oralists do the like? No; they depended on others to do it for them, others who did not know half as much about the deaf and dumb as their teachers did, who could not communicate with them so well by any system, and whose influence over them was in the same small proportion.[42]

Payne's own experiences clearly informed his contribution to the debate, and oralism was here criticized solely for its failure to improve the lives of deaf children. It was a striking rejection of oral educators' inability to understand the workings of the deaf community.

Payne would continue to attend the Headmasters' Conferences, but his arguments regarding oralism varied greatly. On one occasion in 1881, he doubled as a sign interpreter to deaf visitors at the conference. Yet here he used his position as 'the only deaf-speaking member of the Conference' to *praise* the German pure oral system. At that conference, he addressed the prominent oralist St John Ackers, thanking him 'on behalf of the deaf' for 'what he has indirectly done and desirous of doing'.[43] Thus here he acted as a representative for the deaf community while simultaneously applauding the ideology intended to destroy it. Whilst principal of the Cambrian Institution, Payne oversaw the teaching of oral education to what were deemed the most able pupils, and its presence in the curriculum was not hidden. 'Articulation and lip-reading' appeared under a list of subjects taught in the Institution's Annual Reports from the 1880s onwards.[44] Yet letters from Payne to his honorary secretary, Joseph Hall, reveal a deep anxiety about its efficacy. This uncertainty climaxed in 1879 with a lengthy discussion of the system's failings:

> It has been admitted that articulation and lip-reading have generally failed ... that the time and means were found to be insufficient, that all pupils were not capable of developing the faculty of speech and acquiring the art of lip-reading, and that the manual means which were therefore resorted to eventually superseded the first in the affection and practice of the pupils.[45]

Oralism in its pure form appears to have been dismissed. It was costly, time-consuming and exclusionary, thus wholly unsuitable for a charitable institution largely for poor and uneducated children.

Preference for the 'combined system' was, of course, widespread, and it was not unusual for institutions to reject the universal adoption of oralism. Yet Payne's conclusions in the letter suggest a more receptive attitude than first thought:

> We have an oral class of eight. We are ourselves desirous of adding to it. When the Cambrian Institution is supported in the style of the oral schools of London articulation and lip-reading will be taught as extensively as subscribers may desire, compatibly with the education by other means of those who cannot profit from the first.[46]

Oral education here appears to be encouraged as a matter of demand. Wealthier parents with children supposedly able to succeed in articulation would ideally be able to request oral education. Sign language is restricted to the 'other means' resorted to for the weaker pupils. This enthusiasm was not confined to his correspondence with Hall. The following year, Payne enquired for a student from the oralist teacher training school at Ealing to conduct his 'oral class' (though seemingly to no avail).[47] In 1883, an assistant teacher was ordered to spend two months in London teaching the oral method, almost certainly with a view to putting her new skills to use when she returned to Swansea.[48] Payne's attitudes to oralism presented a contradictory opinion; he wrote of oralism's many limits and failures, yet was looking to expand its teaching in the Institution.

It is possible that this varying position stemmed not just from a distrust of the pure oral system, but from a desire to avoid the reliance on sign language. 'We do not teach our pupils to sign', he wrote to the father of a boy taking the oral class, 'It is not the purpose for which they come to us'.[49] A contest of speech against sign was emerging, one which could spill into the children's homes. Responding to her letter concerning a pupil, he wrote to a Miss Maclaran, 'Will you kindly use your influence with her friends in getting them to communicate with her not by signs [original underlining] but orally, or by finger-spelling, or writing?'[50] The request to avoid sign language at home was stressed frequently to parents and guardians, even whilst manual methods were continuing to be used in the school. In other dealings with pupils' home lives and future careers, Payne espoused some of the key methods of social control and normalization associated with pure oralism. The section of the Annual Reports titled 'Hints to Parents and Friends of Deafmutes' made this bluntly clear. Under 'Guidance after leaving school' was written: 'Warn him in time against forming any attachment to a born-deaf person of the opposite sex, and do not be persuaded that a union with "one like himself" is the best for him'.[51] The pupils to whom this would have applied may not have used the oral system at all, yet its sentiment echoed the eugenic motivations of Bell and van Praagh. Payne further confirmed this at the 1885 Headmasters' Conference: 'I have always set my face dead against intermarriages'.[52] Thus aspects of oralism were clearly present as a philosophy, if not as a practice.

Oralism and Experience

Much has been written about the effects of oralism in the classroom and on wider educational policy. There has, however, been little attempt to uncover the children's own experiences of oralist methods. Harry Hendrick notes the general lack of agency given to children in historical work, arguing historians should adopt a perspective which values children as 'social actors and informants in their own right'.[53] This seems particularly appropriate to histories of disabled children. Felicity Armstrong, for example, laments 'the almost total absence of the voices and perspectives of disabled people in dominant accounts of the history of disability and education'.[54] It is, however, difficult to attribute disabled children with the historical voices they deserve when often the only records of their childhood are written from the perspectives of the institutions that educated them. These rarely contain first-hand evidence of the children's thoughts and actions, and details of their lives at home and outside of the school may be completely absent.[55] Yet, Read and Walmsley argue that the 'received' content of sources – the implications about the children's own lives – can contribute towards some understanding of the perspectives of children in special education.[56] Even if they are only seen through the eyes of those in authority, aspects of their lives may still be visible to the careful reader.

This is perhaps the case regarding the Cambrian Institution, whose letter books reveal occasional resistance to oralism from the pupils, and reactions to the Institution's attempts to bring oralism into the home. Payne's letters to children's parents and friends asking them to use speech at home often revealed the pupils' reluctance to participate in their oral education. Concerns about the use of sign language both by children and their parents or friends were sometimes made explicit: 'I found him confirmed in the habit of signing unnecessarily, at all times', wrote Payne to a parent. 'He is certainly making progress now, however, and I hope that no one who can speak or spell and write will ever use signs to him unnecessarily again'.[57] The letters imply that pupils and parents were less compliant with efforts to remove sign language from deaf children's lives than the institution wished, and there were other manifestations of misbehaviour. The same boy was caught using 'bad words' in the school, which he taught to the girls. He had seen the words in the street, which were 'signed to him by vulgar boys'. The boy's use of forbidden signs, combined with a disregard for the 'moral training' given to him in school, suggests signs could be a method of resistance. The boy's punishment was the final move in the contest of communication: pupils were forbidden to talk to him.[58]

Conversely, oralism could be used as a tool to exert power over pupils' home lives and careers. Payne wrote to a mother who wished to remove her son from the school to become a teacher, with a scathing indictment of her plans:

> If Edward remains a pupil for 15 years more he might learn the English language suffi-
> ciently well to teach it by finger-spelling but not by speech. Then if he was a teacher in
> an institution he might earn less than a joiner, and be discontented because he would
> be condemned to a life-long celibacy and never have a home of his own.[59]

Oralism was here used as a standard which the woman's son must attain if he wanted to become a teacher. It is unclear whether Payne's description of deaf teachers was referring to the profession as a whole. However, in other letters he appears more receptive to the idea of deaf teachers using oral methods: 'Our Assistant Matrons are generally aspirant Teachers, and if deaf they should be able to teach orally as well as by manual means'.[60] Yet in the case of Edward, the mother's desire to withdraw the boy before he has finished articulation lessons was met with threats of a life of misery.

Adult Responses

The struggle taking place at the Cambrian Institution to stop its pupils using signs confirms that deaf children resisted oralism. While covert signing did not appear to be a coordinated community effort to keep signs alive, such actions complemented an increasingly visible anti-oralist movement emerging among deaf communities in Britain.[61] The first national conference of Adult Deaf and Dumb Missions and Associations was held in 1890 and spawned an organi-zation, the British Deaf and Dumb Association. At the conference, founder Francis Maginn outlined its intention to defend 'the efficacy of the combined system' and 'defy the conclusions of the Milan conference and of similar packed conventions'.[62] A petition was given to King Edward VII to recognize signing in deaf education, signed by 1,000 deaf people.[63] Though oralism continued to spread across all outlets of deaf education, there was a clear resistance developing from adults as well as the deaf children taught under the method.

The responses of deaf adults are essential to a historical understanding of the effects of oralism. Oral teaching had a profound effect on deaf people, not just in classrooms, but in homes and communities. Their voices were of course rarely documented in institutional records or mainstream media, but the deaf newspapers being printed at the time provide evidence of reaction and debate. Only recently, though, have historians begun to utilize this important source. As Atherton explains in his study of the deaf print media, newspapers are vital insights into the lives and mindsets of deaf communities.[64] Some were written *for* deaf people by missioners or churches, and consequently titles such as *Our Monthly Church Mission for the Deaf* and *Ephphatha* carried a religious and phil-anthropic outlook. Other newspapers contained articles written by deaf people, or were based around links to local deaf communities and schools. The first recorded deaf newspaper, the *Edinburgh Quarterly Messenger* was compiled by pupils of the Edinburgh Institution for the Deaf and Dumb from 1843–5 and edited by its headmaster.[65]

The newspapers revealed a varied and often passionate response to the spread of oralism. Both sides of the debate often found their way into print. The *British Deaf Mute* in July 1894, for example, carried a profile of the Association for the Oral Instruction for the Deaf and Dumb, accompanied by the van Praagh interview.[66] Yet an article in the following issue called 'Mediocrity' suggested the interview caused a debate amongst its deaf readers. It defended the newspaper's decision to print van Praagh's comments, reminding its readers that, 'We have no desire to criticize unduly the opinions advanced by those who have favoured us with interviews'. Though the article went on to highlight some positive benefits of oralism, it strongly criticized the oral schools' encouragement of its pupils to 'ignore their deaf brethren'.[67] Thus the newspapers could reveal oralism's damaging effects on deaf communities, and provided a medium to take a stand.

Articles in deaf newspapers could protest against oralism in powerful and often humorous terms. A piece in *Our Monthly Church Messenger to the Deaf* in the 1890s, entitled 'I don't mix with the Deaf and Dumb!', dealt with interactions between manually- and orally-educated deaf people. The author recalls the visit of orally-educated deaf people to a Mission in detail and with biting sarcasm:

> Then there was Miss Ivy, educated on the *Pure* Oral System. Her folks tell us that we poor Deaf people, with our debates, services and social gatherings, classes, clubs, rambles, and keen interest in current topics, are 'buried alive' ... It does seem so funny to be told that to spell on our fingers or sign is 'so ugly', especially when we see Miss Ivy and her folks pointing about like excited setters, with an expression on their faces as if they were chewing fearfully hot potatoes.[68]

The author is repeatedly told by the orally-educated deaf people he meets that he is somehow beneath them in social status. Yet his response is to mock them, and contrast their elitism to the friendship and discussions he enjoys in his community. The article yielded a response in the following issue, in which a reader lamented 'how very ridiculous some of us are'. He argued, 'If only a little good fellowship could be intermingled, if only we could realise that hearts at least can beat the same time – *If!* IF! IF!'[69] Though this may be an unusual or extreme example, it illustrates the fact that deaf people did not all passively accept the threat to their communities posed by oralism. Indeed, as Jonathan Rée points out, some communities may even have been unified by it: 'the oralist opponents of sign language were helping to bring about exactly the kind of separate deaf society they had always wanted to prevent'.[70]

Other articles about oralism's effects on deaf people surfaced in deaf newspapers. The *British Deaf Mute* in 1895 reprinted an American story of an orally-educated football team fumbling around the pitch and failing to communicate, whose 'ignorance of the rules of the game ... we can only attribute to nothing but the difficulty of explaining them orally to the players'. The purpose of its inclusion, they wrote, was 'to amuse our manualist friends and give our pure oralist friends food for thought'.[71] The magazine also made clear its favour of signs by calling for a sign language dictionary. This would make learning the language easier and avoid the need to 'painfully pick it up at church, in the lecture hall, or in a haphazard manner from our deaf friends'.[72] This article sparked yet another debate. A reader – who lost his hearing at twelve years old – disagreed and asked instead for the time and money to be spent 'remedying the ignorance of the deaf'. Sign language, he wrote, was 'the greatest living obstacle existing to the welfare of the deaf', and ignoring it would force upwards a deaf person's standards of communication.[73] Again, newspapers revealed a fierce and ongoing debate emerging amongst deaf people themselves. This included criticism of oralsim and concern about divisions between manually- and orally-educated deaf people. Most importantly, they demonstrate the importance of sharing experiences. Thus contributors often referred to their own education when discussing developments in schools which concerned them. While the newspapers did not represent the entirety of deaf discourse, they nevertheless confirm that oralism could affect all areas of deaf life.

Conclusion

Oralism's place within the history of British deaf education is deeply complex and multifaceted. This is not to say that it had a weaker impact than first thought: the Royal Commission of 1889, as well as various school boards across the UK, were eager to adopt the method. Likewise, the heads of many British deaf institutions were beginning to welcome its methodology, with cost issues often the only obstacle to its introduction. Its impact as an educational ideology was also significant: the rise of oralism essentially legitimized denying deaf children access to their own language and communities. The aim of this chapter has thus not been to refute oralism's influence in Britain but to understand it as a contest with varying levels of acceptance and resistance. Indeed, many deaf educators showed a level of uncertainty to endorse the bold new practice. This is seen in the cautious optimism of the Headmasters' Conferences, and the fluctuating opinions of Benjamin Payne at the Cambrian Institution for the Deaf and Dumb. Somewhat contradicting himself, Payne declared his dislike of oralism's expensive and exclusionary nature whilst making sure pupils avoided sign language and intermarriage. His attitudes are a reminder that, while oralism may have been influential, British deaf education did not make an immediate and total switch to its ways.

Moreover, the deaf people affected by oralism did not all passively accept it. The lives and responses of the deaf community – both children and adults – are essential to our understanding of oralism, but their voices have only recently begun to be included in historical narratives. This is somewhat understandable considering the lack of historical sources documenting the lives of deaf people in Victorian and Edwardian Britain. Yet the historian can still grant these deaf people agency: their voices can be heard in the deaf print media, and through careful reading of institutional sources. Thus, though many pupils of the Cambrian Institution may have had their language suppressed, this did not stop them bringing in signs and communicating visually with their parents. Adult experiences can also help us understand the question of oralism, and articles in deaf newspapers suggest that deaf people could be critical and dismissive of oral education. Some protested against its attempts to divide their communities, or mocked those orally-educated deaf people who shunned them. The wide variety of opinions in the newspapers also suggests that a debate was emerging in the communities themselves, again with varying levels of receptiveness and opposition. Of course, more needs to be researched on deaf communities' responses to oralism. For example, little has been written about the experiences of children educated on the pure oral system who, in many cases, may have left the school with no sign language and an extremely limited knowledge of English.[74] It is this historical agency given to the pupils and deaf communities, and the interplay between adult and child experiences of deafness, which will truly reveal the complex and contested nature of the question of oralism.

5 EXPLORING PATIENT EXPERIENCE IN AN AUSTRALIAN INSTITUTION FOR CHILDREN WITH LEARNING DISABILITIES, 1887–1933

Lee-Ann Monk and Corinne Manning

Introduction

In January 1887, the *Argus* newspaper reported that the government in Victoria, Australia had initiated a scheme 'to give to the imbecile children of the colony that regular elementary education which is imparted with a gratifying measure of success in England and other countries'. While the want of suitable accommodation had previously presented an obstacle to any such scheme now, the newspaper informed its readers, the government was having four cottages and a schoolhouse constructed in the grounds of the state 'lunatic' asylum in the Melbourne suburb of Kew. The report concluded with the hope that 'as beneficial results will be obtained here as are secured by similar means in England'.[1] When the new institution opened four months later, it was the first purpose-built institution for children with learning disabilities in Australia. Initially known as the Kew Idiot Asylum and later as the Children's Cottages, it remained for the next five decades the most significant state response to the care of children with learning disabilities in Victoria. In this chapter, our focus is on uncovering something of the experiences and feelings of those who lived in the Cottages during this time. This, however, is no easy task.

As other historians have observed, people with learning disabilities have been among 'the most silent, or voiceless of all historical groups'.[2] While this silence resulted in part from the inability of many people with learning disabilities to read and write, it is also the consequence of their historical disempowerment. Past perceptions of people with learning disabilities have seen them both symbolically and actually excluded from 'ordinary life', making it difficult for them to represent themselves and their lives and leaving others disinclined to listen, in the belief that they did not have the capacity to speak about their experiences.[3] In recent years, the voices of people with learning disabilities have increasingly broken this silence.[4] For the nineteenth and early part of the twentieth centuries, however, the only surviving accounts are usually those created by other, more powerful actors for their own purposes.[5]

The extant Kew Cottages archive reflects the historic disempowerment and subsequent silencing of people with learning disabilities. No first-person accounts of life in the Cottages survive in the archive for the period discussed in this chapter. The experiences of the institution's inmates can therefore only be approached through the observations of others, whether visitors to the institution or the officers responsible for its management. A brief consideration of the Cottages' surviving patient case histories provides an example of the difficulties of approaching patients' subjective experiences through such mediated sources.[6]

The law required the institution's medical officers to create a case history for every patient admitted to the institution and case histories are now among the most extensive sources in the archive.[7] However, as with case histories more generally, the content of those from the Cottages reflect the purposes and preoccupations of their authors, tending to be long on accounts of the treatment of physical illness, for example.[8] They only rarely record the direct speech of patients and their actions. Moreover, they privilege 'episodes of behaviour which staff found disruptive', such as escapes or instances of self-harm, rather than day-to-day life, but often without providing the broader context that would make these 'disruptive' episodes fully explicable.[9] Furthermore, doctors' assumptions about their 'patients' and about mental disorders shaped the explanations they did provide about why the 'objects' of their gaze behaved as they did.[10] In 1909, for example, the medical officer attributed John O'Dowd's 'excitement' to 'masturbation', even as he noted that John explained that the reason for his distress was that 'he wanted to go to his father'.[11] As in this instance, doctors' explanations could show remarkably little insight or interest in the feelings of their charges.

Nonetheless, as other historians argue, even given such constraints a careful analysis of case notes can sometimes provide at least a sense of how patients experienced their institutionalization.[12] While what we can know from archival sources may be limited, attempting to discover at least something of patient experience is both a challenge to the silence history has imposed, and a recognition that inmates were people with thoughts and feelings about their experiences, even if these are now mostly lost to us.[13] To acknowledge this is extremely important, given past perceptions of people with learning disabilities as somehow less than human.[14] It is also for this reason that we use 'people-first language' in this chapter.[15]

The chapter begins with a discussion of the history of the institutional care of people with learning disabilities, before turning to an exploration of the everyday life of inmates at Kew and their subjective experiences of institutionalization, using the surviving archival sources. The final section discusses the recollections of Edward (Ted) Rowe. Admitted to the Cottages in 1925, aged five, Ted spent the next eight years as an inmate of the institution. Fascinating in their own right, his recollections emphasize the importance of oral history in recovering experiences of people living with learning disability absent from the archive.

The History of Institutional Care

As the *Argus* article with which we began this chapter reveals, developments in the training of children with learning disabilities in England were an important influence on the decision to build a specialized institution for children with learning disabilities in Victoria. They, in turn, resulted from developments on the Continent. In the early 1840s, the experiments of French physician Édouard Séguin demonstrated that 'idiot children' were capable of individual mental improvement through training, overturning the traditional belief that 'idiots' were ineducable. His work, and that of his 'mentor' Jean Itard, well known for his attempts to teach Victor, the so-called 'Wild Boy of Averyon', encouraged others to establish institutions in Europe dedicated to the care and training of idiot children.[16]

Knowledge of these apparent successes inspired a campaign to establish an institution for idiots in England.[17] This opened in North London in 1848, moving in 1855 to new premises on Earlswood Common. As historian David Wright suggests, the decision to use an 'institutional medium' to train children with learning disabilities was not inevitable. In the case of Earlswood, its founders might instead have established specialized day schools in London or sent 'nurses into the homes of poor families to provide relief or train families in the management and care of idiot children, in a manner similar to the ubiquitous lady visitors of the Victorian era'.[18] Their decision to establish a large asylum in which to train children with learning disabilities had profound implications, reinforcing the 'otherness' of those confined to such institutions and creating a situation in which segregation and isolation were deemed the necessary precursors to their eventual 'integration' into society as '"useful" and productive members'.[19]

By the mid-1860s, a network of charitable idiot asylums based on the Earlswood model existed. Their collective purpose was the training of so-called 'educable idiots'.[20] Through the inculcation of socially acceptable behaviour, classroom lessons, physical exercises and instruction in trades, they aimed to encourage self-control and independence so that pupils would return to their families and communities more self-reliant and better able to contribute to their own support.[21] These ideas and institutions were the inspiration for the Kew Idiot Asylum.

Dr Edward Paley, Inspector of Asylums in Victoria, was the first to propose the creation of a separate state institution for children with learning disabilities. In 1876, he suggested that one solution to the overcrowding of the colony's public 'lunatic' asylums was to build 'a separate small asylum exclusively for idiot children', about fifty-four of whom were then living in the asylums.[22] The government had recruited Paley from England several years earlier, and knowledge of developments there clearly influenced his recommendation. Among the advantages he enumerated for such an institution was the opportunity it would provide to 'initiate a system of industrial training and occupation, like that carried on at some of the home asylums, notably at the Royal Albert Asylum, Lancaster, and at the Earlswood Asylum, Redhill'.[23]

Others in Victoria shared the optimism in the capacity of idiot children for improvement that underpinned Paley's suggestion. In 1885, several witnesses expressed this conviction very strongly at the hearings of the Royal Commission on Asylums for the Insane and Inebriate, appointed to investigate the management of Victoria's asylums (1884–6).[24] Dr Solomon Iffla, one of the Official Visitors to Melbourne's metropolitan asylums, was particularly adamant on this point, declaring that idiot children 'should be all instructed, because they can be taught'.[25] All the witnesses were unanimous in condemning the 'indiscriminate mixing' of the children with adult patients in the asylums,[26] a concern that had helped prompt Paley's original suggestion for a separate asylum for them in 1876.[27] While this conviction derived in part from a particular anxiety about the association of idiot boys and adult male patients, the consequences of which contemporaries only ever hinted at,[28] it also reflected the belief that it was 'utterly fatal to the improvement of idiots that they should be allowed into lunatic asylums'.[29] That an institution was the most appropriate environment in which to train idiot children went completely unquestioned. Given this consensus, it is not surprising that the government's determination to provide for Victoria's 'imbecile children' took institutional form, a decision that would profoundly affect the lives of generations of people with learning disabilities in Victoria.

The Kew Idiot Asylum received its first patients in May 1887 and by year's end there were fifty-four inmates resident.[30] Numbers increased rapidly thereafter; by 1907, there were 292 patients living at the institution.[31] While its officials were determined to model the new institution on the charitable idiot asylums in England wherever possible, its status as a state institution prevented imitation of the selective admission they practised.[32] The youngest patient admitted was only a year old, the oldest forty-five.[33] Nonetheless, Kew Idiot Asylum, like its English equivalents, received a significant number of children and adolescents between 1887 and 1907, a fact reflected in a median admission age of twelve.

While the establishment of the Kew Idiot Asylum reflected the contemporary optimism about the capacity of children with learning disabilities, more pessimistic beliefs about people with learning disabilities were being expressed in Victoria even before it opened. At the hearings of the Royal Commission in

1885 G. A. Tucker, a private asylum proprietor recently returned from an extensive overseas tour of institutions for the mentally disordered, spoke approvingly of a shift in America towards permanent institutional segregation of people with learning disabilities 'to prevent the propagation of their infirmity'.[34] His views reflected a belief that would become increasingly influential, that the so-called 'feeble-minded' were, by virtue of their supposed hereditary 'defect', the cause of a multitude of social problems. As Tucker's remarks suggest, contemporaries believed that the solution to this 'menace' was control through permanent segregation in institutions where the inmates would contribute to their own support.[35]

One of the principal advocates of this view in Victoria was Dr W. Ernest Jones, appointed from England to the post of Inspector-General of the Insane in 1905.[36] As Inspector-General, he was responsible for the administration of the state hospitals for the insane, including the Children's Cottages at Kew. Children with learning disabilities were in fact a particular focus of the anxiety about the feeble-minded, contemporaries fearing the misery, crime and expense they believed must result if such children were 'allowed to reach maturity without being subjected to a system of education and segregation'.[37] Those, like Jones, who were concerned to protect society from the 'menace of the feeble-minded', advocated a series of related measures, beginning with the establishment of special schools. Residential schools, to accommodate country pupils or those of more 'feeble mind', should follow. A colony for adult 'defectives' would eventually be required, to ensure the 'finished products of the schools' remained under control and contributed to their own support. Finally, legislation to allow compulsory segregation might also be necessary.[38] However, governments in Victoria did little to implement such measures until the mid-1920s, with the exception of establishing two special schools in Melbourne.[39]

The Children's Cottages at Kew consequently remained the only residential institution for children with learning disabilities in Victoria, despite the Inspector-General's opinion that it was an entirely inadequate answer to the question of the feeble-minded.[40] Patient numbers rose steadily, from 292 in 1907 to 378 in 1925.[41] As the only institution of its kind, the Cottages continued to receive significant numbers of children and adolescents, but inaction meant that fear of the feeble-minded shaped the everyday lives of inmates less in these years than the parsimony of successive governments.

Reading Patient Experience from the Archive

The initial determination to create a specialized training school for children with learning disabilities, modelled as far as possible along English lines, meant that for many patients admitted to the Idiot Asylum in its first two decades daily life was a round of classroom lessons, physical drill and employment.[42] When journalist Alice Henry toured the institution in January 1898, she observed one class of boys practising a 'simple drill – sitting, standing, folding and extending the arms, turning to right and left' – while in the room next-door 'a troop of girls' marched to music. In another, teachers used the experience of sensation to teach abstract concepts: 'A wooden cube is dabbed on a little one's face. That is "hard–hard". Then a wool ball. "soft–soft"'. Outside, boys worked cutting willow for basket-making, one of several trades established at the institution, while other inmates assisted in the laundry.[43]

For inmates with more severe disabilities, life was quite different. Nineteen-year-old Alfred Walters and seven-year-old Thomas Dunn were admitted within two years of one another, in 1887 and 1889 respectively. Neither was able to walk or talk and in contrast to the patients Henry observed, spent their days sitting in easy-chairs in apparent idleness.[44] To know any more of how patients such as Thomas and Alfred passed their days is extremely difficult. Their experiences are rarely visible in the published accounts of visitors, or in official reports and their case histories tell us little about individual lives or changes within the asylum.

In retrospect, a severe typhoid epidemic in 1907 marked the end of the institution's life as an 'idiot asylum'.[45] The schoolrooms were pressed into service as a makeshift isolation ward and classes suspended. Subsequent attempts by the Inspector-General to have qualified teachers appointed after the epidemic, as a first step in instituting that 'special educational system' he believed would 'be required ... for all the backward and feeble-minded children throughout the state', were entirely unsuccessful.[46] Despite his repeated assertions that there were a small number of children at the Cottages able to benefit from education, successive governments refused to provide the necessary funding.[47] Informal attempts to resume teaching gradually dwindled into nothingness, denying inmates even the slim chance of an education until 1929, when a special school finally opened at the institution.[48] The resulting neglect shocked visitors. In 1911, Arthur Hauser visited the Cottages as a member of a special committee considering 'the question of backward and mentally defective children'. The conditions Hauser observed appalled him, and were in stark contrast to those observed by Henry thirteen years earlier. 'These boys and girls', he declared, 'have been disgracefully neglected. They are untrained in physical habits. Many masturbate openly. Their clothes reek of filth.'[49]

Successive governments also allowed the institution to become increasingly dilapidated. In 1922, an investigation by the *Argus* exposed the 'disgraceful' living conditions to which this neglect condemned patients. The 'mostly wooden and canvas dormitories' were in many places torn and their windows missing, exposing their occupants to the cold, and their wire screens were riddled with holes, leaving the more 'helpless' inmates to be tormented by flies. Defective drainage caused flooding in winter and staff and patients risked injury on the broken asphalt paths. It was, the newspaper concluded, 'a case of housing human beings under the worst possible conditions'.[50]

Two years later, a royal commission appointed to investigate the conduct of the medical officer again revealed the hardships many patients endured. In one example, it described how, for years past, around eighty male patients:

> were taken each day after breakfast to the airing yard on which an old building known as the drill hall, was standing. Almost all of the windows in the building were broken and the doors and flooring were defective. The building contained no fireplaces or heating appliances ... Being contained in a cold, draughty, cheerless drill hall, they were many times found crying from the effect of the cold weather. Some of them huddled into corners to obtain slight warmth from one another.[51]

Many inmates had little to distract them from these hardships or their impoverished surroundings. In March 1923, Dr Springthorpe, one of the Official Visitors, wrote of finding 'some 95 patients lolling about a bare yard some 70 yards square, doing nothing – with as only amusement one unused football'.[52] Five months earlier another of the Visitors, G. T. Howard, suggested that 'something more might be done to brighten the lives' of the patients through the provision of amusements but with apparently little effect.[53] The modest nature of his suggestions provides some insight into the monotony and deprivation of inmates' lives in the first quarter of the twentieth century.

As these examples demonstrate, the accounts of visitors can provide 'insights into the inner world' of asylums and the day-to-day lives of their inmates.[54] Their conclusions about patients' subjective experience are unreliable, however, as Alice Henry's observations show. In 1898, Henry described the feelings she assumed the inmates' basket-making and other trade employments must induce in them, asking her readers to consider 'the sense of just pride that wakes in a poor, useless child when he first discovers that he can create something; what a link with his fellow-beings to be able to give instead of always receiving'.[55] While inmates may well have felt pride in their work, Henry's conclusion rests on negative assumptions about children with learning disabilities implicit to the discourse of 'improvement'. That such training might create a link between the idiot child and his fellow-beings assumes the prior absence of that link. In this, Henry's remark reflects the promise on which Joanna Ryan argues advocates made the case for the training of idiot children in the nineteenth century, that it would lift them from the bestial state contemporaries assumed they occupied.[56] As Dr James McCreery, the first Superintendent of the Kew Idiot Asylum expressed it, training in idiot asylums 'humanizes as far as may be, beings who are often more degraded than beasts of the field'.[57]

As we argued in the introduction, surviving case histories can provide an occasional insight into how individual patients felt about their confinement. In rare instances, this is because the medical officer chose to note the direct speech of a patient in their history. In May 1904, after fours years as an inmate, nineteen-year-old Catherine Hook made her desperate desire for release plain, telling the medical officer that if she was not permitted to leave she would 'commit suicide'. Four years earlier, after several escape attempts, twenty-two-year-old Annie Gately had similarly declared that she would kill herself. In both instances, the doctor interpreted the women's distress as a sign of mental disorder, transferring them to the nearby main asylum, rather than an understandable response to their continuing confinement.[58] More often, though, it is necessary to analyse how patients felt from the actions occasionally recorded in case notes, such as attempts to escape the institution.

Scholars have recently discussed absconding such as Annie's as 'a way of resisting circumstances that the individual found intolerable'.[59] While case notes from Kew record a number of escapes in this period, they usually do little more than note the fact of escape and recapture, so revealing only that the absconder was sufficiently unhappy to attempt to run away.[60] Occasionally, it is possible to speculate on the reason, as in the case of thirteen-year-old Rachael Matthews, who fled the Asylum in 1901, only two days after her admission from home. Given this context, it seems likely that the distress of being separated from her family and confined to an institution filled with strangers prompted her escape.[61] Several weeks later the medical officer reported that Rachael was 'rather more settled', and thereafter she seems to have accepted her confinement.[62]

Other evidence confirms that the separation from family inherent to institutionalization certainly caused some inmates distress. Ten-year-old Agnes Pascoe was reportedly 'very fretful' on the first night of her admission, asking constantly 'for her mother' and wanting 'to go home'.[63] While Agnes was able to 'settle down' other inmates were never reconciled to the separation. A year after the admission of fourteen-year-old Albert Warnak, the medical officer noted an interview with his mother in which he persuaded her not to remove Albert from the institution. Their interview was very likely precipitated by Albert, the notes adding that while his mother acquiesced to his continuing confinement Albert himself was 'constantly asking to be allowed home'. In the following months, he attempted twice to escape, once by climbing through a window in his ward and once by running away from a group out walking. In mid-February 1910, almost two years after the interview with his mother, Albert again climbed through a window in his dormitory during the early hours of the morning and this time evaded detection. Sadly, his desire to go home ended in tragedy when a 'ship-keeper' discovered his body in the Yarra River several days later.[64]

This desire 'to go home' is one of the few motives for escape now discernible in individual case histories. While it was certainly not the only impetus to abscond,[65] the absence of any detail in most case notes makes it impossible to discover the particular circumstances that spurred individuals to do so or that caused the desperate unhappiness of inmates such as Catherine Hook. Nevertheless, it is possible to speculate more generally on their reasons, some of which, as with the separation from family, resulted from contemporary ideas about the treatment of children with learning disabilities. Some inmates may have disliked the regimentation of institutional life. Wright suggests that such regimentation was no accident, contemporaries believing it 'was essential to the amelioration of disabled and disordered minds'.[66] Others may have resented 'the never-sleeping vigilance' officials believed was necessary in the training of idiots.[67] In addition to the classroom lessons, instruction in trades and drilling Henry observed, inmates at Kew received 'moral training', intended to teach self-control and to inculcate socially acceptable behaviour, such as proper conduct at meals. This involved potentially constant observation and correction by staff, both day and night. In the latter case particularly, such surveillance was potentially both intrusive and coercive, extending to control of what the Superintendent called 'sexual vices', the practice of which, he asserted, was 'kept within a very limited compass'.[68]

Other more hidden aspects of institutional life may have motivated escape or caused distress. Some inmates certainly experienced abuse at the hands of staff.[69] In January 1906, for example, the Medical Officer surprised a nurse in the act of striking patient Edith Yorath.[70] In the same year Michael Foley complained to the doctor that he had been 'ill-treated' by an attendant who, he said, in roughly catching hold of him, 'nearly broke my neck'.[71] Such accounts of abuse from patients are extremely rare. One of the very few examples now extant reveals how perceptions of people with learning disabilities disempowered and silenced inmates. In June 1917 patient Frank Dawson told the Senior Attendant that he had seen another attendant 'doing "dirty things" to' a fellow patient the previous evening. The victim subsequently corroborated Dawson's account of the assault in the most explicit terms, and when questioned by the medical officer, both victim and witness 'adhered to their statement'. Despite the clarity and consistency of their account, the senior officers agreed that there was no prospect of successfully prosecuting the perpetrator because:

> the witnesses are of such a low average of intelligence that the court is not at all likely to accept their evidence as sufficiently reliable to convict on & it appears that there is no sane witness to give any sort of corroborative evidence.[72]

Officials consequently took no further action against the perpetrator, having sent him away from the institution shortly after the assault, so avoiding the public exposure of a trial.

For some, the very real prospect of never being released may have precipitated their attempt to escape. Even in the first optimistic decades between 1887 and 1907, when one might have expected residents to return to the community, admission for most marked the beginning of what was effectively institutionalization for life. More than half of the patients admitted in these years died in the institution.[73] Many quickly succumbed to diseases such as typhoid and tuberculosis while others grew into adulthood and spent decades in the institution before their deaths. The status of the asylum as an institution for children condemned others to a similar fate elsewhere. Among the 16 per cent of patients transferred into Victoria's network of public lunatic asylums were those whose temperament and behaviour the medical officers deemed unsuitable for a children's institution.[74] The general asylums could also be the destination of escapees and others considered 'refractory'. Less than 17 per cent of patients admitted between 1887 and 1907 returned to the community.[75] The consequence of admission changed little for most patients entering the institution between 1907 and 1933. Again, more than half died there and the proportion released remained similar. Only the number of transfers changed, falling to less than one in ten.[76]

Thus, admission to the Cottages continued to mark the beginning of a lifetime's institutionalization for most inmates. One of the effects of that institutionalization was the silencing of those subjected to it. Within the surviving archive, we hear the voices of inmates only through the accounts of others and must distil their experiences of institutional life from those accounts. This silence, and the constraints it imposes, makes the memories of Ted Rowe especially important in recovering patient experience from this period.

Ted Rowe's Recollections of Life at Kew 1925–33

Ted recounted his experiences of life at Kew in an interview with Corinne Manning in April 2006, as a participant in an oral history conducted as part of a larger research project on the history of the Cottages.[77] Documenting the experiences of residents was central to the design of the oral history.[78] Among the sixteen residents interviewed, Ted was the only one who had lived in the institution before 1940. His recollections thus provide a rare first-hand account of an inmate's experience in this period. While his experience is not representative of all the patients admitted to the Cottages, his recollections provide a singular insight into how one individual felt about and negotiated life there in the late 1920s and early 1930s.

By the time Ted was admitted in March 1925, conditions were improving. Some renovation and repair of the buildings had followed the 1922 *Argus* exposé,[79] and the government responded to the royal commission two years later by authorizing a more substantial 'plan for proposed improvements and additions, including the erection of two new blocks of buildings'.[80] By the end of 1928, the institution had sewers, electric lighting and power and a hot water system. A new nursery and dormitories provided extra accommodation and an

entirely new dining room reduced overcrowding at meals. New covered walk-
ways connected the various buildings, providing shelter from the elements.[81]
Despite these improvements, Ted's recollections suggest that everyday life in the
Cottages remained bleak, inmates sleeping in crowded dormitories on uncom-
fortable, straw-filled mattresses with a single blanket and quilt.[82] In contrast to
Howard's observation that the food was 'well cooked and good',[83] Ted remembered it as neither appetizing – inmates referred to the porridge as 'the glue'
– nor sufficient. There was no alternative but to eat the meals, however. In Ted's
words, 'You had to eat them otherwise you starve'.[84]

His memories also reflect the continuing regimentation of institutional life.
The day began with the ringing of a bell, signalling that it was time to get up
for breakfast. At the end of the day, after dinner, inmates showered in groups,
timed by the staff, and trooped back to the dormitory 'like brown cows', to be
locked in for the night. In between, the monotony of institutional life Springthorpe observed continued.[85] Other than playing cricket and football, there were
few activities to pass the time. It was this 'sitting around like monkeys', as Ted
described it, that saw him agree to work in the laundry. For inmates like Ted,
who were both willing and able to do so, work provided some relief from such
boredom. Moreover, agreeing to work was a way to gain the approval of staff, an
important consideration given the power they wielded over patients.[86]

This cooperation reflects the way Ted seems to have negotiated institutional
life more generally, by 'behaving himself'. His response to other patients' complaints of mistreatment reflects this strategy: 'Someone said they treated us like
dogs. Well I said it was your fault, I haven't been treated like a dog. I just did what
I was told, see, that was it'. His recollections suggest one possible interpretation
for case notes which describe other 'well behaved' patients or those who sought
to make themselves 'useful'.[87] By his own admission, Ted was a favourite with
the staff, the 'nurses' pet'. In his view, this was because he 'behaved' himself, but
the mild degree of his disability and his responsiveness perhaps influenced their
affection for him.[88] His case notes describe him as 'a happy little chap' and the
photographs in his file, which in their informality resemble family snapshots,
show a 'bright and cheerful' child, smiling back at the photographer. Evidence
suggests that some staff potentially viewed those with more severe disabilities
quite differently. In his autobiography, psychologist Stanley Porteus recalled a
visit to the Cottages in February 1913, accompanied by the Medical Superintendent, Dr Morris Gamble, in which the latter remarked bitterly of a patient,
described by Porteus as 'a hydrocephalic imbecile': '[W]ouldn't you think that
God Almighty would be ashamed of creating something like that?'[89]

While Ted found a way to negotiate life at the Cottages, other inmates continued to find it less bearable, one telling him of his wish to 'get away from here'.
This recollection confirms that absconding was a response to circumstances

inmates found difficult to bear. However, Ted's recollections reveal, where the archive does not, that recaptured escapees faced serious punishment, so much so that he was not 'game to escape'. He warned a fellow inmate contemplating absconding that:

> 'they'll be after you ... find out where you've gone and you'll cop it then, by gee you would'. They do cop it. You could hear them yelling out, 'No, no, no!' They knew they were going [to] get the strap on the backside though. Gee they hit them ...'[90]

Risking such punishment is a measure of how intolerable escapees found their circumstances.

For Ted, friendships with other patients seemingly made institutional life more bearable. Among the handful of 'good things' he recalled about Kew were the many friends he made and the time he spent playing cricket and football with them.[91] His recollections also suggest a sense of shared identity among the inmates of his dormitory. He described the other patients he lived with as 'very good, we didn't have any fights or anything'. He added, apparently in reference to other patients, 'They want a fight we'll give them one'.[92] The importance of such camaraderie is clear from instances in which it was absent. In 1911, fourteen-year-old John Heaney told the medical officer that he had attempted to cut his throat with a piece of tin because 'he wished to die – that boys were unkind & his mother does not want him'.[93] Others endured physical or sexual assault at the hands of other patients.[94]

Despite this, Ted's recollections suggest that inmate solidarity might temper the actions of staff who, as Peter Carpenter suggests, required a certain degree of compliance if the institution was to operate smoothly.[95] Punishments took place in private, Ted explained, because if they were conducted in front of the other inmates: 'We'd start to say "you mongrels" and cause a commotion then and something'd happen, see'.[96] However, the sense of identity and consequent solidarity Ted experienced with other inmates may have been partly an effect of an institution structured around perceived ability. As Ted explained, patients with more severe disabilities 'were in the other part, another dormitory, so we didn't have to worry about them'.[97] Such judgements about the various capacities of children with learning disabilities could have a profound effect on the course of an individual's life, as Ted's experience shows.

Eugenic campaigners had had little success in persuading governments to introduce measures to protect the community from the perceived danger of the feeble-minded before the First World War, but in the 1920s and 1930s their efforts met with more success. The government twice introduced Mental Deficiency Bills into parliament in the 1920s, once in 1926 and again in 1929, intending 'through the use of forced segregation in institutions to deprive a significant proportion of the population of its ability to procreate freely'.[98] Despite apparently widespread community support, neither bill became law, their course interrupted by political events that saw the incumbent governments fall.[99]

While the legislative element of the scheme stalled, the establishment of institutions to provide for the 'different grades' of 'mental defective' envisaged before the war made more progress. In 1926, the government purchased 'Travancore', an existing property in the Melbourne suburb of Flemington, with the intention of establishing a residential school 'for quite young children, who might be described as high-grade mentally [*sic*] defectives'. Those admitted would, if considered suitable, remain in the institution until the age of sixteen when, in the expectation of the Inspector-General:

> it would be possible for them to be so classified that their future could be arranged for by boarding out or being sent on to the next type of institution, which it is intended should partake of the nature of a residential colony.[100]

In 1937, the opening of a Colony for Mental Defectives at Janefield, nearly ten miles north-east of Melbourne, fulfilled the latter intention.[101] The Cottages, meanwhile, were to be reserved for children with more severe disabilities, described by Jones as 'the lower grade of mental defective, that is to say the idiot and imbecile of low type'.[102]

Travancore Residential School opened on 8 February 1933.[103] A month later, Ted was transferred there, presumably because he was deemed, in Jones's words, 'capable of receiving benefit from special instruction'.[104] In February 1937, he was boarded out to a farm near the country town of Stawell, suggesting that the teachers judged him one of the 'small number ... capable of an unrestricted return to everyday existence'.[105] In 1941, Ted enlisted in the army and, stationed in Darwin in the north of Australia, survived the repeated bombing raids inflicted on the city by the Japanese Air Force. After the war, he married and found steady employment before retiring.[106] Ted died in 2008.

Conclusion

Much of the history of learning disabilities has been a history of exclusion, in which the voices of people with learning disabilities were silenced. The extant archive of the Kew Children's Cottages reflects this, containing no first-hand accounts from those who lived in the institution during the first four decades of its existence. In their absence, the historian seeking to know something of patient experience must approach it through the observations of others. The nature of such mediated sources, in which the words and actions of inmates are decontextualized or interpreted according to the observer's assumptions about learning disabilities (that they were mental disorders, for example), certainly limits what we can now know of patient experience. Even so, it is possible to discover something of everyday life in an institution like the Cottages and even a little of the subjective experience of its inmates. Much, however, must remain lost. Such archival silence emphasizes the importance of oral histories and life stories in recovering the experiences of inmates. Recollections like those of Ted Rowe let us see the often hidden world of the institution from a perspective that survives only in fragments in the archive. Moreover, seeking out and listening to the voices of people with learning disabilities, whether in archives or through listening to them tell the stories of their lives breaks the silence history has imposed upon them.

6 FROM REPRESENTATION TO EXPERIENCE: DISABILITY IN THE BRITISH ADVICE LITERATURE FOR PARENTS, 1890–1980

Anne Borsay

Introduction

Twentieth-century Britain was associated with an explosion of health advice. In their important study of texts for women industrial workers, Vicky Long and Hilary Marland found reproductive biology playing second fiddle to 'hygiene, diet, exercise, recreation, fashion and beauty'.[1] At the same time, however, literature on pregnancy and childcare proliferated, targeting professionals,[2] schoolgirls[3] and parents, especially mothers. This material has been analysed in terms of the transition from physical to psychological health,[4] but what it had to say about disability has received relatively little attention. Chapter 6 will address this gap, focusing on the advice directed towards parents with children primarily under the age of one. A lot of information was conveyed in magazines and periodicals,[5] but these are voluminous and sometimes hard to trace. Ephemera – for example, baby product leaflets circulated by commercial companies – were also commonplace, but often undated.[6] And there were information films,[7] but too few to track historical trends. Consequently, we will concentrate on advice books, using their publication dates and the revisions undertaken between editions to locate shifts in the guidance on offer between 1890 and 1980. In exploring how disability was represented, three main themes will be considered: the authoritarian approach to pregnancy and childcare, which gathered momentum from the late nineteenth century; its replacement by an intuitive approach in the aftermath of the Second World War; and the influence of this evolving literature on the experiences of disabled children and their families.

Authoritarian Parenthood, 1890–1945

The authoritarian approach to parenthood has been attributed to the New Zealand guru,[8] Dr Frederick Truby King, whose ideas were taken up by the long-running *Mothercraft Manual* after he visited Britain in 1917.[9] Although his promotion of 'feeding by the clock' exemplified rule-based childcare,[10] there were homegrown precedents in the late nineteenth century. The stimulus was eugenic thinking, fuelled by Britain's relative economic and imperial decline, and an intense anxiety about the quantity and quality of the nation's stock.[11] Infant mortality,[12] which had hovered at around 154 per 1,000 live births since records began in 1838, was used to justify increased medical intervention in pregnancy and childcare. Adapting accordingly, the advice books broke with the discourse of reassurance characteristic of earlier texts,[13] and endorsed the assumption of incompetent mothers that also inspired contemporary schemes set up by the voluntary and statutory sectors to educate women for parenting.[14] In 1900 Dr Genevieve Tucker thus opened her *Mother, Baby and Nursery* with a stark account of how 300,000 children 'perish for want of proper care and nourishment' before the age of four 'due in large measure to the ignorance of those having the care of them'.[15] By the mid-1920s, with infant mortality at half its turn of the century level, the emphasis had shifted from death to disability. Those surviving 'disabled and damaged', argued an honorary physician to the Mothercraft Training Society, were 'many times more than those that die'. Consequently, a lower death rate meant 'a still greater lessening of disease and disability ... and an equivalent improvement in the physique of the nation'.[16]

One of the fiercest advocates of medicine's part in this process was A. R. Dafoe: famous for his role in the birth and management of Canadian quintuplets, born in 1934 and brought up in a purpose-built nursery. Far from lamenting this artificial environment, Dafoe lauded it. Every physician, he observed in the 1936 British edition of his *Baby-Guide for Mothers*, saw 'little children weakened and warped because he could not tell their mothers what to do, or the mothers, if told, would not obey'. The specially designed unit was a cast-iron means of demonstrating to those sceptical of the doctor's value 'the results of medical control'.[17] Although Dafoe's advice was derived from institutionalized baby care, its medical authoritarianism was shared across the literature. Not only were doctors popular authors of the genre,[18] but nurses and midwives stressed the necessity of medical aid and sought medical backing.[19] In the 1910 edition of *Our Baby*, for example, Mrs J. Langton Hewer assured her audience that 'The medical chapters have been specially written for the book, and the whole has had the advantage of being revised by a London physician' (unnamed).[20] Even *What Does My Baby Want?* was less child-centred than the title suggests. Readers were instructed by the author – Mrs E. A. Cocker, a chief welfare worker with connections to the

National League for Health, Maternity and Child Welfare – that 'With doctor visiting you, and nurse in charge, the mother's duty is to obey orders'.[21]

Prevention

The orders emanating from the doctor-led team revolved around prevention and treatment. The campaign for prevention was part of a broader agenda driven from 1919 by the new Ministry of Health under George Newman. At its core was the revival of medical holism: largely confined to the margins of mainstream practice since the late eighteenth century, when localized pathology displaced classical humoralism with an impersonal focus on particular organs. Rejecting such atomistic reductionism, holism advanced strategies in which patients and their environments were envisaged as organic, interconnected wholes and the health-inducing properties of nature were recognized.[22] With both the conception and the rearing of disabled children, these holistic strategies invoked a composite model of heredity in which genetics and the environment were combined. In 1900, therefore, Tucker devoted her first chapter to the hereditary reproduction of social deviance. 'One has but to visit our criminal courts', she proclaimed:

> the jails, almshouses, and all public institutions of charity and reform, to look into the State homes of the feeble-minded, the deaf, dumb, blind, and the insane asylums to fill out the records of the lives of those born under the tyranny of a bad organization, physically, mentally, morally, the sins of the parents visited to the third and fourth generation.[23]

In 1904 an Inter-Departmental Committee, prompted by the deficiencies of recruits for the Boer War, was dismissive of such hereditary causation.[24] However, fortified by eugenics, the advice literature continued to warn against begetting disability. It was 'not right' insisted Dawson in 1912, that 'society should be burdened with inefficient lives', and it was 'cruel to launch upon a difficult world a child handicapped by deformity or disease'.[25] Judicious marriage and a healthy lifestyle were the recommended means of avoiding such risk. Heredity was regarded as 'an exact science', which empowered parents through the 'careful selection of husband and wife' to improve on their genetic inheritance.[26] From the 1920s, regular antenatal supervision was also recommended.[27] Predating this intervention, however, was the advice that a pregnant woman conform to the 'conditions of physical health', which included natural elements like a 'wholesome and nutritious diet', fresh air and sunshine.[28] Harmful substances were equally to be avoided. Silent on the dangers of alcohol in 1891, Hewer was by 1910 advising that 'No alcoholic stimulants should be taken during pregnancy' because 'they seriously affect the health of the child'.[29]

The same regime was marketed as a defence against childhood disability. For babies, the favoured diet was breastmilk, said to maximize progress and confer resistance to disease.[30] For nursing mothers, as for pregnant women, alcohol was outlawed as a 'poison' that interfered with the baby's 'tender, growing cells' and caused stunted growth or degeneracy.[31] Failing to breastfeed carried similar risks. Rickets or 'distorted bones', for example, were among the penalties for artificial feeding.[32] The prevention of such impairments also required a general healthy diet, tailored to age and weight, consisting of milk, eggs, fresh meat and fresh fruit and vegetables, plus Vitamin D in the form of cod liver oil.[33] However, some recommendations were disease-specific: with rickets, correcting the imbalance between starch and fat; with tuberculosis, ensuring that milk was obtained from a reliable dairy and appropriately sterilized.[34] Fresh air and sunshine, delivered through well-ventilated nurseries and daily spells outside, were likewise prescribed, not just for these conditions but also as protection against colds and other ailments, including infantile paralysis or poliomyelitis.[35]

Treatment

In parallel with antenatal monitoring was a growth in inspection or surveillance to identify disabled babies for treatment. At the end of the nineteenth century, advice literature reflected a binary relationship between the normal and the abnormal. In the first 1891 edition of *Our Baby*, Hewer observed that after the new mother had ascertained her child's gender, the next question was often 'Is the baby all right?' In a chapter of that title, she listed 'a few of the commoner forms of abnormality' that occurred on the rare occasions when an affirmative answer could not be given: for instance, spinal tumours, supernumerary digits, harelip, cleft palate, club foot and deaf-mutism.[36] By 1910 this chapter had disappeared, much of its content being absorbed into a discussion of 'Baby's Troubles' under a section headed 'Congenital Defects'.[37] Disabilities were no longer abnormalities potentially associated with all mothers but singled out as signs of physical and moral deficiency. Accompanying this change was the introduction of measurement along a continuous scale.[38] Although Hewer did indicate a normal weight range for newborn babies in 1891, weight gain was not graphically plotted, no reference was made to the 'normal progress' of a child and no milestones in physical or intellectual development were identified.[39] By the early twentieth century, however, both Hewer and other authors were devising standardized graphs and tables to assess the growth and performance of individual babies against statistical norms.[40]

In theory, this transformation had the potential to raise the visibility and accentuate the difference of the disabled child by, in David Armstrong's terms, spreading the medical 'gaze over the normal person to establish early detection ... and to enable the potentially abnormal to be adequately known'.[41] With learning difficulty, there were early signs of the new orientation at work. Whereas in 1891 Hewer merely noted the potential for 'idiocy' to improve with education, she was by 1910 using 'the tests of normal progress' to define a child as 'backward' prior to the recommendation of 'systematic training'. However, surveillance principles were less evident in the coverage of physical impairment. Rickets was identified with a deviation from normal weight gain.[42] Otherwise the mother – assumed to be 'distressed' in accordance with the contemporary tragic view of disability – was expected to recognize the 'sad fact' that her child had been born 'handicapped by physical defect and deformity'. And both parents were pressed to 'realize how great a drawback it will prove should they allow their child to grow to man's estate with an uncorrected defect'.[43]

Advice on the treatment of these 'defects' embodied developments in medical knowledge and practice. The scrofulous hip disease of the late nineteenth century, for example, was rebadged tuberculosis after Robert Koch discovered the tubercle bacillus and diagnostic techniques improved.[44] Medical cures for TB remained ineffective until the arrival of antibiotics in the 1940s.[45] Surgery, on the other hand, was regarded as successful for a growing number of conditions like harelip, cleft palate, club foot, and hip disease.[46] Nevertheless, many treatments relied on the long-term application of splints and plaster casts and parents were urged to play an active part in implementation.[47] With club foot, for example, manipulation and massage were 'very useful' whenever the splints were taken off. Attention was also drawn to the existence of medical equipment. Given 'a few lessons ... the mother at home' was capable of administering electricity to the disabled limb of a child with infantile paralysis. And she would be 'well rewarded for all the trouble if the limb ... [was] only a little weak, instead of hanging as a useless flail, utterly incapable of doing any work at all'.[48]

The 'trouble' of treating disabled children led the literature to raise the spectre of institutionalization. Where the family was poor, the hospital was put forward as the best option for the child with a damaged hip because complete bed-rest was essential. For the infant 'born deaf' who it was assumed would 'grow up dumb', the institution was regarded as the only option because, irrespective of family circumstances, it was 'almost hopeless to teach it [*sic*] successfully at home'.[49]

Intuitive Parenthood, 1945–80

As part of Britain's eugenic mission, the authoritarian literature of the pre-war period drew on a combination of hereditary principles and healthy living to advance strategies for the prevention and treatment of disability. During the post-war period, however, intuition came to displace authoritarianism. In the United States, an 'indulgent, "self-regulated" regime' made 'significant inroads' from 1930,[50] propelled by two particular influences: first, new developments in psychology which stressed 'emotional stability' and 'social adjustment'; and, later, a democratic ideal, framed in opposition to the authoritarianism of Nazi Germany, which lauded reciprocal child–parent relationships and rejected despotic discipline.[51] These trends culminated in the 1945 publication of Benjamin Spock's *The Common Sense Book of Baby and Child Care*. In the wake of the Second World War, Spock reassured parents that 'Bringing up your child won't be a complicated job if you take it easy, trust your own instincts, and follow the directions that your doctor gives you.'[52]

Spock's book was an international bestseller and became the childcare bible for successive generations of parents. In post-war Britain, meanwhile, *The Mothercraft Manual*, mouthpiece for Truby King's ideas, continued to reject the notion that childcare was a 'natural instinct.'[53] Other texts, however, did make overtures to intuition. In the *Housewife Baby Book*, for example – first produced by *Housewife* magazine in 1948 – Anne Cuthbert conceded that 'good mothers are born, not made' and argued that advice had to be dispensed in an 'explanatory and exploratory', not a 'didactic', way to avoid devaluing maternal instinct.[54] Moreover, whereas the authoritarian literature threatened irresponsible parents with disabled babies, post-war publications sought to allay fears. The greater risk of Down's syndrome for women over the age of thirty was demonstrated statistically.[55] For the most part, however, authors noted that while too many babies still died prematurely, infant mortality was 'steadily falling.'[56] Of course, parents still worried whether their baby would be 'normal'; as one mother told childbirth educator, Sheila Kitzinger, 'Things keep running through my mind ... what if it's got no arms or legs?'[57] But such concerns were sympathetically parried. 'Despite the fact that 97 per cent of babies are perfectly normal', observed obstetrician Gordon Bourne in the 1979 edition of *Pregnancy*, 'anxiety over the normality of your own child is understandable.'[58]

Neither the celebration of intuition nor the arrival of the normal baby saw any weakening of the pre-war emphasis on medical supervision. For disabled children and their families, this regulation had a marginalizing effect which in the advice literature was displayed in the migration of impairment from the mainstream. It was at its most extreme in Penelope Leach's 1977 *Baby and Child* where disability retreated to an encyclopaedia 'at the back', reserved for '[l]ess usual circumstances or ones that need extra or more technical information'. In fact, very little additional information was provided, apart from a short section on 'handicapped children' outlining the interconnection between mental and physical impairments.[59] Conversely, Hugh Jolly's *Book of Child Care* had offered substantial coverage when published two years earlier. However, his book was divided into two parts: the first dealing with the healthy child, the second with the sick child. It was in the second part that the seven chapters discussing disabled children were to be found,[60] thus eliding long-term impairment with temporary illness.

The medicalization of childhood disability was also evident in increased classification. The pre-war advice literature had used a generalized language of physical and mental deficiency, mentioning relatively few conditions by name apart from blindness, deafness and rickets. In the 1970s Bourne was still thinking in terms of generic 'abnormalities': 'mild', 'moderate', 'severe' and 'incompatible with Life'.[61] Post-war, however, an expanding number of diagnostic categories were gradually employed. Thus in 1959 the chapter on 'The Child with a Handicap' in *Good Housekeeping's Mothercraft* included eight categories of physically or mentally disabled children: 'deaf', 'blind', 'spastic', 'educationally backward', 'mentally handicapped', 'maladjusted', 'epileptic' and 'disabled', which was described as being 'deprived of the use of a limb or otherwise crippled by ... an illness such as polio, by an accident, or by a congenital deformity'.[62] From the 1970s, conditions like cystic fibrosis, spina bifida and autism were also listed.[63] However, this presentation of disability in terms of diagnostic categories, while simultaneously equating it with sickness, construed disabled children as permanent objects of professional intervention and inhibited family attempts to shape alternative definitions of their lives.

Prevention

Both continuity and change characterized the prevention and treatment of childhood disability in the post-war literature. New was the edict to vaccinate children against tuberculosis, poliomyelitis and measles,[64] but most attention concentrated on parents. Advice books first published before the horrors of the Holocaust were made known continued to tie prevention to heredity, warning 'young mothers and fathers' that they had 'the future of the race in their hands'.[65] By the late 1960s, the infant science of genetics had moved beyond such generalities and specific 'congenital anomalies' had become identifiable.[66] Parents were thus advised that genetic counselling could 'offer considerable help to those who have some abnormality in their family or to anyone who has a handicapped baby and needs to know the possibility of the abnormally recurring'.[67] Once conception had occurred, authors reiterated the pre-war advice that only regular antenatal checks were able to detect complications.[68] However, the difficulty of predicting the disabilities that occurred during childbirth was ignored.[69]

In the immediate post-war period, antenatal care relied for the most part on external monitoring. X-rays were used when an 'abnormality' was suspected but only with caution, which proved justified in 1958 when antenatal radiography was linked with childhood cancers.[70] By the late 1960s, alternative technologies of visualization were emerging, notably ultrasound, which employed high frequency sound waves as the means for locating 'congenital malformations'. This technique was joined by amniocentesis, in which a sample of fluid from around the foetus was tested for types of intellectual impairment and 'abnormalities' of the central nervous. But penetrating the uterus ran the risk of spontaneous abortion as well as 'orthopaedic postural deformities'. Therefore, after alpha-fetoprotein (AFP) was discovered in the sera of pregnant women in 1970, maternal blood samples were increasingly used to screen for neural tube defects like spina bifida.[71] The advice literature dutifully relayed these developments.[72] With abortion legal in Britain from 1968, both antenatal testing and genetic counselling created the option of termination on the grounds of foetal disability. Medical ethics justified abortion with reference to the financial cost of supporting unproductive citizens;[73] the advice literature emphasized parental choice, albeit less than fulsomely.[74] Among disability groups, however, even the right to choose was controversial because it compromised the baby's right to life and implied the invalidation of disabled people's lives.[75]

With environmental as well as hereditary factors there was initially continuity in the advice literature as post-war authors promoted the natural, holistic regime of the early twentieth century.[76] But subsequently the importance of diet was played down and in 1969 obstetrician Geoffrey Chamberlain concluded that its relationship to 'the production of abnormal babies' was uncertain. Writing in *The Safety of the Unborn Child* – a lay guide to his specialty designed to 'appeal only to the more intelligent reader'[77] – he recognized that before the Second World War women who were 'grossly undernourished tended to produce a higher than average number of abnormal babies'. However, this trend was associated with their 'unfortunate genetic background' and not their environmental conditions.[78] Contemporary parallels were also drawn, Jolly observing that 'Perfectly healthy babies are born all over the world to women whose diets seem outrageously "unbalanced" from a Western point of view'.[79] Therefore, in affluent post-war Britain, where women of childbearing age were assumed to have a well-balanced diet, the advice literature emphasized the dangers of excessive weight gain in pregnancy and healthy eating was reduced to dietary supplements: iron to avoid the anaemia that restricted foetal growth and Vitamin D to ensure that adequate supplies of calcium were absorbed for bone-building.[80] Only in the late 1970s did the literature return to its earlier nutrition theme, warning that malnourished mothers and damaged babies had resulted from the 'vague instruction' to only eat for one.[81]

With the discovery that the placenta was not an effective barrier between mother and child, both maternal disease and drug intake joined the prevention agenda. Since the 1920s, insulin had made pregnancy safer for women with chronic diabetes.[82] However, infectious diseases – in particular, German measles or rubella contracted during the first twelve weeks after conception – were now linked to 'congenital abnormalities such as deafness, blindness and ... heart disease',[83] and the advice books urged pregnant woman not previously infected (or later inoculated) to avoid rubella at all costs.[84] The impact of drugs was demonstrated forcefully by the thalidomide disaster of the late 1950s and early 1960s, when just over 400 babies were born with no limbs or incomplete limbs after their mothers had been prescribed an allegedly safe sedative for the nausea common in early pregnancy.[85] The result was closer scrutiny. The parental literature pronounced most antibiotics safe. Steroids for asthma and hayfever, on the other hand, risked foetal abnormalities, anti-epileptic drugs risked cleft palate and the tranquilizer, Largactil, risked eye damage. Even aspirin imperilled the baby's central nervous system.[86] Therefore, women were recommended to spurn all drugs during pregnancy except those that had been 'specifically permitted' by their doctor or midwife.[87]

Like clinical drugs, recreational drugs were increasingly regarded as harmful. The medical literature tended to ignore these substances. By the late 1970s, however, non-medical authors were confronting drug use with stark warnings that if the teratogenic claims for cannabis were unproven, LSD could damage the embryo's chromosomes.[88] Attitudes to alcohol softened over time, the earlier ban on its use by expectant and nursing mothers giving way to an acceptance of moderate drinking. Responses to tobacco were more mixed after it was linked to low birth weight in the late 1950s.[89] However, women unable to control their smoking were urged to give up altogether,[90] and by the 1970s both medical and non-medical authors were warning that heavy smoking 'probably causes both physical and mental retardation in later childhood'.[91] Nonetheless, there were dissenting voices. In a book dedicated to the Association of Radical Midwives, Christine Beels called for 'some degree of proportion': 'Let's remember that bad housing, too many children and lack of freely available abortion facilities, chronic anaemia and poor diet due to lack of money, put mothers and infants at equally great risk'.[92]

Treatment

Social deprivation was not a preoccupation of the advice literature; on the contrary, what counted was 'the mother and her loving skill, not the material surroundings'.[93] Therefore, discussion centred on individual children and not their environments. The graphs and tables that had plotted weight and height before the War, and the accompanying milestones for physical and mental development,[94] continued to flourish after 1945. Parents were told not to be obsessed by these norms and, if worried, to consult a doctor or health visitor who had been trained to assess child development.[95] However, reference to the normal increasingly anchored post-war advice. In 1948, *The Mothercraft Manual* added a new chapter on 'the normal infant, giving hints as to the routine and feeding'.[96] Other authors consolidated this trend, distinguishing the normal baby from the abnormal one.[97] With this divide came more stringent medical examination: in the words of the Consumer Association's 1972 guide to *The Newborn Baby*, to look 'especially for hidden abnormalities which require early detection so that they can be treated'.[98] Jolly extended this argument to justify 'regular checks ... in the early months'. 'Early detection of a handicap', he insisted, ensured that the 'treatment and correct management of the child start as soon as possible'. Cerebral palsy and deafness, for example, could 'now be diagnosed much earlier than before, which improves the chance of preventing deformity in children with cerebral palsy and speech disorders in children who are deaf'.[99] Yet irrespective of the benefits, this scrutiny had the effect of rendering disabled babies pathological.

Their treatment as prescribed by the post-war literature involved natural as well as professional resources and so fresh air, sunshine and a healthy diet, including breastmilk, retained endorsement.[100] By the 1960s, however, 'many parents and doctors had come to believe that breast- and bottle-feeding were all the same to the baby and that the mother had only her convenience to consider in making her decision'.[101] Breast-feeding later regained the ascendency. It was '*physically* better for babies', Leach told mothers. Nevertheless, 'Only you can decide whether to breast or bottle-feed. Nobody has the right to pressure you either way or to condemn you whatever you decide'.[102] The disabled baby was one whose mother might be denied that choice.[103] The child born with a cleft palate, for example, was said to need assistance with bottle-feeding, or spoon-feeding from birth. But such arrangements were temporary because dentists were 'now able to fit ... a feeding plate' and this device helped to 'mould the palate to a better shape' for later surgery.[104]

In the early post-war years, the advice literature portrayed such heroic surgical correction as the mainstay of medical intervention. There were occasions – with operations to close lesions in spina bifida, for instance – when it was a lifesaver.[105] But by the 1950s, surgery for club foot was represented as a last resort after massaging, splinting and plaster casts had failed.[106] And with cerebral palsy, operations were 'seldom advisable', physiotherapy being the preferred option.[107] Drugs, aids and appliances, and education also fed into the treatment equation. Parents were advised that the baby with cystic fibrosis would be prescribed 'the missing pancreatic enzymes, plus antibiotics for the chest infection'.[108] Attention was drawn to the availability of hearing aids for deaf babies, usable from the age of six months.[109] Prosthetic limbs were fitted. And for older children, 'practical' and 'imaginative' devices were recommended to allow them to eat and dress independently.[110] Above all, the necessity of education or 'training' was stressed with mothers playing a central role in accordance with the gendered division of domestic labour.[111]

Simple guidance was accordingly given about how to educate 'mentally handicapped', blind[112] and 'cerebral palsied' babies by compensating for the experiences inaccessible to them. As Jolly advised with regard to cerebral palsy:

Your child ... may not be able to get his fingers to his mouth by himself, [but] he needs to enjoy sucking and to explore his mouth as much as any other baby; knowing how important this is, you can move his paralysed fingers into his mouth for him.[113]

In the case of deafness, compensation took the form of special education. At twelve months, observed *Good Housekeeping's Mothercraft*, 'a child may be admitted with his mother to a hostel for a fortnight's residential training, where the child is given individual lessons and the mother learns how to teach her child at home'.[114] Such family care was benignly pictured. 'In many cases a backward child in the family brings out warm, protective feelings in the other children ... and his family are well able to take the extra responsibility of looking after him at home'.[115] Later literature was similarly effusive. 'All children need to be part of a family', declared Jolly, 'and with a handicapped child the need is even greater'. Relatives were not only capable of coping; they actually benefited from doing so, 'despite the difficulties', because 'caring for a handicapped child gives a new perspective on life and can strengthen family unity'.[116] Contemporary research reporting the financial and emotional strains of caring for a disabled child at home went largely unnoticed.[117]

The appraisal of institutional care was likewise uncritical. In the late 1950s, *Good Housekeeping's Mothercraft* recommended the mental deficiency hospital, set up by local authorities after legislation in 1913,[118] when a child was 'so helpless or so restless that his continued care at home ... [was] not in his own best interests'.[119] Unaware of the humanitarian crisis that was later to erupt through the publication of research evidence and official reports,[120] this guide drew attention to schools and occupational centres within the hospital and maintained that no child was admitted without 'hope of return' because progress was regularly reviewed.[121] By the 1970s, Jolly was more circumspect. Observing that many 'mentally handicapped' children had been incarcerated in the past, he conceded that 'Life in an institution can never be the same as life in a family'. However, it was to be hoped that such care would offer disabled children more 'normal experiences' in the future, in particular a sense of independence and individuality.[122]

Influencing Experience?

Our analysis of the prevention and treatment of disability via parental advice literature for the period 1890 to 1980 paints a disturbing picture of the negative ways in which disabled babies were perceived with a heavy emphasis on burden, professional authority and normalization. The guidebooks relaying these messages existed in profusion. Of course, British authors never matched the phenomenal success of Dr Spock, who at the time of his death in 1998 had sold fifty million copies.[123] Nevertheless, Hewer's volume ran to twelve editions and 70,000 copies in the decade after publication in 1891,[124] while 40,000 copies of the *Housewife*

Baby Book were sold between its launch in 1948 and the appearance of a second edition in 1955.[125] Needless to say, we cannot assume that such childcare manuals are historical evidence for childcare practice.[126] However, by exploring their role within the sociology of parental knowledge, we can examine whether the advice literature influenced the experiences of disabled children and their families.

All expectant and new parents were bombarded with information – from relatives, friends and neighbours; from professionals; and from guidebooks. The roles played by these sources varied over time and in relation to social class. There *were* authors who in the late nineteenth and early twentieth century claimed to be addressing 'mothers who can command little, as well as those who can command much';[127] and it has been said that 'by the Edwardian period the prices of many manuals had fallen to bring them within the budget of working-class parents'.[128] However, the generous references to nurses and nurseries, and to the home deployment of expensive equipment, suggest that the early literature was primarily aimed at the upper- and middle-class woman.[129] In any event, even if accessed via a public library, neither the advice on the nurse, the nursery and the equipment nor the guidance about diet was realistic for parents living in poverty. Therefore, it is reasonable to assume that most of the knowledge deployed by working-class parents emanated from professionals or from informal family and community networks.

Informal advice was at first little touched, either by the development of voluntary and statutory services during the interwar period or by the birth of the welfare state after 1945. Among working-class girls, falling family size did undercut direct experience of caring for infant relatives.[130] However, mothers reigned supreme and in the classic sociological studies of east London, conducted during the 1950s, women favoured their advice over professional guidance.[131] Oral histories from central and northern Lancashire tell the same story.[132] Growing geographical mobility, brought about by slum clearance programmes and improved employment opportunities, undermined maternal authority,[133] and increased the reliance of working-class parents on non-familial sources of information. Encouraged by Medical Officers of Health and their staff, NHS professionals were important in filling this gap, through the growing number of antenatal classes as well as through family visiting after the birth of a child.[134] However, parents also increasingly turned to popular guides as working-class families engaged with a literature previously more consumed by the middle class. In the late 1950s, therefore, only 'a very small minority' in the Newsons' study of infant care in Nottingham had consulted one of the 'appropriate' texts on childbirth, whereas twenty years later all but two of Ann Oakley's sample had read at least one antenatal book or leaflet.[135]

Disability was caught up in this evolving sociology of parental knowledge. The case of Gerald Turner indicates that for some pre-war families there was a dearth of specialist advice. Born with cerebral palsy in 1931, Gerald lived near Rotherham in Yorkshire. He recalled:

> My parents didn't know what to do with me ... At home my dad had to tie me into a chair and tie my head still with a woollen scarf so they could feed me. It was all trial and error.[136]

Before 1945 the paucity of biographical accounts and empirical findings make it is difficult to speculate about whether advice books affected families like Gerald's with a disabled child. For the post-war period, however, we do have enough sources to piece together a fragmentary account of how the advice literature was used.

When Charles Hannam was told that his son was a 'mongol', he 'rushed to the library' in search of guidance.[137] There is evidence of other post-war parents resorting to the written word. Mrs Marsden – interviewed during Caroline Glendinning's in-depth study of seventeen disabled children in the mid-1970s – admitted that she initially 'knew very little about deafness'. 'It was only by reading, once we knew he was deaf, that I found out about the prognosis and things like this, and found out what he could do if he tried'.[138] Moreover, American mother, Clara Claiborne Park – a devotee of Dr Spock for her first three children – found reassurance in his observation that 'babies may prefer very simple toys' when her fourth child, who was autistic, 'did not want to put rings on a stick'.[139] More commonly, however, families relied on medical experts, relatives or personal experience to answer their queries;[140] and on those occasions when they did consult the advice literature, it was not always useful. 'I didn't know about spastic children having feeding difficulties', explained one mother. 'It was confusing because I bought books on babies, but there was no really helpful information in those early months'.[141]

The failure of the advice literature to meet the information needs of parents does not mean that it had no influence on their experiences. This is because thanks to the debate triggered by postmodernism, we now have a more complex understanding of the relationship between social causation and cultural representation,[142] which does not diminish texts like the childrearing manuals to mere displays of 'manual-writing values'.[143] Consequently, in their contemporary study of *Families Raising Disabled Children*, Janice McLaughlin and her co-authors are anxious to 'neither portray parents as cultural dopes nor overemphasize their choices as agents unconstrained by social pressures'. Rather, they are seen as 'active in the creation of their identities and roles associated with the care of their disabled children'.[144]

Historically, advice books were among the resources available to inform this process of emplotment,[145] helping parents to rehearse the experience of having a baby and contemplate childcare strategies.[146] Under authoritarian parenthood, the causes and consequences of disability were integral to the literature, confronting those predominantly middle-class parents who read it with the pos-sibility of impairment. However, the information was relayed in a moralistic way at a time when professionals dominated interaction with patients and women were feared as a threat to the domestic ideology due to the suffrage campaign and the disruptive effects of the First World War.[147] Therefore, the purpose was to train parents thought to be wanting and not to facilitate the negotiation of a bespoke parental role.

As intuitive parenthood tightened its grip post-1945, disability also departed from the main body of the advice book to separate sections and appendices. A decline in the death and morbidity, which had animated earlier texts, was not the only reason for this move to the periphery, though by 1977 infant mortal-ity was fourteen per 1,000 live births compared with a figure of sixty four for 1932.[148] In addition, the cultural function of the guidebook was changing. The intuitive approach was itself a response to growing affluence, greater autonomy for women and a reaction against aggressive medical authority.[149] Parents, free from the strictures of Truby King and the socio-cultural context that upheld them, were thus encouraged to construct more personalized programmes of childcare with a lighter professional touch. For families with a disabled child, the raw materials supplied for this exercise by the advice literature were almost exclusively negative. Not only was disability marginalized within the text, but the heavy emphasis on the normality of almost all babies also intensified the prospect of alienation among parents whose disabled child was depicted stereo-typically as an aberration.[150] What is more, the books presumed to anticipate parental reactions. It took time for 'the knowledge to sink in and become bearable', intoned Jolly, and 'You need ... to be reminded that no parent has con-tinually admirable feelings even about a perfectly normal baby'.[151]

While some families were devastated by the birth of a disabled child, others contested the pessimistic scenario.[152] Not all parents accepted that disability was an abnormality, for example. Margaret Hogg considered that her son, David, was 'a normal baby, minus two arms' when he was born damaged by thalidomide in 1960.[153] Moreover, feelings of insularity motivated families to participate in the local societies for disabled children, which began to spring up from the early 1950s and shifted the focus away from the 'defective' child towards the provision of deficient services.[154] 'I cannot regard my happy smiling four year old mongol boy as a tragedy', one mother commented in the *Newsletter* of the Scottish Soci-ety for Mentally Handicapped Children for March 1970; 'the problem is more due to lack of facilities than to any difficulties in his upbringing because of his handicap'.[155] Yet in challenging the denial of their children proper support, the parents' movement rarely questioned the dominance of the medical profession in the management of disability.[156]

The first specialist advice literature came likewise from the medical stable. Dr Spock led the way with his *Caring for Your Disabled Child*, published in 1965 under the banner of the US Association for the Aid of Crippled Children. The book opened on a gloomy note with the very first sentence commiserating that 'As the parent of a child with a handicap you face all kinds of problems, at times more than you can bear'.[157] By the 1970s, the British literature was adopting a more positive narrative. Despite reducing *The Wheelchair Child* to his or her mode of transport, Philippa Russell from the Voluntary Council for Handicapped Children did frame her book 'with a view to helping and informing parents and professionals about the problems, possible pleasures – and potentials of a wheelchair life'.[158] Unrestrained by a position in the charitable sector, Judith Stone and Felicity Taylor were more militant, introducing their *Handbook* with a statement from parents proclaiming that they were no longer silenced by 'shame and blame' when confronted with poor quality services.[159]

Conclusion

We cannot trace a direct line from the changing tenor of advice literature to the experiences of disabled children and their families. But this is not unusual in the sense that all experience is mediated and even personal testimony does not speak for itself but 'reproduces rather than contests given ideological systems'.[160] With children there are additional complexities, at their most extreme with babies. The baby is an 'experiencing agent – a site of meaning and knowledge of the world',[161] but it is impossible to access his or her voice. Under these circumstances, there is no alternative but to rely on proxies. The advice books are one such proxy. Not all parents read them, but for the increasing numbers who did, they offered a negative narrative in which disability was represented as a deviation to be prevented if possible, but failing that treated to maximize correspondence with normality. To the extent that this pessimistic narrative influenced family behaviour, it affected the experiences of children born disabled; for as Spock counselled in his specialist text, 'If you want your child to develop positive feelings about himself and his future, you'll need to outgrow some of your own anguished feelings'.[162] Only with the arrival of a dedicated literature, produced partly as a result of the parents' movement, did an alternative model with which to challenge the devaluation of disabled children start to emerge.

7 TREATING CHILDREN WITH NON-PULMONARY TUBERCULOSIS IN SWEDEN: APELVIKEN, *c*. 1900–30

Staffan Förhammar and Marie C. Nelson

Introduction

Perched on the coast in the south-western Swedish province of Halland on the Kattegatt, the body of water separating Sweden from Denmark, is one of the country's fashionable spas. A walk around the grounds and among the older buildings leads to a small cemetery, whose 134 graves belong mostly to young children from distant parts of the country who were buried between 1927 and 1948.[1] Immediately questions come to mind. What was this place? Who were these children? How and why did they come to be buried here, so far from their homes? The story is revealed by delving into the health conditions in Europe and Sweden around the turn of the last century. It is a story of social problems, disease, politics, economics, science and dreams of a better world for individuals and society as a whole.

In the late nineteenth and early twentieth centuries, tuberculosis came to be recognized as one of the major killers among infectious diseases and one of the leading threats to health. It is difficult to establish exactly how many people suffered from the disease due to the problems of identifying the infection.[2] Although the pathogen was not identified by Robert Koch until 1882, it is generally acknowledged that tuberculosis mortality peaked in Europe in the late 1800s before beginning to decline; for Sweden this occurred in the 1870s. It has been calculated that at that time the death rate due to the disease in Swedish cities amounted to about three per thousand.[3] Contemporary Swedish doctors, like their continental counterparts, estimated that most of the urban population in the country was infected.[4] The identification of the pathogen and the interest in the disease throughout Europe led in Sweden to the dedication of King Oscar II's anniversary fund in 1897 to combating the disease. One result was a study that first recommended the creation of sanatoria for fighting pulmonary tuberculosis and then presented a detailed plan for the construction and running of such facilities.[5] However, tuberculosis had many guises, only one of which was the pulmonary form.[6] It has been estimated that about 20 to 30 per cent of those suffering from the disease in Sweden were afflicted by non-pulmonary forms, that is, tuberculosis of the lymphatic system, bones, joints and skin. Many of these victims were children.[7]

These non-pulmonary patients, until recently, have been largely forgotten or, rather, obscured by the concentration on pulmonary tuberculosis in major scholarly studies of the disease and its history.[8] The cultural legacy left by what was often termed 'the white plague' has engaged the interest of researchers from many academic disciplines.[9] While notions of the inherent romanticism of tuberculosis have been challenged, to an extent they persist even in literature that emphasizes the realities of both the suffering of individuals and the extension of state intervention affecting groups of patients and potential patients.[10] Such a focus tends to prioritize the experiences of young adults even while acknowledging that they were not the only sufferers. It is the children deemed at risk of contracting pulmonary tuberculosis and the development of 'preventoriums' for them in the first half of the twentieth century, that have received attention from social historians of medicine.[11] Children as sufferers of distinct types of the disease requiring specialist orthopaedic and other treatments as well as age-specific sanatorium provision have only lately received scholarly scrutiny.[12] This implies a need to connect a history of distinctly childhood disability issues to a more adult-centred literature exploring cultural aspects of the human body in various situations.[13] Ideas about sickness and wellness, the normal and the abnormal, have contributed to a rich flora of historical and sociological studies, though the experiences of children are usually noticeable by their absence.[14] This case study is an attempt to begin addressing such deficiencies.

A Swedish example offers not only a useful exploration of provision for children suffering from tuberculosis but also links the emergence of such facilities to wider debates about the development of welfare states. Scandinavian countries have long been recognized as having a distinctive approach to addressing the social needs of their citizens.[15] For many years this led to optimistic assessments by international commentators of the scale and nature of such welfare provision. Yet, there was a darker side to these services, with a strongly eugenic dimension found in some policies and practices.[16] In terms of Swedish tuberculosis services, Marjaana Niemi usefully links social, economic and political debates to public health priorities and municipal policymaking.[17] Neither her approach nor the discussion in this chapter is incompatible with wider efforts to explore how the public and the private spheres, and the relationship between the two, should be understood.[18] The Swedish historian Svenbjörn Kilander has pointed out that the Swedish state was never totally non-interventionist. The key to understanding its actions lies in the changing definitions of the private sphere to which individuals, families and local municipalities had once belonged.[19] In analysing the developments of this period the Norwegian social historian Anne-Lise Seip sees the third of four stages in the development of the welfare state as 'the social help state', a stage during which the cooperation of the private and the public spheres was consolidated.[20]

This study tries to place the Swedish coastal sanatoria within the political as well as medical contexts within which they developed. The chapter concentrates first on the history of one of the institutions, Apelviken, paying attention to its founding principles, governance and funding. It then explores both the treatment options and the lived experiences within such institutions. There is some evidence of shared endeavour between the promoters of the sanatorium project, the staff and caregivers, parents who sent their children as patients and even the children themselves. This development was, however, not without conflict between the different actors and provides evidence of the changing definitions of public and private within the Swedish context.[21] While class and gender have previously been identified as excluding factors, this chapter foregrounds the influence of age and ill-health/disability in casting people as dependent subjects rather than autonomous and participating citizens. This question of citizenship was particularly pertinent in Sweden where political turmoil had both preceded and followed the First World War. This was a period when Sweden experienced comprehensive political reforms that were part of a slow process of democratization.[22] The sanatoria therefore emerged at a time when the roles of various levels of government were being redefined and society was being forced to grapple with huge social and economic problems, often referred to as 'the social question' in the rhetoric of the day.[23]

Building Apelviken

Amongst the many problems facing Swedish society around 1900 was the care of children suffering from non-pulmonary tuberculosis. Following the example of its Nordic neighbours, Sweden created some seaside sanatoria. The first, Styrsö, near Gothenburg, was established in 1890; in 1900 Barkåkra opened and was later renamed Crown Princess Victoria's Seaside Sanatorium in Vejbystrand. Apelviken, the third such institution and focus of this study, began in 1902 when the doctor who would soon be appointed Varberg's city physician, Johan S. Almer, made the first attempt to treat children afflicted with scrofula (a term used to describe tubercular infections of the lymphatic glands in the neck).[24] The Apelviken farm located on the coast just south of the city of Varberg was where Almer initially cared for six children for a period of two summer months. During the two years that followed the number increased to about twenty patients, and in 1904 the first pavilion was built on a lot located on Little Apelviken, a bay on the Kattegatt. The pavilion was called The Seaside Sanatorium Apelviken (*Kustsanatoriet Apelviken*).

In September 1904 Almer initiated the formation of the Association for the Seaside Care of Children with Scrofula (*Föreningen för kustvård åt skrofulösa barn*) with a group of philanthropists.[25] Although Almer remained in charge of the institution, the association purchased the entire sanatorium for 5,415 crowns and assumed responsibility for its operation.[26] The association's expressed goal was 'to prepare seaside care for children afflicted with scrofula and in connection therewith to seek to maintain the coastal sanatorium Apelviken'.[27] In the philanthropic spirit of the day, the association called for financial support to bring 'joy' to the supporters and 'a cure' to those suffering from this disease. Since the disease was particularly found among poor children, it was seen as an opportunity for the better-off to make a contribution to the general welfare.[28]

The association had a seven-member board of directors, one of whom was required to be a medical doctor. Although based in Varberg, it could have representatives from other geographical areas.[29] It is impossible to determine fully either the social background or the relative activism of individual members because the policy of printing membership lists in the annual report was short-lived.[30] Most members were then from the local area, either from Varberg or from the province of Halland, but there were individuals from Stockholm and even Norrbotten, the northernmost province. Among the professionals named were six medical doctors and seven estate owners, as well as pharmacists, factory managers, factory owners, and major merchants. The 1905–6 annual report differentiated between fifty-one standing members (including six women) and the 859 regular members (including 210 women).[31] The former are presumed to have been more active in the running of the association than the latter, though they would also have been recruited for their ability to boost the legitimacy of the association. Limited details about the regular members (who paid an annual membership fee initially set at two crowns) certainly suggest more diverse social backgrounds than are found amongst the standing members (who had paid fifty crowns or more on one occasion). Honorary members, such as the provincial governor in Halland, Axel Asker, were also recruited and in addition there were corporate members sent as representatives from various local government bodies. It is not so much the individuals who are interesting, but rather the interests they represented.

An important question when determining the character of any philanthropic organization is the balance on the board between experts and amateurs. The association, which had a scientific orientation, clearly required expertise in several fields. Medical knowledge was a vital resource, but so were financial and organizational skills. The seven-member board in 1905 included Almer (the founder), four other medical doctors, a pharmacist and a married woman. By

1910 several changes had occurred, most notable of which was a strengthening of the board's economic competence. In 1915 the board was expanded, and the participation of public servants became more noticeable after this date. These officials provided the economic expertise once offered by businessmen. Thus, while board composition changed over time, the balance between those providing medical and financial skills was preserved. The chairman of the board, with the exception of 1905, was always selected from the civil servants. In 1910 the women serving as members of the board were prominent figures who were generally deeply engaged in philanthropic work. Although considered amateurs rather than professionals, these women contributed considerable knowledge and skills. Either on their own or together with their husbands, they provided useful contacts and access to support networks as wives of leading businessmen and major financial supporters of the cause.

The association initially had three main funding streams: membership dues, donations and interest from invested assets. At the outset, the variety of sources of finance probably ensured a degree of autonomy and independence, despite a deliberate engagement between the association and the wider public sphere. As was often the case with philanthropic healthcare organizations, the association soon acquired financial support from the regional government (*landsting*) and the national state. As early as 1904, when Almer was solely responsible for Apelviken, the regional government in Halland voted to contribute 1,000 crowns (raised to 1,500 for 1906–8) to the institution, which was to be used as a subvention of one crown per day for each child from the region that was cared for at Apelviken.[32] At the national level the first decision to support these institutions was made in 1908. Such support was inevitably accompanied by increasing official influence over the association.[33]

The economic reports for 1905 and 1930 provide a picture of the changing scale and balance of different contributions. In 1905 the total membership fees amounted to 2,481 crowns, while the contributions were 5,438 crowns. The majority of the latter included a gift of 5,000 crowns from the Varberg Savings Bank, while 216 crowns came from local activities. The regional government in Halland paid 1,000 crowns, while the patient fees amounted to 394 crowns. Almer provided his services without cost and the local pharmacist did not charge for the medicine provided. The result was that twenty-five of the thirty-five children cared for at Apelviken in 1905 received free care.[34] Financial records show how quickly this picture of strong membership and limited state support was reversed between 1905 and 1930. During the final year of the period studied only 1,114 crowns were received from the membership fees, while payments from several regional governments amounted to 308,712 crowns. The state provided 270,000 crowns for running expenses and another 100,000 for new buildings in 1930 alone.[35]

The use of various funding illustrates the tapestry of public/private support. The 1,000 crown contribution from the county of Halland in 1905 was used to support regional patients. This sum increased in the following years. From 1915 the regional government sought to make a distinction between children without means and children of lesser means. While the costs of the former were to be entirely covered by the regional government, the latter were supposed to provide 30 *öre* (100 *öre* = one crown) per day, which was to be paid by the parent or guardian of the child or by the local government (*kommun*).[36] From the middle of the 1920s, the regional governments did not pay sums directly to Apelviken. Instead, the contributions from the regional governments went to the coordinating organization for the three coastal sanatoria on Sweden's west coast. This organization in turn directed the flow of funds and patients to the three sanatoria. By 1930 the daily cost had risen to 1.75 crowns per patient; the funds were to cover care and two thirds of the costs of the support bandages provided for the patients before returning home.[37] Under these arrangements patients contributed 213,656 crowns in fees in 1930 and an unspecified, though presumably small, number of cases was assisted by the association's own contribution of 992 crowns for patients 'without means'. This sum probably derived from returns on investing earlier donations which had become another significant source of finance, amounting to 101,176 crowns in 1930. While the size of donations was increasingly dwarfed by other sources of funding, they retained symbolic importance and innovative ways were found to solicit them. In his book on Apelviken that was published in 1925, Almer mentions the importance of the Children's Day celebration as an early source of support. The initiative was taken in 1906 by members of the association, both Varberg residents and summer guests. This group made the first concrete economic contribution in 1907, together with the philanthropic organization the Bee Hive Association (*Föreningen Bikupan*), for the construction of a new building.[38] These two organizations were recurring features in the annual economic reports, as was the Varberg Savings Bank.[39]

Treatment at Apelviken

A small coastal farm on the bay Apelviken was rented by Almer in 1902 to test his treatment regime of fresh air, nourishing food, rest, sunshine, sea bathing and exercise for children with non-pulmonary tuberculosis. Such a programme was meant to be holistic.[40] It was informed by the latest scientific thinking and the example of similar facilities in other countries. It also drew on readily available natural resources in the environs of Apelviken. Many tuberculosis experts believed that it was essential to remove the sick child from home as prerequisite to treatment.[41] Since many sick children were also poor, there was great concern about their home environment, which might well be insanitary and overcrowded, as well as exposing them to both urban pollution and close contact with parents and siblings suffering from tuberculosis.[42] While the advocated change of environment could involve admission to a general hospital ward, there was an increasing preference for facilities that offered the promise of fresh air and other treatment. There was some debate about the relative merits of sea and mountain air, although over time any non-polluted air outside of towns was seen as potentially valuable.[43] Swedish doctors who had observed tuberculosis treatment on the continent discussed, for example, their observations of Davos which offered mountain air or Berck-sur-Mer on the French coast, and debated which locations were most favourable in the leading Swedish journals of the day.[44]

Resorts offering fresh air could usually promise the therapeutic benefits of sunshine as well. Heliotherapy was part of the programme that Almer recommended, although its earlier development on the continent had attracted controversy. There was lingering concern that traditional sun verandas, despite being endorsed by an influential national study, had limited utility in a Nordic climate.[45] The answer, a technological solution, came from Denmark where physician Niels Finsen had demonstrated in 1895 that skin tuberculosis could be treated with light. He developed a variety of 'Finsen lamps' for treating different types of tuberculosis under the auspices of the Finsen Institute and was awarded the Nobel Prize in Physiology and Medicine in 1903.[46] Although Finsen died in 1904, the institute continued and variations of his lamps were widely used across the Nordic countries. One treatment at Apelviken consisted of the 'Finsen bath'. Patients, whose plaster casts were removed, sat under the lamps for a specified period of time before entering saltwater showers.[47] Staff at Apelviken also experimented briefly with so-called quartz lamps and local x-rays to treat scrofula and other forms of lymphatic tuberculosis.[48] The problem with x-rays, according to a national study of provision, was that they required skilled personnel to administer treatment while Finsen's lamps did not, hence the adoption of the latter at the expense of the former.[49]

The use of water at Apelviken, both alone and in combination with other treatments such as the lamps above, has received less attention in the historiography than the use of light or fresh air. It was no coincidence that two of the Swedish coastal sanatoria, Styrsö and Apelviken, were developed in places where hydrotherapy was already practised.[50] Existing patterns of health tourism were also important in establishing other sanatoria in that era.[51] Swedish spas had a long history and established links to wider European developments in religious, philosophical and scientific ideas.[52] It is against this backdrop that we need to understand the location of the sanatoria and the development of 'natural cures'. Apelviken was located in an area where people had been 'taking the waters' since 1811.[53] Varberg soon developed as a *kurort* (spa or health resort) and attracted a large number of health tourists. The first bathhouse was constructed in 1822, and by 1866 a new bathhouse offered mud baths and kelp baths, as well as massage and other treatments. This became part of the *Hafsbadkuranstalt* where one could take the cure by the sea. Many of the earliest pictures of the seaside sanatorium patients at Apelviken were taken in the little cove in the vicinity of the first pavilion that was completed in 1904 with children wading in the water under the watchful eye of the nurses and other personnel.[54] According to one patient at the sanatorium some years later, weather permitting, the goal was to bathe in the ocean twice a day.[55] Pools were constructed later for both fresh- and saltwater, and their use became integrated into the treatment of the patients, thus making it possible to bathe during the inhospitable Nordic winter. Although the patients 'bathed' in groups, additional programmes involving water and light (using the lamp treatments outlined above) were individualized by the doctors. Initially these treatments were followed by showers, either saltwater or fresh, but the showers were later deemed unnecessary by some.[56] The showers seem to have been an integrated part of the treatment at Apelviken.[57]

Water treatments have not received the attention given to other therapeutic interventions but just as advocates for fresh air drew attention to the problems of urban pollution, so the focus on water and cleansing underlined the problematic hygiene conditions in slum homes.[58] There always seemed to be scope to criticize the habits of the poor, but there were also sustained efforts to improve access to clean water.[59] Water was often central to Swedish public health programmes, a metaphorical way to 'clean up' both individuals and their environment, but the relationship between clean water and efforts to combat the spread of tuberculosis and treat its effects are still underexplored despite the emphasis some contemporary campaigners and medical experts placed on the centrality of water.[60] A better-known, though controversial, set of debates relates to nutrition. The preventoriums, especially those for children, are usually considered to have put too much faith in the benefits of fresh air and neglected the importance of adequate nutrition.[61] In children's sanatoria, however, close attention was paid to dietary matters and patients were regularly weighed to monitor the desired weight gain. In one of his descriptions of treatment in various European sanatoria, the physician Ernst Lindahl noted the typical diet for children attending the Dutch seaside sanatorium at Loosduinen.[62] At Apelviken, the daily programme in the summer included time for meals, prayers, exercise, bathing and sunbathing, activities and practical work. The youngest children went to bed at 6:30 pm and the older patients at 8 pm.[63]

The regime at Apelviken clearly drew its inspiration from the potential of natural cures, and promoted the idea of conservative treatment. In Almer's eyes the most important form of treatment was 'the direct sunlight in the moving air on the sun verandas and sun decks, and during the summer, even on the beach'.[64] A fundamental part of most programmes included the use of plaster casts and bandages. For example, the treatment of spinal tuberculosis often meant using the plaster cradle where the patient was held in place so that pressure would be put on the 'hump' that had formed, the idea being to slowly increase the pressure and decrease the size of the aberration, producing a straighter backbone. The periods of immobilization were very long: months or even years. Other forms of plaster casts were also used on various parts of the body, but their use diminished during the 1920s when alternative techniques began to be developed.[65]

At Apelviken operations were sometimes performed when necessary, though Almer was not an enthusiast. It was his successor, Robert Hanson, who further developed the surgical side of the work.[66] This was the major change that took place in the institution after Almer's death as those in favour of more 'radical' forms of treatment took over both Apelviken and leadership of the national debate about the future of tuberculosis services.[67] At the time of his death, Almer was serving on the committee appointed by the Swedish National Organization against Tuberculosis to study non-pulmonary tuberculosis and recommend measures for future care. The committee was not convinced that the climatic treatment could be readily transferred to Sweden, although they did point out the importance of a good diet, lots of fresh air, the use of protected verandas, and the importance of well-educated physicians and staff.[68] Almer died before the committee delivered its report but his written reservations to its conclusions were printed.[69] He thought that sceptical members of the committee had been too quick to dismiss climatic treatment. While Sweden had neither the Alps nor the same climate as more southerly latitudes, Almer maintained that these difficulties could be overcome by exploiting the benefits of sea air to increase the resistance of the patient. In any case, he argued, Sweden had its own equivalent of the Alps in the northerly and mountainous province of Jämtland, located on the Norwegian border.[70] Given his conservative approach, it is not surprising that Almer was also opposed to encouraging treatment regimes that would involve building large hospitals with special wards for the care of these patients.[71] Clearly, a number of these facilities were emerging. But for Almer his cherished Apelviken model was sacred and offered in his mind the best solution to the care of child tuberculosis patients.[72] Despite apparently growing opposition, he persisted with his recommendations for generally non-invasive treatment over long periods of time.[73] He remained adamant to the end, although in reality the programme at Apelviken usually used a combination of conservative and more invasive treatments.

Patients at Apelviken

While the discussion above has shown that none of the therapies offered at Apelviken were unique to that sanatorium, the institution was well placed to prosper and demand for care grew rapidly. While initially only Almer and a few of his close colleagues sent children to be treated, after a few years patients were being referred to the institution from all over the country.[74] This required the development of a common admissions process for the three sanatoria, with related funding arrangements.[75] Originally most of the patients came from the surrounding west coast province of Halland, but, as other counties became willing to provide financial support for patients, diversity increased. By 1930 the balance had shifted, and the northernmost counties of Västernorrland, Jämtland and Norrbotten contributed almost one third of all the patients. A number of cities sent patients, but two dominated. Between 1914 and 1922 Stockholm sent twenty or more each year, with a high of thirty-eight in 1916. After 1921 Norrköping sent ten to twenty each year.[76] The number of patients from each area depended on many factors, not least of which was the willingness of respective regional or city governments to provide funding.

The total number of patients grew from the original six in 1902 to 1,268 in 1930. Initially the facilities were open only during the summer months, but the length of the season was gradually extended to the whole year by 1915. By 1930 the maximum number that could be treated at any one time was 500 patients. Originally the patients stayed about 60 days, but in the 1920s the average stay had increased to 140–150 days. Patients suffering from skeletal tuberculosis received the longest treatment, often more than 160 days, while other conditions required shorter stays.[77] Over time, the types of tuberculosis that were treated changed and this impacted on the age of admission as well as length of stay. Initially, the patients were small children suffering from scrofula, but gradually youths (aged 15–20) and young adults were also admitted for treatment. By 1915 only just over 60 per cent of new cases were diagnosed with scrofula, and this figure fell further, to about 20 per cent, by 1924 as a result of a real decline in the number of those affected and a recategorization of some types of cases as understanding of tuberculosis changed.[78] On the other hand, the proportion of patients with skeletal tuberculosis was on its way to reaching one half.[79] The number of patients under five years of age remained proportionately the same, while the oldest patients (aged twenty plus) increased at the expense of the youths.

The goal of the sanatorium was for a healthy, or much improved, patient to return home, a journey that was paid for by the state. However, not all the children survived their stay.[80] If a patient died, then the transport cost of 350–400 crowns fell on the shoulders of the parents, many of whom lived in the far north and could not raise such sums.[81] During the first two decades of the sanatorium's existence patients who died and whose families could not afford to bring them home were buried in one of the local cemeteries. However, complaints of unkempt graves, some of which were those of former Apelviken patients, were among the motives behind the proposal in 1924 to create a special cemetery on the grounds. This was prepared and ready for use in 1927. Ironically, it was Almer, the founder of Apelviken, who was the first to be buried there, and his monument still watches over the cemetery. Of the 134 burials, more than half were children or youths from the northern part of the country (the counties of Norrbotten, Västerbotten, Jämtland and Västernorrland) and about one third were between ten and twenty years of age. A former patient (1938–1940) wrote a booklet about the cemetery and, as far as it was possible to do so, compiled biographies in order to honour his former fellow patients and their predecessors. One example from the early period was Nancy Blom, a six-year-old girl from the far north (Övertorneå in Norrbotten), who died at Apelviken on 30 December 1930. Tragically Nancy, her mother and four of her seven siblings all died of tuberculosis between 1928 and 1930. Her father, a railway worker, was left with just three of his children.[82] From this booklet it is possible to get only brief glimpses into the actors in this terrible drama. Some insight, however, is provided into the earliest period of the sanatorium in the form of summaries of interviews conducted in the 1980s with former patients and personnel.[83]

One of the most extreme and fascinating stories was told by Petter Bernhard Savela, originally from Haparanda, a town at the head of the Gulf of Bothnia, who spent two periods of time (March 1925 to July 1927 and May 1931 to December 1932) at Apelviken. Born in 1905 to an unwed mother (his acknowledged father left for America and never returned), he was auctioned off at the age of six to a farmer who abused him severely.[84] When it was discovered that he had a hip that was broken in several places, the town sent him to Stockholm to the Home for Crippled Children to learn a trade. Tuberculosis was soon discovered, and he was transferred to Apelviken. He describes the sunbaths, air baths, light treatment and ocean bathing, as well as the nourishing diet. The descriptions of meals were lyrical; it must be remembered that this boy had often nearly starved in his home in the north. Because of his poor condition he gained weight slowly, but in the end increased from 35 kg to 76 kg in twenty-eight months. He was returned 'home' to the farm, but was again abused and injured, and, after unsuccessful treatment elsewhere, he was finally returned to Apelviken. Following his second stay there he was sent back to the Home for Crippled Children. Initially taught engraving, he eventually became a typographer and after a few years started his own printing business. This was a considerable achievement for a boy who had spent nearly fifteen years in different institutions, but it was nothing compared to his later successes. Petter became involved in real estate and made a fortune which he donated in time to the municipality in the north that had once put him on the auction block. Petter's story was unusual and he was undoubtedly a survivor. The regime at Apelviken could be beneficial but evidence suggests many children still longed for their own homes and families, even while participating in and often enjoying the social life and education.[85]

Conclusion

The study of a single institution, such as Apelviken, can easily give the impression that the answer to the treatment of non-pulmonary tuberculosis was, if not simple, at least relatively clear. A very different picture emerges from perusing national studies, government reports, medical journals, medical society records, and surviving correspondence. There was in fact a clear division of the medical corps into those who favoured 'radical' (surgical) and those who favoured 'conservative' (natural) treatment. It is also very apparent that the models for treatment came from outside the borders of the country. Swedish experts frequently visited foreign institutions and their findings ignited further controversy. Debates centred not just on the merits of particular treatments, be they old or new, but the way the disease itself should be understood.

One of the roots of the problem was the difficulty in defining the term scrofula. Another source of conflict was inherent within the term traditionally used to describe the non-pulmonary forms, surgical tuberculosis. Techniques developed before the cause of the disease was understood called for the surgical removal of the infected area of the body. The joints and bones were usually the target of the surgeon, as the infection was considered to be localized and thus suitable for an operation. On the other hand, the elusive scrofula was considered best treated by the natural method. Soon, however, the treatment offered by the coastal sanatoria was considered by some actors to be preferable, even for the patients with tuberculosis of the bones and joints. Many of the doctors who advocated this kind of treatment argued for a more holistic approach: the diseased organism, the body, harboured the infection that could break out in any of the organs.[86] Surgery could disable a patient who was still suffering from the disease.[87]

Although in oversimplified form, these were the lines of battle that were drawn up. They exerted great influence over late-nineteenth-century and early-twentieth-century medical discourse. There were two general 'great debates' on tuberculosis within the Swedish Medical Society in 1884 and in 1896, although articles on tuberculosis continuously appeared in the annals of the society.[88] In 1909 a discussion was held concerning surgical tuberculosis that delineated the lines in the debate that appeared and reappeared with the publication of various government committee investigations during the two decades that followed. The questions concerning seaside sanatorium treatment were especially prominent in the journal of the Swedish Medical Society, *Hygiea*, in 1916 and 1917. The cast of characters remained the same throughout these debates in which a number of prominent physicians participated. These included two of the three original founders of the seaside sanatoria and their medical staff, a leader in the development of orthopaedics, and physicians who headed general hospital departments devoted to the treatment of this form of tuberculosis.[89] These sometimes heated discussions display not only different aspects of the subject, but also reflect the rivalries and territorial struggles within the medical corps between surgeons and other practitioners.

This medical debate was just one of many contexts that shaped the development of Apelviken. The history of the institution provides a complex picture of the way part of the struggle against tuberculosis unfolded. Apelviken was not just a medical establishment. It also embodied the political radicalism of the late-nineteenth-century with its fight to improve living conditions through a combination of individual initiatives and government intervention. This combination can be interpreted as a consequence of the 'social help state', which in Seip's socio-political model preceded the 'welfare' state. The 'social help' state rested on the principle of cooperation between public and private actors on different levels. These political relations led, after some hesitation in the beginning of the twentieth century, to a positive decision concerning state support to the private coastal sanatoria, although it also entailed some state supervision.[90]

Acknowledgements

The material on which this paper is based was gathered within the framework of the pilot project 'Unga, krokiga och kroniskt sjuka. Kulturella bestämningar av funktionshinder. Bentuberkulos på Apelviken, 1902–c. 1930. En pilotstudie', funded by The Swedish Research Council. The authors are indebted to Nadja Sehovic, research assistant, and to the archivists Christian Jarnekrantz, Halland County Archives, Halmstad, Sweden and Eva Berntsson Melin, County Museum, Varberg, Sweden, for their invaluable assistance.

8 HEALTH VISITING AND DISABILITY ISSUES IN ENGLAND BEFORE 1948

Pamela Dale

Introduction

At the start of the twentieth century the development of services for disabled children in the United Kingdom accelerated and changed in a number of significant ways. Firstly, there was simply more provision as local councils gradually acquired permissive powers to develop (independently and in partnership with voluntary sector organizations) both specialist services for children and other health and welfare services accessible to people of all ages and utilized by disabled children and their families. Secondly, the new services were not just designed to respond to expressed need; they actively sought clients. This contrasted with the exclusive admissions policies designed to limit access to nineteenth-century residential special schools run by charities and the deterrent principles of the Poor Law. Thirdly, there was a shift away from traditional forms of institutional care to a more complicated network of services delivered in a variety of settings.

These developments have been explored through histories of the school medical service in England and Wales, which draw attention to the importance of establishing both regular medical inspections for school-age children and a number of clinics to diagnose and treat various disabling conditions.[1] Although it has not been a strong theme in the historiography these clinics often worked in close partnership with other local authority services targeted at younger children, and also designed to identify, treat and crucially prevent childhood disability. This chapter concentrates on the contribution pioneering health visitors, working in infant welfare clinics as well as undertaking home visits, made to these agendas. Such an approach is designed to illuminate contacts between a new group of professionals, the health visitors, and sick and disabled children. Emphasis on this aspect of the health visitors' work contrasts with the existing literature focus on the often problematic relationship between health visitors and the mothers of small children.

Assessing the Contribution of Health Visitors

In recent years the historiography has taken a critical view of the aims, methods and achievements of generations of health visitors, with particular condemnation reserved for the pioneers of municipal health visiting in the first three decades of the twentieth century.[2] Yet an earlier literature had celebrated their contribution to the prevention of sickness and disability and attempts to improve the lives of children living with such conditions.[3] In the 1960s, Margot Jefferys suggested that the problems facing contemporary health visitors, explained in terms of role ambiguity, stemmed from their success in tackling serious threats to child health before 1948. This had left the profession without clearly defined responsibilities. Interestingly, Jefferys made little reference to the experiences of client groups, including disabled children and their families. She nonetheless concluded that 'a great deal of the credit' for reduced infant mortality and a fall in the number of children 'permanently crippled by serious illness or nutritional deprivation' between 1900 and 1948 must be given to the 'educative work of health visitors'.[4]

These apparently irreconcilable views of health visiting before 1948 can be explained with reference to three factors. First were changing assessments of contemporary practice, which secondly, over time, encouraged a reassessment of traditional models of health visiting. The third factor is a lack of clarity about which groups of health visitors and their clients were being discussed, with homogeneity often erroneously assumed in contemporary and historical accounts.[5] Most significant however was the developing critique of health visiting as it was practised in the 1970s and 1980s. A number of sociological studies revealed that routine visits to all children under five were failing to deliver measurably better outcomes in terms of child health, with a further concern that the conduct of these visits was provoking client resistance while failing to provide stimulating work for highly trained practitioners.[6] There was also professional and public anxiety that the time devoted to such activities left cases of real need undiscovered and unaddressed. There was for example a sustained campaign to upgrade routine and often inconclusive hearing checks to a sophisticated screening programme that would bring all hearing impaired children into earlier contact with specialist services to support the development of communication skills.[7] Health visitors were also found to have been at fault in several official inquiries into fatal child abuse which raised questions about their handling of other instances of non-accidental injury and neglect leading to preventable sickness and disability.[8]

The developing critique of contemporary health visiting practice, fuelled by the class, gender, and to a lesser extent disability, politics of the 1970s and 1980s, encouraged a more critical historical assessment of earlier interactions between visitors and visited. These were increasingly characterized as paternalistic, and it was client resistance to misguided even sinister professional interference that became celebrated in accounts by Ellen Ross and others.[9] Yet if one model of poor professional practice offers the example of clients resisting the imposition of unwelcome advice and assistance, other clients were let down by a failure to provide support. A third group of clients, not necessarily happy with every aspect of the service they received, benefited from using it. With most critiques of health visiting concentrating on well babies and their mothers it cannot be assumed that parents of sick and disabled children responded, or were treated, in the same way. Here it is worth drawing attention, as Anthea Symonds does, to the emphasis health visitors have traditionally placed on the importance of trust, support and simply being there for vulnerable clients isolated from other sources of support.[10]

There were more frequent contacts between health visitors and clients perceived to have special needs. An ongoing relationship, unlike intermittent checks on well babies, could encourage negotiation leading to mutual understanding and respect. This is the modern ideal with some parents, writing about their experiences of raising disabled children in the 1990s, drawing attention to the supportive role played by sympathetic health visitors.[11] But in the past staff shortages, and the priority given to professional power over parental choice, meant that a period of intensive visiting was often designed to facilitate admission to institutional care. This would support the controlling intentions thesis, but with many specialist educational and medical services only available in institutions parents faced difficult choices. Health visitor advocacy for better access to such provision cannot simply be viewed as an anti-parent strategy. The limited evidence available, from the mental deficiency sector, suggests that in the small minority of cases where decisions about the future care of a disabled child were clouded by an explicit concern to protect the child from abusive or neglectful parents health visitors were less rather than more involved in the process as NSPCC inspectors and employees of social work agencies took a more prominent role.[12]

The health visitors discussed in this chapter showed signs of authoritarianism when instructing parents, but their campaigns for improved child services relied on the power of what Viner and Golden term the 'tableau of distressed parents' desperately seeking treatment for their child.[13] Health visitors could offer useful advice and make referrals to other services. It was the inadequacies of the additional services, as much as the personal or professional limitations of the health visitors, which resulted in problematic experiences for the child and his/her family. Yet, following Viner and Golden, it is worth drawing attention to a strange paradox in the history of child health and disability services; often those most passionately committed to reform used evidence of child suffering to push for service development without making any reciprocal effort to challenge medical practices that all-too-frequently failed to acknowledge either the pain and suffering of child patients or the validity of the child's own experiences and preferences. This means that recognition of increasing health visitor involvement with childhood disability issues does not imply that the quality of health visiting in relation to the care of disabled children improved over time. Instead a series of discrete episodes are discernable, each containing evidence of progress and new constraints on the work.

The Origins of Health Visiting Practice

Health visiting had diverse origins, but none of the classic nineteenth-century or Edwardian case studies have much to say about contacts with disabled children. Scholars have certainly prioritized other aspects of the health visitors' work but practitioners may have deliberately avoided such potential clients, either on their own initiative or following instructions from their employers and/or professional leaders. This interpretation allows for significant variations in practice across time and place, with different health visitors following a variety of policies coloured by their own personal preferences. There were for example opportunities to divide the workload in ways that allocated tasks to staff with particular skills and interests when teams of municipal health visitors operated in the interwar period. On the other hand the prevalence of sickness and disability before 1948, with all children viewed as being at significant risk of developing these conditions, meant that all staff had responsibilities for the identification and care of disabled children. This suggests that existing research has misunderstood this crucial aspect of health visiting.

It certainly seems likely that staff and volunteers connected with organizations like the Ladies' Branch of the Manchester and Salford Sanitary Association, widely credited with pioneering health visiting in the voluntary sector and then encouraging statutory activity, encountered many disabled children and adults in the course of their work.[14] However, any personal or professional concern with individual suffering witnessed and/or the wider social and economic costs of disability was unlikely to have encouraged a positive view of disability. In the case of pioneer health visitors this problem was compounded by the background of the personnel recruited and the scientific theories circulating when professional education began.[15]

As health visiting professionalized in the 1890s, but before trained nurses gained ascendancy within the profession in the 1920s, the principles of the Charity Organization Society (COS) had a definite influence over the work.[16] Disabled children and their families could be presented as both victims and threats,[17] with a question over whether or not they were part of the 'deserving poor'. Sympathy for certain individuals was combined with a determination, that crossed traditional political divides, to reduce overall levels of dependency and break the link between various forms of deviancy and disability. Thus moral purity campaigns aimed to reduce the incidence of venereal disease and thereby the number of children born showing signs of the multiple disabilities associated with, for example, congenital syphilis. In some quarters eugenic theories encouraged the idea of introducing punitive measures aimed at eradicating certain types of disability altogether.

Even when the highly questionable impact of eugenic ideas is discounted, there is every reason to conclude that Edwardian health visitors were not encouraged to develop a positive view of disability issues.[18] Instead their work was framed by a narrative of personal tragedy and an emphasis on the social and economic burdens imposed by physical, mental and/or sensory impairment. This narrative had not been developed by health visitors, but neither was it systematically challenged by staff who found themselves on the fringes of what Viner and Golden present as a quantitative and qualitiative shift in contacts between children and medical services. With no unified disability service health visitors made sporadic contact with disability issues in a variety of settings and circumstances. Any health visitor's understanding of disability issues was going to be coloured not just by the type of cases they met but the context for the encounter.

Although contemporary and historical practitioners of health visiting point to the independence enjoyed by such professionals this was always somewhat circumscribed in the case of disabled children. Rather than start from the premise that all children, regardless of any disability, had very similar needs there was a view amongst health professionals that special expertise was required to address any aspect of the care of a disabled child. The evolution of separate services, stressing different client needs, arguably undermined health visitors' confidence in their own skills and increased their reliance on medical guidance. Municipal health visiting was originally organized on the 'patch' system and in any given year it was unlikely that many, let alone all, different kinds of disability would be encountered in a small geographical area. Yet, even experienced health visitors accustomed to working with physically disabled children might well be viewed as unqualified to work with blind or deaf children.

Rather than draw attention to the excellent work done by health visitors there was a consistent concern that health visitors who were primarily concerned with the care of well babies lacked the specialist training necessary to work effectively with children with special needs. The key health visitor role quickly became one of referral to appropriate medical staff, leading clients almost inexorably towards specialist services remote from the day-to-day work of the health visitor. This meant that the knowledge health visitors gleaned from their home visits about the social causes and consequences of certain disabling conditions, that in some senses anticipated aspects of the social model of disability, was subordinated to medical concerns. Health visitors, as municipal employees primarily tasked with domiciliary visiting, had limited access to and no influence over doctors working in the voluntary hospitals. The public health doctors planning and staffing the municipal infant welfare clinics, where health visitors spent a considerable portion of their time, also deliberately limited the work of the health visiting staff in relation to the formal identification and ongoing care of disabled children in various ways.

This doctor-defined service must however not be viewed as inevitable. In some places an earlier generation of health visitors had discovered the special needs of disabled children for themselves. Yet even during a period of comparatively independent practice, such staff tended to organize their concerns and activities in a way that facilitated later medical dominance and created other problems for the future. There was a failure to establish a unified community-based disability service. This privileged institutional care despite its unsuitability for many disabled children. A strong practitioner commitment to campaigning for better care also tended to detract from work with individual clients, and even unnecessarily stigmatized families as staff used the worst possible examples of neglectful care to advance their own agenda for change. These issues are explored with reference to the situation in Edwardian Bradford.

Pioneering Work in Bradford

At the end of the nineteenth century there were competing models of health visiting practice.[19] Employment as a sanitary inspector rather than health visitor gave most autonomy to staff. There was scope for these officials to define as well as manage their own caseload. This was a powerful vehicle for discovering and addressing unmet need, but the encounter between visitor and visited carried risks as well as opportunities for both. Pressure to improve services in the Edwardian period went hand-in-hand with increased official powers of surveillance and coercion.

In Bradford, the female sanitary inspectors (FSIs) were originally tasked with controlling nuisances. It was during their house-to-house inspections that they discovered many sick and/or disabled people living in intolerable conditions. Faced with evidence of people living in dilapidated accommodation without heat, lighting or the most basic of furniture let alone special equipment that would assist with nursing care, the officials unhesitatingly recommended admission to institutional care and used various powers to coerce the frail elderly into the workhouse.[20] Yet over time the FSIs found, as a result of their discussions with the slum dwellers, themselves advocating the development of more services that would better meet the needs and preferences of vulnerable groups.[21]

While the inspectors remained pessimistic about their ability to improve the situation of disabled adults they gained a better understanding of the way poverty was a cause and consequence of various disabling conditions and they showed increasing determination to protect children from the toll exacted by the social, economic and environmental problems of the city.[22] Although the FSIs made no explicit reference to the work of Margaret McMillan and other pioneers of better child services in Bradford they shared common goals and approaches.[23] The education of parents went hand-in-hand with efforts to develop comprehensive municipal health and welfare services designed to optimize child development. This led to attempts to prevent disability, treat all remedial conditions, and offer specialist support to those living with a significant impairment.

In Bradford the School Board, later Education Committee, was famous for its wide-ranging reforms before 1914. Its programmes of school feeding, school medical inspections and provision of special schools addressed all the agendas above.[24] The FSIs experienced more difficulties when defining their responsibilities, and this hindered service development. They had to balance the needs of a number of client groups with their inspection duties and the burden of increasing infant welfare work. In many cases, where the FSIs seemed powerless to act, they could only use their reports to recount the human misery they witnessed in the hope of encouraging a response from other agencies. For example, a 1905 home visit revealed,

> In a very dirty home, a boy suffering from an injured spine slept on a sofa with a hard wooden seat covered with a filthy rug; there were no bedclothes whatever – his covering at night consisting of clothes worn during the day.[25]

The FSIs deliberately narrowed their interest in childhood disability to the management of just a few conditions where their work promised to make a significant difference.[26] One of the most important, but hardest to evaluate because of problems calculating how many people were either at risk or assisted by official intervention, was an educational campaign to help parents nurse their children through common but potentially serious childhood illnesses. Measles was identified as a disease that could easily kill and leave survivors either blind or partially sighted. Practitioners viewed this as entirely preventable and worked tirelessly during epidemics to take the latest advice to all households in affected neighbourhoods. Cases of measles leading to disability quickly reduced to the point where they became sufficiently unusual to serve as examples of parental negligence rather than evidence of the dangers of the disease. The following case appeared in a report dated 25 March 1906.

> ... three of the children were suffering from measles. In each case their eyes were in a very tender condition. The sight of an elder girl, who had suffered from the same complaint some years previously, was seriously impaired, yet in spite of this no attempt was made to isolate the sufferers...[27]

The prevention of blindness was also the successful outcome of a very different programme led by the FSIs. Ophthalmia neonatorum was viewed as a significant cause of blindness, but its problematic association with venereal disease called for tact when dealing with parents. Attention turned to instructing local midwives to bring patients forward for treatment, usually at the eye and ear infirmary.[28] Statistics on cases identified and treated are not given consistently before 1912 but the Bradford FSIs appear to have shared the view of Dr Hope, Medical Officer of Health (MOH) for Liverpool, that following the full implementation of the 1902 Midwives Act the 'diminution of Ophthalmia Neonatorum' would be 'considerable'.[29]

Another condition that seemed amenable to prevention and treatment, which attracted the sustained attention of the Bradford staff, was rickets. The severity of cases in Bradford cannot be overestimated. It was not unusual for the FSIs to discover children aged two or three who were incapable of walking at all.[30] At first the practitioners were simply critical of the poor diet of the youngsters they met, but as the FSIs came to fully appreciate the poverty in the slum areas, and the difficulty of finding safe and nutritious supplies of milk even when funds were available, the tone of the campaign changed. The FSIs used their reports to encourage voluntary groups to provide free milk and other foodstuffs, and when the scale of the necessary expenditure became prohibitive demanded that the council take responsibility for the service. Although interwar health visitors pursued the medical treatment of severe rickets, the Edwardian FSIs simply argued that hungry children should be fed.[31]

The problem was that unless a safe supply of milk could be guaranteed and storage problems in the home remedied, then there was a significant danger of spreading disease.[32] Contemporary practitioners were perhaps more alert to the risk of fatal infantile diarrhoea from unclean milk than the threat of tuberculosis from unpasteurized milk. When the FSIs did discuss tuberculosis it was pulmonary tuberculosis, and sudden death rather than long-term disability, that most concerned them. FSI reports describing the horror of watching one family member after another quickly succumbing to fatal disease fed into shifting cultural images of tuberculosis which in turn facilitated new public health campaigns. To take just one example, the FSIs reported:

> Another instance of the way in which tuberculosis is spread, was found in a case where every ordinary precaution had been neglected; an adult son suffering from the disease was lying upstairs in bed – a healthy brother sleeping in the same room. And in the kitchen, where the other members of the family were congregated, lay the corpse of the other son, who had already fallen a victim to this dread scourge.[33]

Such cases encouraged the idea that children, as a group in need of protection by the local and national state, were quite different from adults, who might act as a source of physical and moral contagion. The Bradford FSIs were keen to remove all children from close proximity to infected adults. They initially addressed sleeping arrangements within the home but also encouraged the development of 'preventoriums'. It was however in the years after 1918 that these pioneering, but piecemeal, initiatives for prevention and treatment became part of a more comprehensive service for disabled children.

The Expansion of Municipal Health Services

The management of patients affected by, or simply at risk of developing tuberculosis, rickets, and blindness from untreated disease were major tasks for the municipal health services that evolved between 1918 and 1948. Health visitors had roles in many of the separate campaigns directed at these agendas but their work was different from the FSIs in Edwardian Bradford. The health visitors were more closely concerned with infant welfare work, and their independence was further limited by the direction their work received not just from Medical Officers of Health but a number of medical officers serving different local authority clinics and hospitals. The actual work of health visitors was largely determined by the scale and scope of local authority services, their internal organization and the relations they enjoyed with complementary voluntary sector provision. In places like Halifax, where municipal enterprise was celebrated, health visitors staffed important new public health services but found their work with disabled children was hampered by the controls exercised by the MOH and a lack of cooperation from and coordination with medical services provided by the education committee and the local voluntary hospital.[34]

Models of health visiting that emerged from infant welfare work rather than sanitary inspection tended to exclude many disabled children. In discussions about an influential Edwardian model of municipal health visiting introduced in Huddersfield, Hilary Marland makes it clear that the aim was to reduce preventable infant deaths and preserve the health of well babies rather than all newborns.[35] Infants, born with severe congenital deformities, or at risk of developmental problems because of difficult, delayed or premature birth were expected to die without becoming clients of infant welfare services.[36] This position did not change much before 1948, and the major advance evident in municipal records was in the classification rather than care of such infants.

Records compiled by the Halifax MOH, based on data supplied by midwives and others, and collated by the health visitors and the woman medical officer, became increasingly detailed. In 1908, when the first Halifax health visitor was employed, a general category of 'atrophy, disability and marasmus' was applied to a large proportion of infant deaths, but twenty years later records kept by the team of health visitors were more specific.[37] Cerebral haemorrhage, hydrocephalus, congenital tumours and congenital syphilis appeared in a list of twenty assigned causes of death, but with forty of the fifty-two deaths analysed

occurring within the first week (indeed often hours) of life the scope for municipal intervention was limited and seen as undesirable.

It is a strange omission that in an otherwise exhaustive survey of the fairly
comprehensive municipal services provided by Halifax Corporation following
the 1929 Local Government Act, officials from the Ministry of Health made no
mention of what happened to those infants whose condition at birth required
medical attention. Midwives provided medical aid certificates in cases where
doctors were summoned but their main task was assigning cause of death.[38] It
is only at the end of the 1930s that medical aid certificates in relation to surviv-
able and potentially treatable conditions such as club foot appear in the records,
but even then there was no formal scheme to prioritize the admission of such
patients to local hospitals or any mention of ongoing health visitor contact with
the child or his/her parents.

Health visitors in Halifax found themselves excluded from the long-term
care of other disabled children. A subcommittee of the education committee
made all the decisions about admissions to day and residential special schools
and claimed jurisdiction over all local 'educable' disabled children aged from
three to nineteen. The operation of this special committee was unhelpful. Firstly,
it prevented continuing care by the health visitors, who met disabled children
aged from a few weeks to five years at home and at the infant welfare centres,
which unusually in Halifax offered medical care. More significantly, the multi-
purpose education subcommittee conflated the care of disabled children with
the council's responsibilities for destitute and delinquent children. The committee had a long tradition, established before 1914 but continued to 1948,
of sending children away from Halifax for specialist institutional training and
rehabilitation.[39]

Yet, when community services were developed in Halifax there was no clear
role for health visitors either. Mental deficiency work in Halifax was undertaken
by male sanitary inspectors; male school attendance officers reported on the
nourishment of school children; the education committee employed a separate
staff of school nurses; tuberculosis aftercare was largely left to voluntary workers
and welfare of the blind work was contracted out to a voluntary organization.[40]
In other places, like Exeter, health visitors had interwar responsibilities in all these
fields, although the possible benefits of coordination were overshadowed by the
problem of lack of resources and chronic overwork.[41] Municipal services for sick
and disabled children were very weak and it was only after 1948 that the frag-
mented provision originally developed for tuberculosis work in Exeter became
a showpiece National Health Service for disabled children and their families.[42]

In Halifax the health visitors were, despite the problems outlined above, in a
better position to assist disabled children. Although less independent than the
Bradford FSIs they gradually discovered similar client groups for themselves and,

where the MOH agreed, developed new initiatives for them. Ophthalmia neonatorum (ON) was an important concern. The MOH regularly warned about
the danger of ON but vigilance by the health visitors and others had reduced the
number of cases of the disease since the first statistics were collected in 1914.[43] A
special campaign against ON was initiated in 1922 and after that date no surviving child was left permanently blinded.[44] The success with this work, together
with the woman medical officer's concern about syphilitic babies and unease
about the role of male clerks at the venereal disease clinic, prompted the Ministry of Health to recommend that health visitors staff the women only VD clinic
sessions to make patients feel more comfortable.[45]

In Halifax, as in Bradford, the health visitors did not treat ON, which was left
to midwives and hospital doctors though they had a role in preventative work,
following up cases and collecting statistics. The health visitors did, however, take
responsibility for the treatment of rickets. There had been a prolonged campaign to improve nutrition through the provision of subsidized milk and food to
pregnant women, nursing mothers, babies and toddlers. Yet the Halifax MOH
believed such endeavours, and advice to parents, were insufficient to tackle the special geographic and climatic problems of the town. Industrial smog was believed
to cut out the light necessary for health, and an artificial sunlight clinic was provided to counter the ill-effects of living in Halifax. Many children were treated
successfully, though it is noticeable that as the total number of rickety children
declined the condition of the children was discussed more in terms of parental
neglect than environmental perils. The health visitors had aimed to cure the severe
rickets existent and then trust their educative work to limit the number and severity of future cases. Instead they found parents came to rely on the artificial sunlight
clinic, bringing sibling after sibling forward for treatment. The clinic opened in
1928 and, in 1930, 131 sessions catered for 291 children who made a total of 4,399
attendances. The artificial sunlight clinic was run in conjunction with orthopaedic
clinics for preschoolers and schoolchildren, with all three assessing and treating
children affected by rickets and non-pulmonary tuberculosis.

Halifax Corporation had made arrangements to send children needing
surgical treatment to Bradford, and a very small number of orthopaedic cases
were treated in Oswestry at the council's expense in the 1930s. Yet the preferred
choice, for a Halifax child sick or disabled by a variety of conditions, was admission to the open air school. This was developed before 1914 by the education
committee but the site also included specialist facilities run by the public health
department for the long-term care of certain children including, against the
specific instructions of the Ministry of Health, a growing number of cases of
pulmonary tuberculosis.[46] The health visitors had a variable level of involvement
with these patients, with change noticeable over time and different approaches
evident in different cases. Linda Bryder took a snapshot view of the Halifax

open air school in 1912 through the lens of an article published by its medical officer.[47] She emphasized the surveillance function of the health visitors, but this is not the whole picture.

It is correct to note the frustration of practitioners who believed that the long-term health of children was unnecessarily impaired because of some omission or neglect. Taking the grim environmental conditions pertaining in the town as a starting point, the Halifax public health staff constantly made the case for enhanced municipal services to combat their ill-effects. Then, with an often unwarranted belief in the efficacy as well as appropriateness of the treatment they were able to offer, they put pressure on parents to bring children forward for lengthy and frequently painful treatments. It took time to appreciate the very real difficulties this presented for working-class families. There was limited discussion about the rights of patients to reject the expert advice available and make their own adjustment to long-term sickness and disability before 1948. Instead efforts to 'sell' the benefits of treatment were redoubled, with parental sacrifices balanced against the benefits accruing to children saved from long-term impairment. Some of these issues are captured in a lengthy discussion about orthopaedic services in the 1928 Halifax MOH Report.[48]

Conclusion

The work of health visitors with working-class families before 1948 has often been criticized for being both authoritarian and ineffective. Such analysis can be applied to their care of disabled children but it is also valid to follow Margot Jefferys and conclude that many children avoided long-term impairment because of the interventions of health visitors. Where the impact of their work was more ambiguous, it remains important to recognize that there were many constraints on the work of the health visitors besides the personal and professional limitations of individual practitioners. Health visitors identified many people living with disabilities. This could lead to the provision of useful advice and material aid, though wittingly or not the health visitors' own actions in terms of identifying and quantifying need served to increase the stigma and surveillance attached to disability issues. The health visitors also seemed unable to view disability as anything other than a personal and family tragedy or conceptually separate their work with disabled children from other child 'rescues'.

Health visitors came to believe that many of the disabling conditions they encountered before 1948 (which are not the same as today) could be avoided altogether. With the success of their work bound up in evidence of well babies there was a tendency to blame parents for any signs of impairment. Disabled children became evidence of health visitors' professional failure as well as opportunities to develop and practice professional skills. This helps explain why so many disabled children found their experiences of growing up blighted by intrusive official assessments, and lengthy, painful and often disappointing treatments. Many health visitors were alert to the social and economic causes and consequences of disability, but a social approach to the problems of daily living was only possible once the person's condition was stable.[49] This frequently required medical intervention and continuing healthcare. Heath visitors concentrated many of their earliest campaigns on improving access to treatment without acknowledging the limitations of the medical model.[50] This meant that the expansion of services went hand-in-hand with increased professional power and all the problems that created for service-users. The role of the interwar health visitor was conceived as identifying child 'cases' and bringing them forward for expert medical diagnosis and treatment rather than offer a distinctive service to families located in their own homes or community.

Acknowledgements

The research for this chapter was generously supported by a Wellcome Trust personal fellowship, grant 074999.

9 SPANISH HEALTH SERVICES AND POLIO EPIDEMICS IN THE TWENTIETH CENTURY: THE 'DISCOVERY' OF A NEW GROUP OF DISABLED PEOPLE, 1920–70

José Martínez-Pérez, María Isabel Porras, María José Báguena and Rosa Ballester

Introduction

On 19 April 2010, representatives of the Spanish federation of people affected by polio and its late effects (FEAPET) met with political leaders of the Spanish social security. The meeting provided an opportunity to discuss Article I of Royal Decree 1851/2009. This changed eligibility for early retirement in cases of disability in a way that disadvantaged some polio survivors. It was agreed to look into the possibility of retrospective reviews of cases where assessments had previously been inadequate (in the sense that no account was taken of the distal axonal regeneration of the motor neuron and neuronal loss due to the aging process of a damaged motor unit). To properly understand this issue, and the attention it has recently received in the Spanish media, we need to turn to historical analysis of polio in Spain and its social and cultural meaning in the context of both the history of childhood and disability studies. Health, disease and childcare provide paradigmatic case studies in modern history. The history of childhood in particular reveals the strategic character of health in the modern industrial world. Indeed, medical care of children is one of the elements defining the status of children in the contemporary period.[1]

A study of poliomyelitis (polio), as it affected Spanish society, allows us to analyse a set of interesting problems for a better appreciation of the social, cultural and medical perspectives on children and youth in the twentieth century. It enables us to delve into an understanding of how the connection was established between the biological aspects; the perception of disability among victims, family and health professionals; and the strategies implemented by the community to cope with the problem. This case study helps demonstrate the potential of

'new disability history' which, in the words of Longmore and Umansky, 'rec-
ognizes the corporeal dimension of human experience and its consequences for
daily functioning, while striving to understand the contingencies that shape,
reflect, express and result from that dimension'.[2]

Traditional histories of polio have taken three main forms: biographical
studies lauding 'great figures' such as Jonas Salk or Albert Sabin; empirical studies assessing the effectiveness of national strategies to combat the disease; and
papers written by polio sufferers about their experiences. All these approaches
agree that feelings of compassion were aroused by the vision of crippled children and this led to the mobilization of wide sectors of society. The worldwide
crusade against polio in the twentieth century was a fine example of this type
of 'humanitarian wave'. From the 1990s, publications by E. Sass, Daniel Wilson and Marc Shell introduced a new era in the historiography of the disease.[3]
Polio survivors themselves, they put the 'polio narratives', or memoirs of people
who suffered polio, at the centre of their studies. Their work gives an insider's
view of the polio experience while drawing on insights from disability and cultural studies. Shell certainly investigated the broad cultural implications of polio
epidemics and found the influence of polio in every area of twentieth-century
western cultural expression including literature, cinema and music.

The historical study of disability requires us to take into account not only
medical knowledge and practice, but also the patient and their family and community support network. Polio, as a life-changing illness affected every facet of
human experience, became inexorably part of the life experience of sufferers and
those close to them. There is, therefore, a particular knowledge of the disease
that can and should be 'interpreted' by doctors, but that cannot replace the first-
person narrative. After Sigmund Freud, psychology has defined the victim of
illness not only as a patient but also as a spectator and interpreter. Thus we put
ourselves in the place of the patient and learn, in the first person, the experience
of falling ill in the past and what it meant for the patients; experiences perhaps
coloured by the religious sense of transcendency, ideas on destiny and fate, and
on life and death. Memory recall, in this case the memory of trauma, may be
achieved by recourse to oral sources. This chapter draws on the narratives of
twenty-five Spanish polio survivors who acquired the disease between 1940 and
1970. Interviews cover the entire life experience from the first alarming diagnosis to the most recent development of post-polio syndrome (a condition in
which the symptoms of the disease may return two or three decades after they
originally appeared). Through the narratives of polio patients, and the doctors
and physiotherapists who treated them, we have been able both to analyse these
experiences and contrast them with written records created by local, national
and international organizations concerned with the polio epidemics in Spain.
These sources include legislative records, hospital and rehabilitation centre

archives, scientific papers, newspapers and World Health Organization (WHO) reports. Recourse to multiple sources, approached using anthropological methods, reminds us of the useful distinction between the different categories in the ethnography of experience, the delimitation of the term 'experience' and its application to human suffering.

The Emergence of Polio in Spanish Society

In order to comprehend the national framework in which measures to combat the impact of polio took place, we need to know the place that a child affected by polio occupied in that society. Spain, like other countries in the last decades of the nineteenth century and first decades of the twentieth century, had witnessed the rise of a movement devoted to securing the health and welfare of children.[4] This concern with the physical, mental and moral wellbeing of children encouraged the development of numerous institutions and professional groups. Compulsory schooling revealed the problem of children who were unable to fit in with educational norms. These children were labelled 'abnormal'; an unspecific category that embraced children with physical impairments (including sufferers of musculoskeletal system illnesses such as polio), the mentally handicapped, and children exhibiting problems of adaptation and bad behaviour.[5]

In Spain, polio played a key role in the growth of specialist health services and the new professional groups that staffed them. In parallel with these developments, child polio victims emerged as a special category of disabled people. Yet, disability services in Spain owed much to the wider political environment and the prevailing economic situation. Spain underwent a series of dramatic changes in this period. The constitutional monarchy was followed by military dictatorship (1923–30), a brief attempt by the crown to restore constitutional monarchy (1930), the Second Republic (1931–6), the Civil War (1936–9) and, finally, Franco's dictatorship (1939–75). This led to a series of legislative initiatives establishing (and/or changing) various provisions for healthcare including specialist institutions where child victims of polio were treated. Such developments tended to consolidate the 'medical model' of disability in Spain.[6] There were, however, two distinct periods. Polio emerged as a problem in the first decades of the twentieth century and by the 1920s and 1930s new institutions were being created for the disabled. The second period, associated with the main epidemics, lasted from the 1940s until the 1960s. This chapter considers how medical, social, political, economic and cultural factors served to define agendas, establish priorities and create new identities for patients and professionals.

Sporadic manifestations of poliomyelitis in Spain from the end of the nineteenth century spawned medical publications about the disease.[7] In 1913, Ramón Gómez Ferrer (Professor of Paediatrics in the Faculty of Medicine of

Valencia) conducted the first survey of polio in Spain.[8] This led him to conclude that, given the increasing frequency of poliomyelitis, the government should establish the obligatory notification of cases. Gómez Ferrer's demands should be understood as evidence of the growing medical attention given to poliomyelitis, and other 'avoidable' infectious diseases, in Spain in the second decade of the twentieth century. The country was then in the midst of serious social, political and economic upheavals linked to a parliamentary crisis. Doctors (especially hygienists) showed increasing awareness of the need to carry out a complete reform and modernization of the health system.[9] Unsurprisingly, under the pressure of the great epidemic of New York in 1916, the General Inspector of Health decided to undertake a 'health campaign against infantile paralysis in Spain', and asked the Royal Academy of Medicine to include poliomyelitis (an 'avoidable disease') among the notifiable diseases in Spain.[10]

There was, however, no evidence of modern epidemiological research until the 1920s. Such developments awaited the introduction of the health reforms prompted by debates which took place during the influenza pandemic of 1918–19. These pointed to Spain's backwardness in healthcare and the need to undertake important health reforms.[11] An epidemic of poliomyelitis in Madrid in 1929 then encouraged the establishment of the Central Epidemiological Service, a modern institution created during the dictatorship of Primo de Rivera. Research quickly, and importantly, showed that 91 per cent of cases occurred in children under five and 99.5 per cent in children under fifteen. The modernization of the health system, carried out during the Second Republic, led to the creation of the Health Statistics Service in 1930 and the implementation of the system of compulsory notification of diseases, including poliomyelitis. These measures facilitated new epidemiological studies, but offered no immediate solutions to the polio problem.[12]

During the first six decades of the twentieth century, polio epidemics challenged medical science and public health institutions, and represented one of the most important global health problems.[13] Furthermore, it was of considerable significance that widespread epidemics of polio first occurred in Scandinavia, northern USA and Australia, countries with high standards of living and hygiene.[14] In developed countries, during the 1940s, 1950s and early years of the 1960s, poliomyelitis underwent a gradual transition from an endemic state to a phase in which there were severe outbreaks of the paralytic type of the disease. The most frequent hypothesis used for understanding this phenomenon is that before the late nineteenth century, all infants were exposed to the common virus and, as a consequence, developed lifelong immunity against polio. However, sanitary improvements in some western countries provided a healthier environment which made the virus less common. This increased the proportion of unexposed individuals susceptible to polio later in life. Since improvements in hygiene were frequently initiated in areas of relative affluence, it was the higher social classes who proved most susceptible to the virus. For this reason, polio was considered a disease caused by civilization. Unlike other causes of physical disability in childhood such as rickets and tuberculosis, that were associated with the slums, polio was less class specific.[15] Internationally, methods used to control polio before the 1950s appeared to be unsuccessful. Measures such as quarantine, used to combat other infectious diseases, did not appear to work. However, the WHO, which played a vital role in the fight against polio, stressed the importance of a number of traditional policies such as the notification of cases, monitoring contacts (in families, nurseries, schools) and encouraging communities to protect themselves with frequent hand-washing, covering food from flies, delayed opening schools after the summer holidays, and careful maintenance of swimming-pools.

New Developments from the 1920s until the 1950s

The social and economic upheavals of the interwar period in Europe gave rise to significant unrest in Spain, with an upsurge in strikes and revolutionary movements following the success of the Bolsheviks in Russia. In this climate, the workplace became central to reform efforts. There had been long-standing criticism of the legislation covering industrial accidents, dating from 1900, and in 1922 a new *Occupational Accidents Act* came into force. This played a key role in determining how the problem of physical disability was addressed in Spain. It gave priority to the re-education and rehabilitation of accident victims with the stated aim of enabling people 'to earn a living'. This was the first step towards establishing the Institute for the Occupational Retraining of Disabled Victims of Work-Related Accidents (Instituto de Reeducación Profesional de Inválidos del Trabajo, or IRPIT), which became the main agency for dealing with disability.[16]

From the outset the work of the IRPIT was driven by two distinct considerations; to improve conditions for those affected by a disability, and to help solve the economic and labour-related problems that the high rates of occupational accidents brought to employers and the state. The creation of the IRPIT was also influenced by surgeons' growing interest in occupational medicine (including traumatology and orthopaedics), with the institution later fostering such specialisms.[17] A medical model then provided a framework for dealing with physical disabilities in Spain, as in other countries.[18] The IRPIT experienced difficulties following the 1929 economic crisis. Its failings were highlighted by legislative reform aimed at regulating occupational accidents. After a period of uncertainty, it was renamed the National Institute for the Retraining of Invalids (Instituto Nacional de Rehabilitación de Inválidos, or INRI). Two developments were crucial. The new INRI extended its remit beyond injured workers and concerned itself with the recovery of all disabled people. The institution was also dominated by doctors, as the medical side achieved ascendancy over the administrative and technical staff inherited from IRPIT. Indeed, the INRI was established as 'a charitable-teaching body of a predominantly medical nature', and in accordance with this policy a doctor was required to head its management and take responsibility for its administrative as well as scientific functions.[19] The first director of the INRI was Manuel Bastos-Ansart, a prominent specialist in traumatology and orthopaedics.

In a significant departure from the work of the IRPIT, the INRI's *Rules* established preferential admission for the youngest applicants.[20] This concern with child health extended the institution's work to cases of tuberculosis, congenital malformations, and particularly the sequels of polio. The INRI aimed to correct the functional and/or anatomical defects of such patients. This was an entirely medically determined view of 'normality'. In so far as social issues were considered at all, it was believed that the successful social integration of those affected by physical defects depended on the possibility of making such defects disappear. Therefore, orthopaedic and traumatology specialists played a key role in addressing the problem of physical disability in Spain. Medical experts were quick to grasp the importance of their position within disability services, and used their experience with 'correcting' the bodies of children with sequels of poliomyelitis to enhance their professional prestige and skills (especially operative orthopaedic techniques).

These reforms, like many others initiated during the Second Republic in Spain, were threatened by Franco's dictatorship. A period of international isolation following the Second World War also meant that Spain was excluded from the United Nations and its technical agencies until 1955. The period 1945–50 was one of great hardship, poverty and hunger. Spain was one of the poorest and most underdeveloped countries in Europe. Awareness of these problems created the conditions for limited reforms in 1951, which gathered momentum after 1957. The Compulsory Health Insurance, created in 1944, was developed. Within this framework, provision for maternal and child health drew on earlier attempts to use such services to increase the birth rate and inculcate the values of the Franco regime following the Civil War. Such measures had included the *Auxilio Social* (Social Aid), modelled on Hitler's Winter Aid.

There had been some measures to combat polio in the 1940s and 1950s, although the extreme politicization of healthcare in Spain proved problematic. In 1947, four centres were set up to fight the illness in Madrid, Barcelona, Seville and Santander. In 1951, an anti-polio service was founded under the auspices of the General Health Board, and this was followed in 1954 by the creation of the Society for the Fight against Infantile Paralysis within the framework of the same Board. Epidemiological work increased and revealed both a progressive increase of morbidity from poliomyelitis and the epidemic presence of the disease in Spain.[21] There were major outbreaks in 1950 and 1952, but the most important epidemic was in 1959, when 2,132 cases of paralytic poliomyelitis were officially reported.

The Faculty of Medicine in Valencia conducted some research into polio but the main centre of excellence for combating the disease was the National School of Health in Madrid.[22] This group of public health professionals performed their tasks along pre-Civil War Republican-style lines. Prominent within this institution were pre-war Spanish fellows of the Rockefeller Foundation.[23] They were keen to develop a model of comprehensive and preventive medical care similar to American health centres despite the Francoist authorities' mistrust of innovations from abroad (especially from the Second World War allies). In fact, the polio epidemics in Spain in the 1950s and 1960s overlapped with the gradual re-engagement with the international community. The WHO became an increasingly important player in efforts to understand and control the disease.[24] A number of WHO experts visited Spain in the 1950s and 1960s, although the national archives retain practically no trace of any of their reports owing to the political situation. Therefore a complete understanding of polio in Spain requires access to the WHO archives.[25]

Interestingly, active participation in the international fight against polio offered Spain an excellent opportunity for alignment with other European nations. While Spanish provision for many aspects of healthcare lagged behind other countries, its fight against polio was on an equal footing. Polio appeared to be an illness of developed countries, with Spanish officials noting that 'as in nearly all the countries with a high level of healthcare, polio cases tended to rise in Spain while infant mortality fell'.[26] These remarks were made to the European Poliomyelitis Symposium, held in Madrid in 1958. This event showcased the Francoist government's efforts, then unfamiliar to the international community, to combat the disease. They were presented as a great technical advance by the regime, although each element was imported from abroad and close examination reveals that the five front programme (research; vaccination campaigns spreading gradually over wider areas; propaganda systems designed to reach most of the population; treatment for those affected and a network of iron lungs in all provincial capitals and some towns; and rehabilitation services) mostly existed on paper. Yet the Francoist regime was turning its attention to a plan to create social peace (and compensate for the lack of democracy) by stimulating economic growth and providing new services to the people. In the 1960s there was spectacular economic growth in Spain and a rapid expansion of population. This was accompanied by the beginnings of a welfare state, albeit one that was run on authoritarian lines and lagged behind comparable provision in Western Europe. One of the significant political measures was the introduction of the new Social Security Law (December 1963) unifying the different systems of prevention and public protection (sickness, old age and widowhood benefits) and widening the mechanisms of social cover provided by the state.

The First Mass Campaign with Sabin's Oral Vaccine

We have already noted the politicization of healthcare in Spain and this had a major impact on the adoption of vaccines to combat the scourge of poliomyelitis in children. There were two rival vaccines, both produced in the USA. Jonas Salk's killed-virus vaccine (IPV) had been tried in the USA in 1951, while Albert Sabin's oral vaccine (OPV) was first trialled in the USSR in 1953.[27] Oral testimony from Spain suggests ideological objections to OPV were further encouraged by Sabin's Polish ancestry (he had US citizenship) and the fact that Poland fell within the Soviet sphere of influence.[28] Spain was technically ready to undertake a national campaign of polio vaccination in 1961,[29] but despite a press and public awareness campaign its implementation was delayed until 1963 when ideological objections to OPV appear to have been overcome.[30] In fact, two anti-polio vaccination campaigns coexisted in 1963. There was a pilot project using the oral Sabin vaccine. This was the work of the National School of Health, but lacked resources despite its promotion by the General Health Board of the Ministry of the Interior. The Salk vaccine belonged to the Ministry of Labour. It was used by the better-resourced Compulsory Health Insurance, but it tended to favour therapeutic activities (for example the acquisition of iron lungs) over preventive measures. Delays over the implementation of an effective immunization programme meant polio epidemics continued to claim child victims. Indeed the highest rates or morbidity and mortality were recorded in Spain from the mid-1950s until 1963. Witness testimony records the frustration and suffering associated with these 'lost years'.

It is useful to compare the anti-polio strategies adopted in Spain with those used in other developed countries. Medical journals are an excellent source for detailed reports about the 1960s.

> The national campaign was carried out in two phases, the first between 20th November and 20th December 1963 and the second in April 1964[...] A little before each of the phases a propaganda campaign was carried out in which all the proper means collaborated (press, radio, television, etc.) [...] The organization of the campaign was planned with great thoroughness in order to ensure it reached the most remote corners of the country, through the introduction of mobile units made up of a doctor and three nursing assistants who carried the vaccine from the provincial health departments to all urban, suburban and rural areas.[31]

In February 1963, Sabin himself attended a conference in Madrid and, in March, Pierre Lépine (head of the virology service of the Institute Pasteur of Paris) also visited Madrid. Press coverage of these events aimed to win public support for mass immunization with OPV, as in other countries. The main message was that the Sabin method was 'thoroughly scientific', and also that it represented a chance to 'eradicate polio'.[32]

In Spain the campaign against polio was presented as a sign of modernity and a vital part of the regime's development plans. Key to this was the idea that the nation was on an equal footing with countries abroad in the worldwide fight against polio. The NO-DO (an official documentary service that preceded feature films in cinemas during Franco's dictatorship) gave detailed reports of this global initiative, not only in western countries, but also in the Soviet Bloc.[33] This active propaganda, at the national level, was targeted at families with the aim of reducing fears about immunization. Ill-informed parents were understood to believe that sickly children should not be immunized and even fear that children could catch polio from the vaccine. The mass pro-immunization campaign was evaluated after a year and found to have been successful. Polio cases fell from an annual average of 1,733 in the years 1955–63, to just 155 in 1964. The last case of polio in Spain was reported in 1988 and the WHO certificate of eradication was published in 2002.

The Patient Perspective: Spanish Polio Experiences

The life stories of Spanish people who contracted polio in the 1940s, 1950s and 1960s share a number of common features with those of survivors and sufferers in other western countries despite the obvious political, economic and social differences. The following testimony is drawn from interviews with polio survivors in the Valencian Community, a Spanish region on the Mediterranean coast.[34] The 'lost years' mentioned above, when there was no vaccine then duplicity of vaccine and ongoing confusion about the administration of the scheme and the dosage required, caused particular anguish and condemnation of the authorities. Joaquín M. recalled:

> I had polio in 1962. I was 20 months old and my mother has always talked of the feeling of desperation because I received a shot of vaccine and nobody gave her information about what the problem had been. Therefore, my brother and sister were not vaccinated. I am sure that the health system in those years was really bad.

The narratives capture the nightmare of polio and its aftermaths. No two experiences with polio are alike but they all follow the same progression: diagnosis, acute symptoms, rehabilitation and life in the polio ward, going home, living with limitations and coping (in some cases) with post-polio syndrome. As the onset of the disease usually occurred at a very early age (usually under five years) most patients cannot remember on their own this first stage of the disease and, thus, it enters the family collective memory which is assumed and shapes the patients' interpretation:

> The disease appeared after I had suffered an infection of the nose and throat for two or three days in April 1960. I was one year old. I had already begun to walk but in the

morning of the third day, my mother noticed that my legs were weak and I couldn't stand up. I was taken to hospital which was more than five kilometres from my village. The Doctor was reluctant to give an accurate diagnosis but although he never pronounced the terrible word, the disease had already taken possession of me. (Carmen H.)

When I was 3 years old (1951), I began having symptoms, a high fever for 24 hours. When I recovered, neither my legs nor my right arm could move. Before the doctor made a diagnosis, my mother suspected that it could be polio because there had been several cases in the neighbourhood. The news was worse than a bomb of the war but we had to struggle to go forward. (José V.)

Amongst doctors a sense of discouragement at the lack of efficacy of treatment was common. 'Infantile paralysis is, without doubt, the most unfortunate illness that doctors know; its outset, symptomatically so imprecise, is usually an unpleasant surprise for the practitioner who often crosses his arms and limits himself to discussing the sad prognosis'.[35] What stands out in Spanish publications is the wide variety of treatments that were available, although most were criticized by observers for their lack of verified efficacy. One author claimed that 'nowadays, there is still confusion and a diversity of opinion on this question and when we review the bibliography we can see the multiplicity and polymorphism of the treatment of infantile paralysis'.[36]

Patients tend to have clear memories of hospitalization, surgery and orthopaedic treatments.[37] Since there was no effective remedy to fight the infection once the clinical illness had developed, treatment was still mainly palliative and directed towards the prevention and observation of complications. Electrotherapy was commonly employed and, in severe cases when respiratory muscles were affected, iron lungs. Other treatments came to include climatotherapy, balneology, masotherapy, kinesitherapy, and thermotherapy. Following recommendations from international experts, hydrocinesitherapy was another techniques adopted in Spain. Most of our patient narratives (Ana S., Pascual S., Leonor G., Manuel B., Angela G., Josefa C., María P. G., Isabel C., and José M.) recollect more than one of these physiotherapy treatments and describe the daily life within institutions such as the Sanatorio Maritimo de la Malvarrosa, at the Valencia Beach. Rest and warmth were believed to be essential. Testimony from a professional nurse, herself a polio survivor, underlines this point.

As part of my treatment I had complete rest during the febrile period and the days immediately afterwards, in which pain in the affected limbs was a very important symptom. Rest and immobility were necessary in order to ensure the normal curve of the spine and to prevent deformities but it was a real trauma for both child and family. But, at the time (1945), it was the only possibility. The presence of spasms in infantile paralysis patients was understood as the result of incorrect treatment, which, whether it was late, erroneous or insufficient, was the clear responsibility and fault of the doctor. (María P. G.)

There were, however, alternative views. Interestingly the ideas of Sister Elizabeth Kenny began to take root in Spain from 1940. Kenny had no formal training but was a popular as well as controversial physical therapist. She pressed for a new understanding of polio and a different treatment regime. Arguing that muscle spasticity (observed in the first stage) rather than paralysis was the main symptom of the disease, she considered that polio was more a disease of the muscles than the nerves. Kenny therefore attempted to fight the spasms through postural treatment and the early mobilization of affected limbs. This involved the application of homemade hot packs (strips of wool dipped in boiling water) to the damaged limbs, and 're-educating' the loosened muscles to enable them to function again.[38] Her methods were initially condemned by the medical profession but its 'common sense' approach and apparent efficacy came to find support amongst doctors, including those in Spain. Spanish authors give very detailed accounts of the practical ways to carry out the postural measures including the type of mattress (sprung mattresses were discouraged in order to avoid stretching the posterior horn cells of the spinal cord) and the positioning of pillows on both sides of the body or the placing of a rolled-up sheet to maintain the lumbar lordosis. Some institutions in Madrid (Institute for the Retraining of Invalids) hosted exhibitions of Kenny's work and she herself treated some of their patients. Dora O. (a doctor specialized in rehabilitation and also polio) provided witness testimony about Kenny's visit to Spain in 1947. This visit was called 'The Embassy of Hope' and patients from all over Spain came to Madrid in search of relief for their complaints.

Advocacy of home-made and unsophisticated remedies gradually changed the role of the expert. Direct intervention became less common, and the role of the expert became one of guidance to patients and their carers. Pascual S. remembered that 'my mother learnt quickly how to apply hot packs and my father made an original bicycle specially designed for me'. Many interviewees experienced episodes of hospitalization for acute care and corrective surgery, but an important part of their narratives discussed the lengthy process of rehabilitation as well as the orthopaedic devices used. Since the paralysis mainly affected the lower limbs an important goal (for patients, families and professional carers) was aiming to walk again, often with the assistance of braces or crutches. Carmelo F. reported:

> For more than two years I tried to follow all types of exercise and professional advice from the doctors and nurses but, finally, I failed ... At first, it was very hard but then I learned to live with my disability.

There are important similarities here with the situation in the USA, where Wilson found that both physicians and polio patients placed great emphasis on recovering the ability to walk and experienced feelings of failure when this did not occur.[39]

While most patients received little or no psychological assistance, their narratives make it clear that they experienced significant emotional as well as physical difficulties as a result of their illness and its treatment. Isolation, separation from family, loss of quality of life and problems overcoming/adjusting to disabilities are all strong memories. Even more significant were the problems of living with the long-term effects of polio including the seriousness of the sequels and the presence of post-polio syndrome, characterized by the exacerbation of existing or new health problems (most often muscle weakness, fatigue, and pain) after a period of stability subsequent to acute polio infection. The memories of interviewees are no doubt shaped by their current situation. Since 1980 a number of associations for polio survivors have emerged. This collective action has been encouraged by the ongoing problems experienced as a result of emerging post-polio syndrome but also permitted by a more favourable political climate. After Franco's death, the 1978 Spanish Constitution marked the transition to full democracy. Prior to 1964, laws had made it difficult to constitute societies and there was no social movement for people affected by polio.[40] Instead, work on behalf of polio victims had been conducted under a philanthropic model dominated by aristocratic ladies.

Images from this period tended to stereotype polio sufferers, like other groups of disabled people, as victims.[41] Polio patients were entitled (and expected) to receive social welfare, compassion and medical treatment but this was because they were not able to conform to 'normality'. Following this thinking, doctors contributed to the identification of polio patients as a group of people with *specific* needs that were best served by a medical model of care. Polio was seen as a matter of physical and intellectual dysfunction that needed permanent medical supervision. The psychological profile and the psychosomatic problems caused by the illness in very young patients also helped to define specialized care for the polio child within their family environment.[42] Over time 'polio children' acquired a distinct identity, and expert and official attention turned to the question of making them useful workers and citizens of the future.[43] Here great importance was attached to overcoming the inferiority complexes which the young patient might develop.

Conclusion

The polio epidemics of the mid-twentieth century in Spain seemed out of control and caused widespread fear. They also encouraged the development of a health service to combat the disease and its effects. Social, political and cultural factors all served to define agendas, establish priorities and contribute to the creation of new identities for sufferers and professionals. Between 1920 and 1950, the development of the 'medical model of disability' was clearly encouraged. By demonstrating an ability to correct the physical defects that helped differentiate 'invalids' from the 'normal', orthopaedic surgeons suggested that medical treatment was the key to making people 'useful' members of society. Impairment was viewed as a sign of a specific disabled identity, that was dependent and a recipient of medical treatment and social welfare. There was a focalization on the polio sufferer as a person subject to medical control. Only at the end of the study period did a new debate about the integration of people with polio begin to take centre stage. Identity was at the heart of the drive for integration. Images designed to arouse pity were discarded in favour of more dignified ones based on the person's possible contribution to society.

Witness testimonies from those affected by polio allow a comparison between the official record and personal experiences. Thus we can identify the shortage of healthcare resources for polio patients and the lack of policy coordination. Narratives also highlight the difficulties of integrating into school and work. Families, who received no financial compensation from the state, are shown to have carried the burden of care and rehabilitation. Alongside these issues, we should, however, stress that the majority of witnesses faced their lives with courage and are proud of their efforts. Children who contracted the disease between the 1940s and 1960s are now claiming their rights. In particular they have won the campaign for official recognition of post-polio syndrome. Activists have established the requirement to assess and meet needs based on the current degree of disability, with polio survivors treated as full and equal citizens rather than beneficiaries of charitable actions.

Acknowledgements

This research was supported by the Spanish Ministry of Science project '*Enfermedades Emergentes y Comunidades de Pacientes. La Poliomielitis en España y Portugal a lo Largo del Siglo XX*' (HAR2009-14068-C02-01-02); Fundación de Investigaciones Sanitarias de la Junta de Comunidades de Castilla-La Mancha (CTCS-2006_E/04) and *La Asistencia Antipoliomielítica en España en el Siglo XX (los Casos de Madrid, Valencia y Castilla-La Mancha): Aspectos Médicos, Sociales y Políticos* (PII1I09-0114-0843).

10 CURED BY KINDNESS? CHILD GUIDANCE SERVICES DURING THE SECOND WORLD WAR

Sue Wheatcroft

Introduction

The Second World War arguably marked an important watershed in approaches towards the care of sick and disabled children in Great Britain. While wartime conditions could, deliberately or otherwise, permit the neglect and mistreatment of some vulnerable groups children were the intended beneficiaries of carefully expanded statutory and voluntary sector health and welfare provision.[1] Such services tended to be framed more by a concern about the health of the nation and its future citizens than close attention to individual needs but they nevertheless were used by large numbers of children. Thus the Second World War, like earlier twentieth-century conflicts, encouraged investment in new facilities for diagnosing and treating children who either had, or were at risk of developing, a disabling condition.[2] To an extent such specialist services were subsumed into the wider development of the welfare state after 1945 and have perhaps received less attention from historians than either the school medical services that emerged after the Boer War, or the maternity and child welfare provision established after 1918. They merit a closer look however because although it is certainly true that many of the post-1945 services had their origins, or at least inspiration, in pre-1939 provision the war years encouraged an important change of emphasis as well as an expansion of the scale and scope of provision.

An examination of the child guidance movement provides a useful example of services that, despite being highly influential in some intellectual circles during the interwar period, were far from universal in 1939 but became an important part of post-war plans for many local authorities. Perhaps more than any other service at this time the child guidance movement (with a long-standing interest in how treatment should be tailored to the child's individual needs and behaviour pattern) was well-placed to both develop what came to be seen as a much-needed new focus on the emotional health of children and explore the connections between mental and physical health. By the late 1940s, largely through the work of leading child guidance experts, it was increasingly accepted that: the special needs of sick and/or disabled children made them more vulnerable to emotional disturbances and these problems were exacerbated by institutional stays associated with different treatment regimes; the condition termed 'maladjustment', recognized in 1944 as an official category of disability, could have significant and long-term disabling effect on individuals, families and communities; and certain 'minor' childhood conditions, that had perhaps been previously overlooked by medical services accessible to the mass of the population, such as stammering or bed-wetting, were both the cause and consequence of emotional trauma that unless resolved was likely to cause permanent damage to the mental and/or physical health of patients.

Such thinking obviously had its origins in the interwar work of the Child Guidance Clinics (CGCs). These however were few in number, and despite the best efforts of their promoters, tended at least in England to address the needs of a rather elite (or at least carefully chosen) clientele. Under wartime conditions far more children, with very different needs, fell within the orbit of these specialist services, especially where these were developed alongside other evacuation arrangements. Wartime conditions also appear to have facilitated child guidance experts' access to government and increased their influence over a number of policy areas. John Bowlby's work is credited with using evidence from the mass wartime evacuation of children to develop new theories of attachment and mother–child bonding.[3] He, and other theorists, then encouraged a new approach to care, with the pre-war practice of separating the sick and/or disabled child from his/her home and family for extended periods to facilitate medical treatment increasingly seen as undesirable. Following the 1959 Platt Report on children in hospital there was an almost overnight revolution in the organization of some children's wards and departments,[4] although it took far longer to recognize let alone meet the emotional needs of all institutionalized children.[5] This change of approach owed a significant debt to the wartime child guidance movement, although clearly other influences were also important.[6]

Influential studies by Deborah Thom and John Stewart have concentrated on the origins and early history of the child guidance movement.[7] These findings are briefly summarized to provide a context for the wartime developments that are the focus of this chapter. The Board of Education and the Ministry of Health had raised concerns, before the war, about the emotional difficulties children might face as a result of air attacks and enforced separation from parents if evacuated. This chapter explores how child guidance provision evolved under wartime conditions, with particular emphasis placed on the contested nature of care and how treatment was made possible both on an outpatient basis and in residential establishments. Close scrutiny is given to the wartime work of leading practitioners such as Dorothy Burlingham and Anna Freud, Susan Isaacs, Clare

Britton, and John Bowlby. The chapter shows how lessons were learned about the complexity of emotional disturbance as attention switched from children whose behaviour (perceived to be delinquent or aggressive) caused distress to others to a variety of individuals thought to be nervous or merely withdrawn. As a result the boundaries between the normal and abnormal were redrawn as new groups of children were brought forward for investigation. This process had an important impact on post-war health and education services.

The Child Guidance Movement before 1939

In her study of the interwar period, Thom examined the growing interest in the treatment of disturbed children and the conflicting theories and practices that influenced techniques within CGCs. With no unified system in place, clinics were influenced by one or more of the three main schools of thought: the British child-study tradition,[8] psychoanalysis from Vienna,[9] and American psychological medicine.[10] In 1927 the Child Guidance Council was established 'to encourage the provision of skilled treatment for children showing behavioural disturbances and early symptoms of nervous disorder'.[11] The Commonwealth Fund of America, which financed the work of the Council, was responsible for much pioneering work in London, and asserted a certain amount of influence over the clinics and staff training. Consequently, many clinics tended to be run along similar lines to those in America. In 1929 the Fund financed the Diploma in Mental Health course for social workers at the London School of Economics (LSE).

In contrast to the work carried out by the Commonwealth Fund of America, local education authorities (LEAs) were slow to develop CGCs. Depression-era public spending constraints meant LEAs were prevented from financing CGCs until 1935 when they qualified for grants from the Board of Education. By 1939 there were fifty-four CGCs, twenty-two of which were provided, wholly or in part, by LEAs. Many of these were concentrated in the London area leaving much of the country with little or no provision despite the careful dissemination of key child guidance principles to a variety of practitioners. A situation that led Thom to conclude that, with the possible exception of London, 'it would be ludicrous to suggest that a culture of child guidance clinics arose during the interwar period'.[12]

There had however been a gradual proliferation of services, in part explained by the wide definition of behaviours that could and should be treated within CGCs. While such behaviours did not obviously apply to any pre-existing notion of disability, perhaps explaining why both CGCs and the emotional problems of disabled children have tended to be overlooked by mainstream historical studies of disability issues, they were nonetheless relevant to the care of all sick and disabled children, and more significantly still helped shape an entirely new category of disability termed 'maladjustment'. As early as 1920, George Newman, the Chief Medical Officer, identified not so much childhood behaviours requiring the intervention of CGCs but a set of characteristic behaviours and health problems that made an individual child a candidate for investigation and treatment. These behaviours included: 'a tendency to quarrel; to make violent friendships; to engender bitter dislikes; to attend unduly to his bodily functions; to night terrors; to unreasonable fears, grief, abnormal introspection and self-examination; and to separation from family and friends'. Such behavioural traits were especially significant when accompanied by physical characteristics such as 'loss of sleep, constipation, diarrhoea, sickness, stammering, fainting, and resentment of change of diet and scene'.[13]

Such a catch-all definition was possibly particularly applicable to the treatment of children who fell into some previously recognized official category of physical or mental disability but it was work with the 'delinquent' child that became the interwar focus of many CGCs. Shortly before the outbreak of war the *Times Educational Supplement*, in an article entitled 'Cured by Kindness', reported:

> London child guidance clinics have treated and often cured children and have helped to educate public opinion in the theories that lie behind the treatment. The difficult child is not merely naughty but suffering from some unconscious disturbance causing asocial or neurotic behaviour.[14]

It would not be completely unfair to say that theorizing about the potential benefits of child guidance, and the search for a client population to treat, had progressed much further than practical arrangements to provide services. Yet, through work with 'delinquent' children there was already a tendency to view residential provision as a necessary adjunct to the work of the clinics although early experiments with this proved disappointing. In 1931, the Northamptonshire Home for Difficult Girls in Dallington became the first such establishment to be approved by the Board of Education and consequently, the first to accept girls sent and paid for by LEAs.[15] Soon after, the Red Hill School, one of the few private boarding schools dedicated to treating such children, opened in West Chistlehurst, Kent.[16] However, neither school was deemed successful by the education authorities and, on the whole, residential schools for emotionally disturbed children before 1939 were few and relatively unsuccessful. This was despite clear recognition by the health and education authorities of the need for such places, especially in a time of national crisis.

Warnings and Responses

In April 1939, the threat of war prompted the five national organizations for mental health, including the Child Guidance Council, to create the Mental Health Emergency Committee (MHEC).[17] The MHEC aimed to co-ordinate policy in regard to mental health problems, and to assist government departments, local authorities, community groups, and even individuals with cases of mental and nervous disturbance during wartime.[18] One of the first actions of its Secretary, Evelyn Fox, was to write to the Director of Education warning of the expected increase in nervous disturbance among children in the event of war.[19] The MHEC immediately compiled a register of salaried social workers trained and experienced in mental health, along with details of their geographical distribution, to facilitate their transfer to reception areas to assist psychiatrists, school medical officers, teachers and other social workers working with evacuated children. In particular, such staff would help with the boarding out of evacuated children who, in their first billet, displayed behavioural problems.[20] In May 1939, the MHEC also offered the services of educational psychologists.[21]

The mass evacuation of children revealed that re-billeting and/or treatment on an outpatient basis would not be sufficient to meet the needs of many of them. To an extent this problem had been anticipated by the government, with hostels established to take evacuees unsuitable for ordinary billeting, but the accommodation was overwhelmed by the numbers requiring it.[22] In September 1939, at a meeting at the Board of Education, John Bowlby was already expressing concern that the separation of children from their parents (and especially the mother) at an early age would lead to delinquency and went as far as to suggest it was preferable for children to stay with their parents even if this meant remaining in danger zones.[23] At this meeting, two types of 'difficult child' were identified. The first, and largest, group were children whose problems resulted from separation from home, aggravated by mal-billeting. The second group were those who had suffered problems before the war, some of whom were already attending a CGC. Both groups of children were believed to need residential care but the latter group would require more specialized treatment, in a small residential home or school with experienced staff.

Although the concept of residential accommodation for disturbed children was not entirely new, the type and scale of the hostel system developed for evacuees was unprecedented. Inevitably problems developed. These are captured in a February 1940 memorandum the Ministry of Health published detailing the results of a survey of the existing hostel scheme, highlighting areas which needed attention.[24] It marked a turning point in the treatment of hostel children. The worst difficulties apparently arose when hostels accepted children of all ages, both sexes and many different kinds of problems. Such hostels were believed to institutionalize the children making them harder to re-billet. Therefore the importance of only allowing short-term stays was re-emphasized, not least to facilitate the treatment of more children.

At this stage of the war the contribution of the CGCs was somewhat ambiguous as relocations, closures and other upheavals detracted from the genuine concern for wartime child mental health.[25] Yet, by August 1940, many clinics outside London had reopened, while five new CGCs (including one at a London hospital) and four temporary ones had been established.[26] It was the CGCs' role in relation to the 'delinquent' rather than the 'disabled' child that seemed to provide the necessary impetus for creating new clinics, and under the auspices of the Joint Committee of Working Women's Organizations there was a sustained campaign to increase provision.[27] By the end of 1942 there were sixty-two CGCs' in reception areas. Many were organized according to the American system, which employed three full-time professionals: a psychiatrist, a psychologist and a psychiatric social worker (PSW). Acting as liaison between the clinic and the child and its family, the PSWs were integral to the success of the clinics and this was acknowledged by their inclusion in the list of reserved occupations issued in March 1939.[28] Their role expanded even further during the war and most found themselves combining clinic work (sometimes running the CGC until a full-team of staff was established) with general assistance in billeting.

While CGCs were well-established in London, they were relatively unknown in the reception areas. This left the transferred PSWs struggling to cope with referrals from billeting officers, doctors, nurses, teachers, social workers and the courts.[29] Their heavy workload was further complicated by a certain ambiguity in attitudes towards the disturbed child at this time. Some children from urban areas attracted the label delinquent merely because they acted differently from their rural counterparts. In April 1940, David Wills addressed the Howard League for Penal Reform on the practical difficulties and cultural barriers faced by potentially delinquent evacuees. It was obviously harder to escape detection when stealing from the village shop than from a stall in the street so previously unknown thieves were likely to be exposed. It was also probable that foster parents would frown on conversation allowed at home. These different standards were likely to confuse children, and even cause emotional disturbances.[30]

One of the most frequent problems reported amongst 'disturbed' evacuees was enuresis. A study of 155 evacuated children referred to the Cambridge CGC found that over 60 per cent suffered from some kind of incontinence. Stealing/pilfering was the next most frequently recorded complaint (16 per cent), along with other 'bad' behavioural habits including quarrelling, disobedience and temper-tantrums. The more 'nervous' children tended to experience homesickness, sleep-disturbance, crying, anxiety, speech difficulties, babyishness, worrying and fearfulness.[31] The attention given to these problems reveals a broadening of the pre-war CGC agenda, since in the beginning 'the existence of problem children, as distinct from children with problems' was appreciated by few.[32] Consequently, it was children whose behaviour presented problems for others who were likely to be referred.[33] Gradually, the teaching and medical professions, and parents, came to recognize that the unnaturally quiet, withdrawn, child also required psychiatric help. The extent of this problem, however, was not realized until the evacuation.

Finding the children experiencing difficulties was, however, only part of the problem. There remained many barriers to successful treatment. The movement of children and personnel, coupled with severe staff shortages, interrupted the work of many clinics and prevented continuity of care. These problems were most acute in urban areas, but the operation of rural clinics suffered from transport difficulties and the inability as well as unwillingness of foster parents to travel long distance for regular attendances. Since it was believed that it was essential for staff to know the patients well as a first step to understanding the cause of their disturbances, residential treatment came to be encouraged.[34] This marked an important policy shift as Bowlby's early reports on the evacuation experience in Cambridge had endorsed a model of utilizing carefully selected, experienced foster carers in preference to large homes which seemed to encourage children to behave like 'wild little hooligans'.[35] Bowlby criticized the Government's evacuation scheme for failing to make any attempt to enlist the services of social workers who had the necessary skills, training and experience to successfully place children in foster care.[36] In the absence of such a scheme, residential care – however problematic – appeared the only realistic solution to finding accommodation for children with complex needs.

Lessons in Residential Care

In 1944, the Ministry of Health published the results of a July 1943 survey of hostel experience under the evacuation scheme.[37] It aimed to examine how the hostel system had evolved between September 1939 and July 1943 and to assess the ways in which children had been affected. It was hoped that the results would be of benefit to statutory and voluntary organizations, and looked to peacetime as well as wartime service needs. The forty-eight hostels surveyed, accommodated children aged five to sixteen with a variety of problems. Some hostels only admitted boys or girls while others were mixed-sex. Interestingly, the survey reported that in general hostels 'do not specialize in one type of problem, and it has been found unsatisfactory to have too many children who, say, pilfer or behave aggressively'.[38] Other lessons had been learnt. The most important was the requirement to get a detailed assessment of the child, as well as his/her background. This had been impossible in 1939, but by 1943 it was this assessment that determined which hostel a child should go to. Some children were believed to respond best in a small hostel where the matron could give individual attention and 'mothering', whereas others might be more suited to a larger hostel where there were many interests and activities, and perhaps a male warden acting as a father figure. The main purpose of the hostels was to help the child reach the stage where he/she could be billeted out with a family, and the hostel staff aimed to provide a sense of community where the child could develop a sense of self-respect and responsibility. The children were encouraged to mix with local children and to join organizations such as the Guides, Brownies, Scouts and Cubs.

A successful hostel depended on its staff but in these early and experimental times it was not clear what if any specialist qualifications were required. The hostels attracted staff with practical qualifications in catering or household management, and some employees were qualified nurses, teachers or social workers, but the most important skills were deemed to be sympathy and understanding. The Ministry of Health organized courses and conferences for hostels. These concentrated on the causes of children's difficulties, advice on occupational activities and forms of play, and other related subjects. It was also advised that, although the children suffered from some form of behavioural problem, the hostel should be run on a relaxed basis, giving the children as much freedom as possible. Some hostels were able to send their residents to local schools and thereby potentially aid community integration. Other hostels, for a variety of reasons, provided their own education programmes that were perhaps better-tailored to the needs of the children but were also somewhat isolating.

The hostels were treatment as well as residential centres, with all but eight (which could transfer patients to more specialist centres) offering differing degrees of psychiatric treatment and/or advice. By the time of the survey, most children were being sent to hostels from ordinary billets rather than straight from home. The decision to send an evacuee to a hostel depended on whether or not the foster-parents could cope with the child's 'abnormal' behaviour. For example, although enuresis was one of the most common symptoms of emotional disturbance it did not automatically result in being sent to a hostel. According to the Ministry of Health, 'a boy who wets the bed should not be moved for this reason alone as it gives no clue to the real nature of the problem, and moving him might make more problems for the hostel and for the child'.[39] In these cases, if the foster-parents were agreeable, the child could remain in the billet and attend a CGC. In reality, though, most children suffering from enuresis were, in fact, sent to one of the hostels for 'difficult' children.

In addition to the state-run hostels, the LEAs provided funds for children to attend hostels run by private or charitable organizations, or to attend one of the newly established special schools for difficult or maladjusted children. These schools and hostels had mixed results. The Chaigley Manor hostel, opened by the Friends Relief Society in 1941, for maladjusted children from Liverpool, was seen as a success.[40] On the other hand, the Little Beckett's Farm School for Maladjusted Children at Saffron Waldon, Essex, had its approval, only issued in June 1942, withdrawn by the Board of Education and the Home Office in March 1943.[41] This followed a negative report from a hospital doctor who had also been acting as the school's medical officer. He claimed:

I have only paid occasional visits but I feel I want a bath when I go there. I cannot think the boys will improve. One of the boys was in my hospital for a few weeks. Supposed to be a hopeless enuretic and also incontinent of faeces. When in hospital he never wetted the bed and was the brightest boy in the ward. As soon as he returned to the school all the abnormalities returned and he was as bad as ever.[42]

The schools, like the hostels, clearly had mixed results. Other new, and previously established, facilities also attempted to treat emotional disturbance during the war years. A good example is provided by Brambling House, an open-air school and children's centre (essentially a CGC) in Chesterfield, Derbyshire. Initiated by the Board of Education in 1936 and opened in July 1939, the school was the first to accommodate side-by-side the physically disabled, the delicate, and the emotionally disturbed. Mental health workers at Brambling House worked on the premise that emotional disturbance could result in physical defects such as asthma, enuresis and eczema which, in turn, could develop educational retardation. The school and CGC worked closely together in order to discover whether the child's disturbance was caused by something physical, intellectual, emotional or a combination of all three. Subsequently, the treatment could be carried out simultaneously along any or all of the three lines.[43] It is difficult to ascertain how successful Brambling House was. It was found that a classroom of twenty-five, which included children with a variety of problems, worked well so long as noisy and/or uncooperative pupils were limited to three. In the children's centre there was praise for the teamwork carried out by the psychiatrist, psychologist and play therapist.

Evaluating the Experiences of Child Evacuees

Brambling House practised play therapy on the lines devised by Dr Margaret Lowenfeld.[44] The Lowenfeld technique was just one of several methods employed in wartime CGCs and this section explores the contributions made by some of the better-known theorists and practitioners. The evacuation presented child-guidance workers with an unprecedented opportunity to study the behaviour of children, and their parents. In the interwar period, Stewart found a 'fixation on the home' among mental-health practitioners,[45] and it is important to evaluate if and how this changed. Many experts were seriously concerned about the impact of evacuation on children exhibiting emotional disturbances.

In 1945, when Katherine Wolf described the separation of around three-quarters of a million children from their parents at the beginning of the Second World War she termed it a 'cruel psychological experiment on a large scale'.[46] She was fearful that while the 'percentage of neurosis formation caused by evacuation is relatively low considering the deep trauma which we would have expected separation from parents to constitute' the long-term effects of the evacuation were unknown. Subsequent research, recently illuminated by powerful witness testimony, reveals that although many evacuees coped well with their experiences and suffered no psychological damage there are many harrowing accounts which testify to the long-term psychological damage and 'deep trauma' suffered by many children.[47] Such findings suggest Wolf, and the psychologists whose opinions she surveyed, were rightly concerned. Yet even these contemporary actors appreciated that it was difficult to evaluate the evidence contained within disparate wartime publications. For example, Susan Isaacs based her report on children in foster homes in the reception area of Cambridge, whereas Freud and Burlingham's material came largely from the observation of preschool age children in a nursery on the outskirts of London. There was however one notable point of agreement between the different researchers; a child's ability to deal with the evacuation experience seemed to depend on their prior relationship to their parents.

For Bowlby, the real problems lay with very young children who were unable to understand why they had been separated from their parents. He believed that this could lead to the child bearing a grudge against both the parents and society in general.[48] Yet despite the special problems faced by the very young there was even less provision for them than older children experiencing difficulties. Only two establishments explicitly offered residential nursery facilities for 'difficult' under-fives. The Caldecott Community[49] in Dorset was a long-term project while the Church of England's Waifs and Strays Society's new institution in Wiltshire resulted from a specific request for assistance from the Ministry of Health.[50] This extremely limited provision was in part due to officials making two key assumptions. The first was that 'normal' babies and toddlers would be evacuated with their mothers as part of the official government scheme and the second was that mothers would be especially keen to accompany young children with special needs since 'the mother tends to cling to them more than to a normal child'.[51]

Such thinking dictated that only a limited number of residential nurseries existed for unaccompanied young children, and these naturally became the focus of research work exploring the effects of wartime evacuation and separation. An important study by Anna Freud and Dorothy Burlingham drew on experiences of children aged one week to ten years at the Hampstead War Nursery between December 1940, when the facility opened, and February 1942.[52] In line with Bowlby's theory of early-age attachment, Freud and Burlingham found that the conditions of war held comparatively little meaning for young children. Changes in their safety, material comfort and food provision were insignificant compared with being parted from the person (usually the mother) with whom they shared the strongest emotional bond. These young children tended to express a desire to cling to memories of their previous lives by refusing new clothes and/or hanging on to torn and dirty clothes or other items from home. The older children reacted in different ways. Those who regarded their new homes as a drop in

social status may have interpreted it as punishment for their former ungrateful-
ness at home. Those whose standards of hygiene and other forms of behaviour
deteriorated in their new home were seen as expressing hostility against their
own parents. On the other hand, children who were urged to adapt themselves
to a higher level of cleanliness and behaviour often regarded these demands as
criticism directed against their parents.[53]

Freud and Burlingham saw the problems associated with the evacuation not
in terms of the 'fact' of separation but the 'form' in which it had taken place.
Rather than suffering the sudden loss of family and home, the new primary carers should have been introduced beforehand and the separation should have
been effected slowly so that the child could be 'weaned' from his/her old life
and there would be no empty period where the child could turn inwards.[54] At
the Hampstead nursery, the damage caused by sudden separation led to many
children developing secret fantasies of, say, being stolen.[55] The propensity to
fantasize was a theme found among many evacuees during the war and was not
limited to children of a particular age. According to Clare Britton (later Winnicott), a social worker who supervised five Oxfordshire hostels during the war,
some children, especially those from the worst backgrounds, tended to create
the ideal home in their mind, a fantasy that they would never be able to find. In
response to those who believed that all a child needed in order to be good is a
good home, Britton wrote:

> ... the answer is not so simple. They cannot enter into a good home and become part
> of it until the idea of a good home has first been created or revived in them.

She regarded an important function of the hostel as helping the child to recon-
struct the past, however good or bad it had been.[56]

Regardless of the successes and failures of individual residential establishments, much was learnt during the war about the emotional needs of children.
Awareness was raised of the objective reality of children's losses and traumas, and
how their behaviour reflected the sense of loss and rejection they experienced
when parents failed to write or to visit.[57] Children who were sent to hostels from
billets rather than straight from home suffered a second rejection and Britton
noted that those children often brought with them a deep sense of failure and
guilt. She found that some people believed that adjustment to hostel life would
be easier if the child's contact with the past was severed. Many parents rarely
communicated with their child and social workers were often their only link.
The children's expectant, almost desperate, reaction to any kind of contact with
their parents, however, made social workers realize the need to respect the child's
attachment to the parents, no matter how distant or problematic.[58]

The apparent stress among practitioners during the war on the role of the family in the emotional state of children was a continuation of what has been found

by scholars of the interwar period, not least by Stewart who found that '... child guidance, through the medium of the psychiatric social worker, became less concerned with the child per se. Rather the emphasis was on the child in its domestic setting and, thereby, on the parents'.[59] Reports of children suffering from poor hygiene and a lack of morals and discipline in their own homes, thereby leading to insecurity and unhappiness, was largely blamed for children being unable to adapt to their new surroundings. The idea that a child's home life determined how he/she would handle the evacuation was shared by Bowlby who wrote:

> The child who feels happy and safe in his own home is the child who settles best in a foster-home. It is the child who has felt unhappy and insecure at home who finds it most difficult to leave it.[60]

Officials at the Board of Education also blamed the children's home life for their problems: 'The largest single factor in the causation of delinquency and social maladjustment in children is no doubt the unsatisfactory home'.[61] However, it was acknowledged that the problem could not be adequately dealt with under the current economic and social system.

As with many aspects of children's welfare, real change for the emotionally disturbed came about through post-war social policy. Under the 1944 Education Act, 'maladjustment' became an official category of disability for the first time with the result that the education authorities could now approve special schools and boarding homes for maladjusted children.[62] Consequently, there was a relatively rapid growth in both education and child guidance provision 1945–55.[63] The other significant piece of legislation that benefited maladjusted children was the 1948 Children Act, which Harry Hendrick regards as 'a significant piece of child welfare legislation, which has been unjustly neglected in standard histories of the welfare state'.[64] The act created a care system for children who could not live in their own homes, advocating a preference for boarding out rather than institutional care. Such an approach drew heavily on the input of experts who had considered the impact of the wartime evacuation, including John Bowlby, Susan Issacs and Clare Britton.

Conclusion

Mental-health practitioners had anticipated that the mass wartime evacuations, and other war traumas, would have a significant negative impact on many children.[65] Wartime arrangements to promote child guidance were meant to alleviate these difficulties, but also created a lasting framework for post-war health and education policies. Between 1939 and 1945 the CGCs acted as both treatment centres and as a locus for diagnosing various types of disability. Children with special needs came to be viewed as especially vulnerable to maladjustment. Paradoxically while this finding encouraged efforts to keep families together and involve parents more closely in the care and treatment of their sick and/or disabled child, it also reinvigorated certain models of institutional care for other groups of disturbed and/or disabled children. In some respects the post-war period showed an increasing tendency for this distinction to become blurred. This worked to the detriment of some groups of disabled children, while other youngsters benefited from the new emphasis given to promoting and protecting the emotional health of children as a vital first step to securing the mental and physical health of the individual and thereby maximize the health of the nation. The war years and the special arrangements made for all children, tended to crystallize new identities for the 'disabled child' and helped protect such individuals from the neglect and mistreatment suffered by some vulnerable groups (including adults with mental health problems and the frail elderly) between 1939 and 1945.

Acknowledgements

This chapter is dedicated to Vicky Eller.

11 EDUCATION, TRAINING AND SOCIAL COMPETENCE: SPECIAL EDUCATION IN GLASGOW SINCE 1945

Angela Turner

Introduction

In the period from 1945 to the early 1970s, special education in Glasgow expanded as part of general developments in education born out of a post-war concern for the health of the nation. The Education (Scotland) Act of 1945 made it the duty of education authorities to ascertain which children might require 'special educational treatment' and to provide this.[1] However, the ascertainment of handicap was, until the Education (Mentally Handicapped) (Scotland) Act of 1974, also used to discover those with 'severe' learning disabilities who were excluded from educational provision because of their perceived lack of 'educability'. The publication of the Warnock Report in 1978 heralded a new era of special educational policy in the whole of the UK. Its publication and the passing of subsequent education acts sought to promote integration and inclusion. Furthermore they stressed the need for structuring understanding of handicap around the idea of a continuum of needs and the movement away from designated categories of impairment.

This history has received relatively little attention, although lately developments in special education have been scrutinized at the national level.[2] Recent studies of community care have also directed attention away from traditional institutional histories of disability.[3] Such research suggests renewed interest in exploring the experiences of disabled children outside of hospitals. French's study of education for visually impaired people also helps provide new perspectives on education for those outside the mainstream. Her focus on experiential accounts provides significant new evidence of the impact of segregated schooling on individuals and groups.[4] Studies by Hurt, Cole, Armstrong and others have explored different aspects of the history of special education in Britain.[5] However none of these authors extensively cover provision in Scotland.

A case study of Glasgow allows insight into the ways in which national policy developments shaped local authority provision, and how in turn these impacted on pupils' experiences. The chapter demonstrates how medical understandings of disability continued to dominate policy and how, particularly in the case of Glasgow, many pupils with learning difficulties continued to be segregated from the mainstream even in an era of supposed integration. It highlights the continuing centrality of intelligence testing as well as the increasing emphasis placed of vocational training and citizenship within special education. These factors are evaluated with an emphasis on the experiences of those receiving special schooling. This provides a story of change, and sometimes progress, but all too often one of continuing isolation and segregation for disabled children.

Medicalization and Intelligence Testing

Medical involvement and control, key characteristics of earlier policies for dealing with impairment and 'mental deficiency', continued to be evident in special educational policies after 1945. Medicalization involved 'defining behaviour as a medical problem... [therefore] mandating or licensing the medical profession to provide some type of treatment for it'.[6] This helped to create a wide and negotiable set of capacities and behaviours that could be portrayed by medical professionals as 'scientifically objective and benevolent'.[7] The process also extended the regulating power of medicine in society by removing individuals with particular learning difficulties, low IQs or nonconforming behaviours from the mainstream educational system.

Special education provided in special schools or occupation centres therefore operated within a medical framework demonstrated by the use of clinical language. One early report described special education as a process of 'diagnosis, proper grading and continuing treatment'.[8] Teachers who provided special education also adhered to a medical model. In 1963 for example, Mrs Choiko, a teacher working in a school for 'non-communicating' children stated that 'I think that the school, or the classroom if you like, should be an important part of the whole treatment set-up'.[9] Teacher training played an important role in developing this medicalized understanding of special education. One teacher recalled that during her time at Jordanhill College in the 1960s in Glasgow the training 'was very rigid ... the colleges of education don't teach you to go in and deal with specific things ... they give you lists of what impairments the children may have'.[10]

In addition children deemed to require special education were felt to be 'handicapped by ... disability'.[11] Educational handicap therefore was understood to be caused by diagnosed impairments which required treatment. The social characteristics of 'the patient' were secondary concerns.[12] Treatment could begin at an early age, particularly after the Mental Health (Scotland) Act of 1960 promoted the 'ascertainment', training and care of 'mental deficiency' in pre-school children.[13] Child welfare clinics and nurseries were set up throughout Glasgow to facilitate the early detection of defects in children. When 'mental handicap' was diagnosed young children were often placed in segregated special schools.

In 1963 the Scottish Society for Mentally Handicapped Children (SSMHC) highlighted the dangers of medical dominance within special education. The organization was concerned that in some local authority areas the educational future of a child was settled by the medical officer without the assistance of an educational psychologist and experienced teachers.[14] The medicalization of special education was further promoted by the development of child psychology and child guidance. The Education (Scotland) Act 1945 empowered local education authorities to establish child guidance services in Scotland to undertake assessment, treatment, prevention, advisory services and research. The Education (Scotland) Act of 1969 made it mandatory to provide such child guidance services.[15] Stewart demonstrates how medicalization was 'embedded in the very language of the child guidance' with children always referred to as 'patients'.[16] Psychological examinations were also used to provide 'appropriate diagnostic and remedial measures'.[17] Since they were central to efforts to both discover and understand 'abnormalities of behaviour' in 'retarded individuals' such examinations were also used to provide 'methods of correction for these handicaps'.[18]

Psychological and intelligence tests were used throughout the school system to identify pupils with mental handicaps.[19] Psychology was also given prominence in teacher training institutions and shaped the curriculum for special education. As a result, when child guidance clinics were established in Scotland they became part of the education service and not another branch of medicine.[20] Tests utilized by clinics and medical professionals were significant in providing legitimacy and scientifically measurable categories which related to medical diagnoses and educational categorization. A popular measure of educability remained the IQ test, which had a major impact on classification and school placement.

Policy-makers consistently stated that the difference in ability to learn came from the inherited or innate nature of dullness in children with low IQ levels. Commentators, such as Munn, stressed that 'a congenital idiot, whose idiocy results from defective inheritance ... will make relatively little of the opportunities for development offered by a human environment'.[21] Indeed he even went as far to say that in the case of an 'innately dull' child, 'his mental growth may be no more influenced by the educational opportunities than would be that of a chimpanzee'.[22] IQ tests were therefore often utilized to discover which children could benefit from usual instruction, with the rest excluded from mainstream schools.

Professional literature, however, made a distinction between those considered 'innately dull' and those who were merely 'backward'. Thomas Ferguson (who served on the Advisory Council for the Employment of the Disabled for the Ministry of Labour in 1945) argued that 'dull children are born with inferior mental equipment', whereas backward children were 'hindered in their normal development by external agencies'.[23] This led the Ministry of Education to state in 1946 that 'retardation due to limited ability ... is not likely to be ... overcome by even the best forms of special educational treatment'. Underpinning this assessment was the assumption that if children were so 'retarded' as to be unable to do work designed for children half their age it called into question 'whether [they are] educable at school at all'.[24] This led to the commissioning of large scale surveys to identify children requiring special instruction.[25] The unattractive aim was to relieve 'teachers of some *dead weight*' (my emphasis).[26]

Much of the discussion above reflected widespread concern about the mental and physical health of the nation in the post-war period. The *Glasgow Herald* used a 1952 article to welcome a new focus on mental hygiene at the Department of Health for Scotland. The article noted that average intelligence is 'now tending to fall about one point in each generation' and placed part of the blame on a 'differential birth rate' which was 'highest in the lowest social classes'. This prompted concern that in effect 'we are breeding from the least intelligent and least socially efficient stock and failing to breed from the best'.[27] Eugenic concerns may help explain the continuing adherence to educational selection and segregation.

Citizenship and Vocational Training

Special education in this period was strongly influenced by wider health and welfare policies. The trend towards medicalization outlined above encouraged a variety of professional groups, including teachers and other educationalists, to shift their focus from the immediate needs of special-school pupils to a longer-term vision of the roles vulnerable people could and should play in the society. An economic contribution was presented as vital to the future of individuals and the nation. For example, in 1944 the Association for the Directors of Education in Scotland (ADES) stated that the 'future is entirely dependent on what we make of our people' leading to a claim that '[it is] primarily the job of the educational service of the future to produce a people, a working population to fit into this state of affairs'. Children in special schools therefore needed 'training in order to render them competent to undertake employment'.[28] Elsewhere overt encouragement to 'oil the wheels of industry' led to a new focus on vocational training.[29] According to the *Glasgow Herald*, special education in 1950 aimed to 'help the child learn something of the ordinary education system' and 'equip them for after life'. This was because 'securing a useful job was of supreme importance to the handicapped'.[30]

Other actors were more concerned that 'the uneducated mentally retarded child' would become 'an unemployable or unstable casual worker' whereas an 'educated one [could become] ... a more dependable and useful citizen'.[31] This new special education required emphasis on 'practical things'.[32] Ferguson argued that educational authorities needed to realise the 'educational need and future potential' of these children.[33] However, the children were often trained for 'suitable' jobs at the low-paid menial end of the labour market. Indeed the ADES suggested that it was:

> In that part of industry where repetitive processes predominated that there was excellent opportunity for the employment of the less mentally equipped person who would be perfectly happy under conditions which would be quite soul destroying for the more gifted boy or girl.[34]

Steps were taken therefore, in special schools and occupational centres, to instil the required knowledge and skills. In a 1962 article about Dalton School (Glasgow) the head teacher (Mrs Broadly) and the principal guidance teacher (Mrs Rogerson) explained that the general aim of the school leaver's programme was to prepare pupils for adult life. They went on to explore how the curriculum could be tailored to promote self-discipline, social competence and employment skills. Lessons might address topics such as wages, factory language and safety at work. Even religious studies could be utilized if bible stories were used to illustrate the importance of 'honesty at work' and the need to avoid petty pilfering, boy–girl relationships and alcoholism.[35]

Another newly qualified teacher recalled her use of 'practical education' in special schools in Glasgow in the 1960s and 1970s. She explained that such programmes were heavily gendered.

> The girls were then taught laundry, sewing, cooking, how to care for a baby and we based a lot of the reading on practical things. One of the girl's baby had died, a former pupil, because she couldn't read the instructions on, whatever it was, a tin or something that she was using and we had a brilliant head of domestic science Mrs McMurtry who said we will never have that again. So we taught them to read from recipes from tins, from soap packets.[36]

Research by the Scottish Education Department (SED) suggested that such a gendered programme of activities was common to many special schools.[37] The importance of these vocational and practical lessons was reaffirmed in the 1980s by Gilbert MacKay (Lecturer in Special Educational Needs, Jordanhill College of Education) who summarized recent research addressing the education of 'children affected by extremely severe degrees of mental handicap and emotional disturbance'.[38] Emphasis also continued to be placed on preparing pupils for adult life, with employability given particular attention. A 1981 report from the Scottish Education Department highlighted the importance of pupils showing a readiness to learn, being reliable and 'having an awareness of what going to work involves' as a first step to playing 'an active part in the community'.[39]

However, anecdotal evidence collected from interviews pointed towards the unsuitability of some of this teaching. One headteacher noted that the material used in special schools was not always age appropriate, perhaps reflecting an old belief that such individuals were unsuitable for education. She recalled an inspector's visit to her school stating:

> The thing that he noticed, and until he said it I should have been aware of it and I always blame myself for this, but the reading material was geared to younger children ... We changed over right away. We did teen reading and magazines and things and that was a big improvement ...[40]

Flagship vocational programmes promoting work skills and active citizenship continued, however, to be tainted by official fears that untrained students would add to the ranks of the delinquent and the criminal.[41] In Glasgow it was also seen as important that 'as a future citizen the pupil should be trained to develop proper pride in his own city'.[42]

A resource pack, 'The Kerr Family', was produced in Glasgow in the 1970s as a method of delivering 'social education' in special needs schools.[43] It was designed to help teachers prepare pupils 'to take their place in society'. The social background of this fictitious working-class family was constructed in such as way as to localize wider social issues. In an industrial city like Glasgow urban poverty was a reality for many people, with the disabled probably disproportionately affected in a way that fuelled negative stereotypes. An article looked at the way 'The Kerr Family' was used in St Aidens School, noting that 'many of these children come from less well-off families, often with a tradition of unemployment and consequently housing conditions tend to be poor'.[44]

In 1978 HM Inspectors of Schools surveyed 1,000 pupils who had entered secondary schools in Glasgow with poor performances. It concluded 'the picture was depressing, one of impoverished homes ... the stamp of failure on them'.[45]

A former teacher described her time in Rottenrow, a special needs school in Glasgow, in the 1970s. She expressed serious concern that both the diagnoses of handicap and the types of educational provision children received were directly linked to their social status. She recalled:

> It was a special needs school, girls only when I arrived and these girls were classified as mildly mentally handicapped, but in fact most of them weren't ... Most of them came from the east end schemes and they just needed [to be] nurtured. There were three girls in my class who shouldn't have been there who all went on to get jobs in offices but you couldn't say anything to influence either the doctor or the psychologist who said they are better here, they are looked after.[46]

The decision to educate children in special schools did not therefore necessarily relate to their ability to learn or diagnosed handicaps. The Rottenrow teacher noted:

Rottenrow had been there since a way back before 1945, and the children were being signed in and there were bad things. If you came from a family with one child who was in a special school and classified as they used to say then it was likely that the brothers and sisters would be considered seriously for it even if they didn't exhibit the same problems.[47]

Girls attending the school were only too aware of the stigma attached to the institution. A teacher recalled meeting former pupils in town who begged her 'don't say to anyone … that I was in a special school'.[48] She knew the girls had their own strategies for concealing their special-school status, and tried to live normal lives outside school hours.[49] There appeared to be growing official concern about a situation where entry into special schools appeared to depend on both a diagnosis of mental handicap (based on IQ scores) and an assessment of the social status of the child's family. When a 1977 report revealed a third of children admitted to special schools in Glasgow had IQ scores of over 70 commentators said 'it is pertinent to enquire whether the social and other factors which led to such labelling offered a justifiable basis for classification of this kind'.[50]

Segregation and Regionality

Commitment to separate educational facilities for the mentally handicapped and the 'severely mentally handicapped' went further in Scotland, where education authorities provided instruction in occupational centres, than England. It appears that segregated classes had long been supported on the grounds that they benefitted the less able and others in the classroom.[51] To underline this point Ted Cole (until recently a Director of the Social, Emotional and Behavioural Difficulties Association)[52] highlights a 1951 Scottish Advisory Council report which first discussed the 'ruthless unconcern for the less able' within mainstream provision and then described the 'mortifying and hurtful experience for children to be perpetual failures' which encouraged 'a sense of crippling inability which magnifies the task of recovery'.[53] Cole attributes separate facilities to a contemporary belief that 'a child cannot be more cruelly segregated than to be placed in a room where his failures separate him from other children who are experiencing success'.[54] Continuing this theme he found special educational provision was informed by a 'genuine wish to help such children achieve the dignity of self-supporting, integrated adulthood'. He went on to argue that employment was 'the most potent touchstone of "normality" to the handicapped person'.[55]

The expansion of special education, from 15,173 children ascertained as moderately educationally subnormal in England and Wales in 1950 to 66,836 in 1976, was also noted by Armstrong. He concluded that 'the rationale for this expansion had largely been humanitarian' and linked segregated schooling to a progressive agenda that attempted to meet individual needs through specialist provision. For Armstrong, this was about inclusion not exclusion as 'the post-1945 political ideal was centrally concerned with extending both opportunities and citizenship for people who in the past had been marginalized and disadvantaged in their own society'.[56] Professionals argued a lack of facilities disadvantaged both the individual and the community, although old fears about uncorrected behaviour also lingered. In 1971, W. Brennan, President of the National Association for Remedial Education similarly noted that the 'backward child who does not enter the special school is left in the most hazardous situation'.[57]

The provision of special schools went even further in Glasgow than other parts of Scotland.[58] In 1962 there were 372 schools in Glasgow serving 178,852 children. The total included twenty-five schools for 'handicapped children', and in addition there were eleven occupational centres for the 'trainable mentally handicapped'.[59] The number of places available tended to increase. Glasgow's Medical Officer of Health (MOH) found 18 schools providing education for 2,509 'educable' mentally handicapped children in Glasgow in 1963, and in 1964 19 such schools served 2,620 pupils.[60] In 1970 no less than 21 day schools provided education for 3,231 'educable' mentally handicapped children with a further 429 'trainable' mentally handicapped children catered for in occupational centres.[61]

This expansion of segregated facilities appeared to conflict with central government policy. Cole noted that in 1965 the Labour Government's 'declared objective was to end selection and separatism in secondary education', while the Scottish Education Department was arguing that 'special education should be a last resort'.[62] Moves towards integration were boosted by the development of comprehensive education and the publication of the Warnock Report in 1978. This described a 'continuum of needs' in preference to using several different categories of handicap and called for all children to be educated within mainstream schools. However, only some of the recommendations were incorporated into subsequent legislation.[63] This disappointed many observers who also expressed dismay that the government made no additional funding available to help implement the 1981 Act, thereby limiting progress towards integration.[64]

At a national level the rhetoric of integration became important but local and regional provision depended on a number of contradictory factors. A 1981 SED report highlighted diversity in local authority policies on teacher training and funding. This meant that 'placement in a special school became dependant to some extent on where a pupil lived'.[65] Cole similarly noted that for a mentally handicapped pupil 'his educational future is at the mercy of completely fortuitous circumstances which may differ not only from area to area but also from school to school'.[66] Cole identified an apparently 'adventurous' and 'integrationist' policy in Glasgow, where the Regional Study Group in 1982 called for abolition of special classes for those with moderate learning disabilities. He saw a trend in Glasgow 'away from separate remedial provision and towards mixed ability organization', although other evidence points to a continuing reliance on and investment in impairment-specific schools.[67] There was significant distance between national educational objectives and the reality of the special educational sector in Glasgow, which continued to expand in the 1970s and 1980s.[68] This was both a cause and consequence of a culture of segregated education for mentally handicapped children. Indeed the SED estimated that, in 1981, 75 per cent of 'mildly mentally handicapped' pupils of secondary school age attended special schools.[69] A diagnosis or categorization of 'mental handicap', later termed 'learning disability', therefore often resulted in a segregated educational experience.

This growing provision of special education for the mentally handicapped was, however, slow to take account of those designated as 'ineducable' and 'untrainable'. The 1962 MOH report stressed that, under Section 65 of the Education (Scotland) Act of 1962, the local health authority (LHA) had to be notified of children of school age who were considered as unsuitable for education or training in a special school. Under Section 12 of the Mental Health Act the LHA had the duty to provide training and occupation for these children but in Glasgow such provision remained at 'the planning stages' and was identified as a major unmet need in the city.[70] An excessive emphasis on categorization hindered integration, even within the special education sector although it took time for official reports to recognize and respond to this problem. In 1971, *A Better Life* argued that since 'very few children fall easily into tidy compartments' local authorities should begin to recognize the 'varied nature of individual educational needs'.[71] However, the Association of Directors of Social Work (ADSW) had some reservations about this new type of approach which abandoned old categorizations in favour of new individualized approaches.[72] In 1979 they stated:

> The Executive Committee view that one of the difficulties in the Warnock Report is that too many children would be treated as handicapped, and that there required to be a narrowing of the criteria for ascertainment as handicapped, with the resultant continued process to integrate handicapped children into normal educational life and schools.[73]

There is no doubt that new ideas such as integration and the 'continuum of needs' could result in practical difficulties, especially in cities like Glasgow which had developed impairment-specific facilities. Arrangements in Glasgow were discussed in a 1975 paper by the Scottish Council for Educational Technology. This concluded that the city's special education provision was a rational response to the needs of its population. The report went on to argue that 'the reasons for such choices are not always educational ones; it is obviously easier to operate a separate school system in districts where there is a greater concentration of population'.[74] An earlier report from the Secretary of State for Education in Scotland in 1967 had similarly noted the distinctive scale and nature of provision in Glasgow:

> Glasgow and Edinburgh have been the only authorities able to establish consider-
> able numbers of medium sized schools, with limited catchment areas for mentally
> and physically handicapped pupils ... in most industrialized lowland counties the
> tendency has been to build considerably larger schools which cater for a wide variety
> of handicaps and bring in pupils from a wider area.[75]

The growth of impairment-specific facilities in Glasgow was not just driven by
officials. One teacher suggested that parental pressure and wider assumptions
about 'mental handicap' were also important. She recalled that:

> One of the PH [physically handicapped] boys in a Catholic school [in Glasgow] ...
> his parents sued the Corporation, as it was then, because they were bringing Charlie
> up, they were educating him with pupils who were mentally handicapped and Glas-
> gow was forced to set up a school for children with physical and visual impairments.[76]

Glasgow struggled to resolve the tension between the new integration agenda
and its own legacy of segregated facilities. Extensive, and expensive, specialist
provision encouraged a tendency to send children with even 'moderate' learning disabilities to these institutions rather than trying a mainstream setting. A
report, produced by Jordanhill College in 1989, found that this could harm
pupils with moderate learning difficulties. This was because the transition from
special school to work became harder over time and there was increasing risk
that people would be caught in the system as 'open employment prospects are
negligible'. The report noted:

> Young people staying on at school appears to be a Strathclyde phenomenon, and is
> particularly true of Glasgow. It would seem that where there are large special schools
> with extra accommodation currently available, there is a greater tendency to retain
> young people beyond the school leaving age.[77]

Over time the goals of special education became somewhat confused and
perhaps less ambitious. Protecting the mainstream rather than nurturing the
special needs child was a key theme identified by Tomlinson who argued special
education was used 'a safety valve for the mainstream, allowing it to function
unimpeded by these troublesome deviants'.[78] Elsewhere, remedial education was
increasingly viewed as a 'safety net', although approximately 7 per cent of primary school and 8 per cent of secondary pupils (in years 1–4) received special
education in Scotland in 1976. This amounted to 42,687 primary school and
25,074 secondary school children.[79] New children continued to enter the system with the SSMH (previously SSMHC) reporting 1,742 admissions (1,273
classed as mentally handicapped) to special education in Scotland in 1973–4.[80]

The work of the urban special schools continued in Glasgow but tensions
between official objectives and children's experiences were apparent. A 1978
article describing such a school stressed that many of the pupils could not cope

in a mainstream setting. [81] This meant the school had a perceived protective as well as nurturing function. The article suggested that in such an environment the teachers can 'detach themselves to the extent that they can treat the children as nearly normal' and the pupils can 'widen their horizons and add to their skills for personal enjoyment as well as survival in the outside world'. This fulfilled the school's objective to 'produce young men and women who are socially acceptable and competent'. Yet, the very operation of the school led to feelings of isolation and exclusion. The article noted that the 300 children 'arrived on a special bus', and one pupil told the author that 'they think we are all daft in here'. Testimony from other formal pupils of special schools in Glasgow in the 1960s and 1970s also recalled feelings of difference. One interviewee said, 'I went to Middlefield you know the special school ... she [her sister] went to an ordinary school, I didn't, I went to special schools ... I didn't study anything'.[82] Another respondent similarly remembered how in the 1960s his brothers had gone to the local primary school while he 'went to the special school' recalling how 'they had reading and writing where we had things like plastersine'.[83]

Oral testimony therefore reveals a number of different perspectives about the impact of the segregated educational experience. One teacher recalled how some of the pupils responded to this special treatment noting that 'the children disliked being either pitied, patronized or treated in too soft a way'.[84] Another former pupil stressed in her testimony that she rejected the label of 'handicapped' given to her as a child. She stated 'I dunno I just don't like the word handicapped, I'm not blind, right, I can walk and there is nothing wrong with me, there is nothing wrong with me at all that's how I'm not handicapped'.[85] She also remembered how her father organized for her to go to college as he felt she had come out of school with little basic education when she recalled how 'a long time ago I went to college as well cos my father he flared up cos I didn't know anything about money'.[86] One respondent recalled how he was keenly aware that it was a 'special school' stating 'my brothers and sisters all went to the ordinary school, I have to have a special bus and it didn't feel nice'.[87] Similarly another argued that 'because I have been to a special school sometimes people out there give people a sort of label. I feel angry about that'.[88]

Policymakers seemed disengaged from such concerns but there was a genuine debate in official circles about the future of special education and the number of pupils who required segregated provision in the 1980s. On the one hand there was support for breaking down rigid classification boundaries. The White Paper *Special Educational Needs* suggested the implementation of a record of needs (as opposed to categorization of pupils with special needs), which was estimated as 1.3 per cent of pupils in Scotland.[89] This and many other ideas were incorporated in the 1981 Education Act which set out to undermine 'previous terms associated with handicap ... breaking down boundaries between the normal, the remedial, the maladjusted and the handicapped, making them all in one sense 'special'.[90] On the other hand the legacy of segregated provision cast a long shadow over attempts to objectively evaluate the past, present and future of special education in Scotland.

In 1984 a Glasgow Council for Remedial Education working report recounted some of the changes that 'remedial' education had gone through since the 1960s. It presented the evolution in the 'treatment' of pupils with learning difficulties as a story of progress. The report highlighted the transition from separate schools founded on categorizations of pupils by IQ tests, to the contemporary situation of extraction classes in mainstream schools.[91] However, complete inclusion of children with learning disabilities was rarely presented as an objective in educational sources. Indeed the Scottish Council for Educational Technology argued in 1975 that 'no-one would ever claim that complete integration could ever be a possibility'.[92] The continuing segregated special educational system meant that this view was shared by many educationalists.

Such thinking went against the conclusions of the Warnock Report. This had suggested that, since about 20 per cent of all children had some kind of special educational need, 'the notion of the handicapped and the normal as two distinct parties has, I believe, been effectively overcome'.[93] Yet although teachers had anticipated the closure of their special schools very few pupils transferred to mainstream provision. One former Glasgow headmistress recalled that:

> What happened really was that when the children were moving from primary to secondary those that could started to go into the secondary schools, the psychologist would place them. You wanted the children who could cope, you didn't want the children to go who could not cope.[94]

This has led commentators such as Cole to argue that 'in national terms, although integration was much talked about ... DES statistics did not indicate substantial movement towards it beyond what already existed in 1965'.[95] Cole noted that many special schools continued to flourish, while parent activists saved others from closure and some new segregated facilities opened. In 1978, Milne identified that twenty-four new purpose-built special schools had been completed in the last five years, with most of the provision designated for 'mentally handicapped' pupils.[96] Glasgow certainly continued with its segregated provision, with a 1980 HMI report concluding that 'few severely and profoundly handicapped pupils are educated in units in ordinary schools'.[97] It is therefore unsurprising that a 1989 survey found there were still at least ten segregated secondary special schools in the city and similar number of primary schools for children with special needs.[98]

Integration remained a distant goal, though a much discussed ideal. An article in the SDSA magazine in 1990 noted that 'arguments in favour of integrated provision for all children derive their moral force from the belief that any selective model of education will inevitably undermine the social status of some groups in the community'.[99] Similarly, the 1992 report *Every Child is Special* laid out the key principles of the educational authority in Strathclyde. These included positive discrimination, the non-segregation of children with special needs and recognition of individual learning needs.[100] However, it is significant that the report continued to see a place for special schooling and did little to suggest that the trend for segregated education facilities in Glasgow was in decline.

Conclusion

It is clear that there was often a gap between the aims of educational policy at a national level and the practice of special education in the local context. Intelligence testing and medical classifications continued to play a significant role in special-school placements. At the beginning, if not at the end, of the study period there was significant exclusion. Yet, Cole, Armstrong and others have shown that the expansion of the special educational sector owed much to concern about the welfare of mentally handicapped children. This can be seen in Glasgow, where specialist schools were promoted as the best way to offer suitable 'treatment' and 'training' for these pupils. However, this chapter has demonstrated that a problematic segregation resulted. By the late 1970s 'the majority of intellectually impaired special school leavers were transferring to local authority adult training centres' rather than moving into employment or further education.[101] In Glasgow the creation of a large special educational sector did much to explain its subsequent failure to develop a more inclusive approach. Neither the advent of the comprehensive school system in the 1970s nor the publication of the Warnock Report had a major impact on the number of pupils educated in special schools.

Oral testimony has demonstrated the ways in which placement in special schools could affect pupils and impact on their experiences inside and outside of school. Numerous reports highlight the way special schools concentrated on teaching 'practical' things and neglected to focus on age-appropriate materials or traditional reading and writing skills. This approach hindered rather than helped former pupils to find jobs and achieve the independence and 'integration' that both officials and service-users associated with paid employment. Developments in special education in Glasgow in this period therefore again demonstrate the gap between policy initiatives and the practical realities of segregation felt by many mentally handicapped people. Thus, despite the introduction of new ideas such as inclusion and the 'continuum of needs' into educational legislation there continued to be a reliance on segregated provision and outdated categories of impairment.

12 HYPERACTIVITY AND AMERICAN HISTORY, 1957–PRESENT: CHALLENGES TO AND OPPORTUNITIES FOR UNDERSTANDING

Matthew Smith

Introduction

In 2007 the Centers for Disease Control and Prevention (CDC) reported that 4.5 million American children, roughly 7 per cent of the school-age population, had been diagnosed with hyperactivity, or what is currently referred to as Attention-Deficit/Hyperactivity Disorder (ADHD).[1] Characterized by impulsivity, inattention, over-activity, defiance and aggression, hyperactivity has been the most commonly diagnosed childhood psychiatric condition in the United States since the 1970s and stimulant drugs, such as Ritalin, have been used to treat the disorder since the 1960s. Hyperactivity has also been among the most controversial and most discussed disabilities to emerge after the Second World War. This is partly because of the powerful stimulants used to treat hyperactive children, and partly because of what the disorder implies about childhood, the education system and the way in which we perceive mental health. While many physicians have argued that hyperactivity is still underreported, critics have claimed that its existence is merely a myth constructed to curtail the natural development of children so that they conform to society's demands.[2] Similarly, while some parents have resisted the diagnosis, believing that it labels their child unfairly, others see hyperactivity as a powerful heuristic, explaining a great deal about why their child has struggled to achieve educationally, socially and emotionally. Due in part to the notion that hyperactivity is genetic, many parents of hyperactive children have also been diagnosed themselves, adding to the increasing numbers of adults with the disorder.[3] Such controversy has even extended to the question of whether or not hyperactivity was a disability. Although it was not listed specifically in the United States as a disability in the 1975 Education for All Handicapped Children Act, or the renamed the Individuals with Disabilities Education Act (IDEA) of 1990, a 1991 Department of Education memorandum directed schools to include it as a disability.[4] As such, American children

with hyperactivity can receive special educational services set out in Individualized Education Plans (IEPs).

Putting the emergence of hyperactivity as a medical condition in its historical context helps us to understand why the disorder has been so controversial.
Although a number of sociologists have investigated the disorder, often providing
insightful analyses of how parents have conceptualized hyperactivity, most features
of its history have been left unexamined.[5] When the history of hyperactivity has
been explored or represented as such in medical literature, there has been an unfortunate tendency to focus on what could be called the prehistory of hyperactivity:
the years prior to when the disorder became a medical and cultural phenomenon
in the late 1950s.[6] Included in this prehistory is the story of Fidgety Phil, a character from a mid-nineteenth century German nursery rhyme who might be seen
as a precursor to Bart Simpson.[7] While the prehistory of hyperactivity provides
some insight into the scientific, pharmaceutical and intellectual developments that
paved the way for hyperactivity – for example, the slowly hardening thesis dating
back to the late nineteenth century that children's behavioural problems could be
caused by neurological injury or dysfunction – it fails to shed much light on why
the disorder has become so ubiquitous and so controversial in the last fifty years.[8]
In contrast, such accounts suggest that hyperactive behaviour has always been seen
to be pathological, thus reinforcing the perception that the disorder is universal,
fixed and timeless, and therefore an ontological entity that is beyond questioning or contestation. As such, these approaches do little to help historians, parents,
physicians or politicians understand the numerous factors that contribute to the
emergence and proliferation of psychiatric conditions such as hyperactivity.

It is useful to provide a brief overview of the history of hyperactivity, from
the year in which it was first identified (1957) to the present day, focussing on
three broad themes that underlie its history. These are: concerns about the education of American children; profound changes within the field of psychiatry;
and the experiences of parents of hyperactive children. By doing so, I hope to
demonstrate how historical explorations of contested disabilities such as hyperactivity can not only provide helpful insights into such conditions and how to
deal with them, but also present ways in which to approach American history.
Within the history of hyperactivity, key aspects of the histories of childhood,
education, parenting, mental health science, patient activism, the pharmaceutical industry, environmental medicine and occupational changes in the United
States are also revealed. The story of how hyperactivity has been understood by
physicians, addressed by educators and, most importantly, experienced by those
diagnosed with it and their families helps reveal how American thinking about
intellectual and mental disability has changed markedly during the past half
century.[9] In turn, any exploration of hyperactivity demands consideration of the
broader features of American history if it is to have any meaning or substance.

The Problem of our Schools

In 1957, Maurice Laufer, Eric Denhoff and Gerald Solomons, a team of Rhode Island psychiatrists, coined the term 'hyperkinetic impulse disorder' to describe children who exhibited 'hyperactivity; short attention span and poor powers of concentration; irritability; impulsiveness; variability [of behaviour and school performance]; and poor school work'.[10] The team stated that 'hyperactivity is the most striking item' in this list of problem behaviours, thus explaining their name for the disorder.[11] According to paediatrician Howard Fischer, there are few differences between Laufer and his colleagues's description of hyperkinetic impulse disorder in 1957 and what is believed about hyperactivity today.[12]

Unlike those who had previously associated childhood behavioural problems with brain trauma (following head injuries or disease, such as encephalitis), and even those who recognized that such problems could occur in the absence of neurological damage, the behaviours the Rhode Island psychiatrists working at the Emma Pendleton Bradley Home for mentally ill children described were a common occurrence.[13] Specifically, Laufer and his colleagues saw such children as presenting behaviours found to various degrees in most children:

> One striking point is that the characteristics which have been described are to some extent normally found in the course of development of children. That is, as compared with adults, children are hyperkinetic, have short attention span and poor powers of concentration, and are impulsive.[14]

As such, hyperkinetic impulse disorder could be applied to a significant proportion of the child population and, soon, it was.

It takes more than an easily applied label, however, for a new childhood behavioural disorder to become accepted and readily diagnosed. As historian Joan Jacobs Brumberg has demonstrated with anorexia nervosa, and anthropologist Allan Young has shown with post-traumatic stress disorder (PTSD), emergent psychiatric disorders often reflect broader social concerns and changes.[15] In the case of hyperactivity, concerns about American scholastic achievement were paramount in prompting interest in hyperactive behaviour. Such concerns were crystallized in 1957 when the Soviet Union launched two Sputnik satellites, thus signalling to Americans that they were no longer ahead in the 'Brain Race' that was central to Cold War anxieties and politics.[16]

The American education system was under considerable stress prior to Sputnik. The baby boom generation, the 75 million children born between 1946 and 1964, overloaded a school system already suffering from infrastructure deficits incurred during the Great Depression and the Second World War. Schools also struggled to cope with teacher shortages, caused in part by the resignation of many female teachers who left the profession to marry and become mothers.[17]

As contemporary educator Paul Gardner described, 'in these days of crowded classrooms, expanding enrolments, and the rapidly changing world ... teachers across the land are hard pressed to deal adequately with their responsibilities for the welfare of their students'.[18] Laufer, along with others, asserted that over-crowding contributed to academic difficulties:

> in the crowded classrooms of today, the teacher often becomes hostile to the child who, despite seemingly good intelligence, can not sit still, can not keep his mind on his work, hardly ever finishes the assigned task and yet unpredictably may turn in a perfect paper. ... The child frequently fails to gain a proper foundation for the fundamentals of schooling so that each successive year he falls progressively behind.[19]

The child of 'good intelligence' who struggled to reach his/her academic potential was also singled out for attention by critics of the education system, such as James Bryant Conant. He advised guidance counsellors to 'be on the lookout for the bright boy or girl whose high ability has been demonstrated by the results of aptitude tests ... but whose achievement, as measured by grades in courses, has been low'.[20] Conant and others, such as Admiral Hyman Rickover, Max Rafferty, Asa Knowles and Lloyd Berkner, also blamed the prevailing education system, namely, progressive education.[21] Envisioned by philosopher John Dewey, progressive education was democratic, experimental, egalitarian and above all, child-centred, and by the 1940s was considered 'the dominant American pedagogy ... the conventional wisdom, the lingua franca of American educators'.[22] In theory, it sought to provide children with practical, tangible experiences in which they would learn skills and knowledge to prepare them to be productive Americans. In practice, however, many progressive classrooms were thought to be disordered and aimless, leading critics to call for a return to more strict, subject-centred, authoritarian and demanding classrooms.[23] Responding to such calls, legislators passed the National Defense Education Act in 1958. This invested 1 billion dollars in an effort to improve science, mathematics, English and foreign-language instruction. The aim was to improve student achievement at all levels and this also involved hiring guidance counsellors to work in schools.

Increasingly, the behaviours associated with poor scholastic achievement were symptomatic of hyperkinetic impulse disorder. While, on the one hand, treating such behaviours as disabling, and seeking to correct them, made sense and could be seen as being in the best interests of children, on the other hand, why certain behaviours, and not others, were seen as problematic was related to broader political and educational issues. As Katherine Reeves described in the education periodical *Grade Teacher*, concern shifted from shy, neurotic children to children like 'Charles' who 'slips from one interest to another, intense in his preoccupation of the moment, absorbing the essence of each, but moving insatiably from one activity to the next'.[24] The politics of this shift was also illustrated in a study intended to address the 'great concern about the use of talent in our society' and the 'wastage in the [educational] system'.[25] The authors compared impulsivity in 'underachievers' and 'future scientists' (students who had been accepted into a summer space camp), discovering that the 'future scientists' were not only much less impulsive than the underachievers, but also less hyperactive.[26] They concluded that the impulsive, hyperactive behaviour displayed by underachievers distinguished them from the 'future scientists' desired by education critics. Educational success was inseparable from larger geopolitical goals, meaning that children were very much seen as means to scientific, political and economic ends, rather than ends in themselves.[27] The notion of disability, when it came to hyperactivity, was connected, therefore, with an inability to contribute to the goals of the state.

Cold War fears about scientific inferiority, combined with demographic pressures on the education system, therefore, meant that considerable attention was devoted to 'smoking out and stimulating the efforts of the under-achievers', whose hyperactivity, inattentiveness and impulsivity were believed to be hampering American technological and political ambitions.[28] Although analysis is still required to determine how other historical developments influenced the emergence of hyperactivity, dissatisfaction with the American educational system and the academic performance of American children provided the foundation on which concerns about hyperactivity flourished. The process by which an educational problem became a psychiatric disorder and an educational disability, however, also involved developments in the medical community.

Psychiatry and Hyperactivity: the Search for Magic Bullets

Hyperactivity emerged at the same time as many other psychiatric disorders. Psychiatrists came to believe that a large percentage of the American population, particularly children, was mentally ill. Such thinking coincided with the development of the first widely prescribed psychoactive drugs to treat such conditions.[29] The relationship between new drugs and new disorders is, however, a complicated one. Building on the success of antibiotics and antihistamines during the 1930s and 1940s, pharmaceutical companies began investigating the psychoactive properties of various compounds.[30] The resulting anti-psychotics, anti-depressants and tranquillizers were seen by many psychiatrists and patients as magic bullets, allowing psychiatrists to see almost immediate improvement in their patients and helping institutionalized patients return to their communities. But alongside the development of such drugs came the proliferation of the disorders they were meant to treat. While David Herzberg has emphasized the role of advertising in raising the profile of psychiatric drugs, and therefore psychiatric disorders, David Healy goes further, claiming that pharmaceutical companies not only marketed antidepressants, but also the idea of depression.[31] Similarly, Ritalin (methylphenidate) was a drug in search of a disorder. Although the link between amphetamines and improved scholastic achievement had been recognized as early as 1937, Ritalin was first marketed by Ciba, relatively unsuccessfully, as a pep pill in 1954 for depressed and geriatric patients.[32] After it was approved for use in children in 1961 it became one of Ciba's bestsellers.

Ritalin's success was due, in part, to Ciba's advertising campaign. Significantly this included presenting not only its product but also the concept of hyperactivity to physicians, teachers and parents at Parent-Teacher Association meetings and medical conventions.[33] Although it was banned from such direct marketing in 1971, Ciba continued to advertise aggressively in medical journals, making Ritalin 'the treatment of choice [despite] ... very little empirical basis for its supposed superiority' to other drugs.[34] Effective marketing strategies, however, cannot explain fully the popularity of Ritalin. For many parents and psychiatrists, Ritalin did what behavioural therapy and psychotherapy could not do; it calmed down children within minutes. It also reinforced what an increasing number of psychiatrists were claiming by the mid-1960s, that hyperactivity was primarily a neurological condition best treated with drugs.

This is not to say, however, that other theories about hyperactivity did not exist. Psychoanalytical and social explanations and treatments for hyperactivity competed with those of a biological nature throughout the 1960s. Indeed, the first mention of hyperactivity in the second *Diagnostic and Statistical Manual of Mental Disorders* (*DSM*) in 1968 as 'hyperkinetic reaction of childhood' had a decidedly psychoanalytic ring to it.[35] While psychoanalysts believed that hyperactivity could be triggered by unresolved familial conflict, social psychiatrists saw its origins in social problems, such as overcrowding, exposure to violence and poverty. Yet, despite the plausibility of such approaches and the likelihood that hyperactive behaviour had at least some social and emotional aspects, they failed to influence conventional understandings of hyperactivity by the 1970s. Although the preventive elements of social psychiatry were believed by many during the 1960s, including President Kennedy and many presidents of the American Psychiatric Association, to be the solution to increasing numbers of children requiring psychiatric care, social psychiatric theory did not provide immediate answers to parents with hyperactive children. Psychotherapy, which was expensive, time-consuming and often levelled blame on parents, was also seen to be an impractical method for dealing with hyperactive children, and some accused psychotherapists of rejecting hyperactive children.[36] Perhaps more importantly, however, was the fact that, by the 1970s many psychiatrists saw the future of their discipline not in psychoanalysis or social psychiatry, but in biological psychiatry, where brain dysfunction explained the cause of mental disorder and drugs were central to treating it. Long encumbered by the opinion that psychiatry occupied the lowest rung of the medical ladder, many psychiatrists believed that the newly developed antipsychotics, antidepressants, tranquillizers and amphetamines held the key to establishing psychiatry's scientific legitimacy. Ritalin, according to Maurice Laufer, provided psychiatrists with 'one of the few situations in which you can do something quickly for people'.[37] Laufer's colleague, Eric Denhoff, was so impressed by Ritalin's efficacy that he considered 'it as "sort of criminal" to withhold treatment from those who can use it'.[38]

Also important in establishing the scientific validity of hyperactivity was the development of psychological tests to use in the diagnosis of the disorder. The most influential of these were the Conners scale, developed in the 1960s by C. Keith Conners, who, with Leon Eisenberg, directed the first major trials of methylphenidate in 1963.[39] The Conners scale was timely, in the sense that it provided an apparently more objective way to diagnose hyperactivity and fitted into a broader trend within psychiatry, whereby clearer and simpler ways by which to diagnose psychiatric disorders were sought. *DSM-III*, published in 1980, represented the fulfilment of this goal. It included a description of Attention Deficit Disorder (ADD), and a checklist of its symptoms. The *DSM-III* split the disorder into ADD and ADD with hyperactivity (ADD-H) subgroups, suggesting that inattention, rather than hyperactivity, was the key characteristic of the disorder. Although ADHD would replace ADD as the preferred term for hyperactivity in the revised version of *DSM-IV* in 1994, the focus on inattention helped to increase the number of people who could be diagnosed; hyperactivity was no longer seen primarily in rambunctious boys, it also could be found in girls and adults, who tended to be more inattentive than hyperactive. The *DSM* criteria also made it easier for children with hyperactivity to be identified as disabled and receive support under disabilities legislation.

Parents and Alternative Approaches

Developments within psychiatry, therefore, were important in understanding how hyperactivity came to be perceived as a common neurological condition that was best treated with stimulants. Such explanations also found a ready audience among parents trying to cope with hyperactive children. Unlike psychoanalytical and social explanations, biological psychiatrists stressed that hyperactivity had nothing to do with parenting skills. Nor was it explained by educational practices or social conditions; it was a neurological glitch, sometimes caused by brain injury, but typically genetic. For many parents, particularly mothers, this was a shift from previous trends in parenting advice.[40] As sociologist Ilina Singh has noted, 'weary of mother-blame ... the news about drug treatment and the emphasis on the organic nature of children's behavior problems appears to have been very welcome'.[41] Indeed, the formation of Children and Adults with ADD

(CHADD) in 1987, which lobbies on behalf of people with the disorder, was due in part to the perception that parents were being blamed for their children's behavioural problems. Lesley Freeman (a pseudonym), for example, was continually blamed for her son's behaviour problems. Her interactions with both mental-health workers and people in her neighbourhood made her believe that, 'whatever is wrong with the kid, obviously, it's the mother's fault. She feels like a failure, like a bad parent'. But when Freeman was first told that her son's problem was genetic, neurological and had little to do with her parenting, she 'was happy; I was off the hook, it wasn't my fault'.[42]

But despite feeling 'off the hook', Freeman, along with many other parents and children, found that hyperactivity drugs had disturbing side effects. Although her first impression of Ritalin was that it 'was amazing' and 'a wonder drug', she became concerned that 'after a little while they couldn't get it [the dosage] right'. Her son 'was either a zombie or as it wore off he was crazy and throwing furniture'.[43] When Freeman's physician recommended switching to another stimulant, Cylert (pemoline), which also lacked the anorectic side effects of Ritalin, her son became much calmer and quieter, but he also began hallucinating. Freeman finally took her son off all medication when he was nine and expressed that he did not 'want anybody to mess with my brain anymore'.[44] Not all physicians, however, agreed that the benefits of stimulants outweighed their side effects. While California paediatrician Sidney Adler admitted 'I don't know what the drug will do in twenty years ... but I have to try to do what we can do now to keep the kid from winding up in juvenile hall', Richard Young, an Indiana psychology professor, stated that 'I shudder when I hear my colleagues suggest you can go ahead and give drugs to children ... We really don't know what are the effects of a lot of these drugs on a lot of processes over the long run'.[45] Due to such concerns, some physicians advocated prescribing caffeine instead of Ritalin since it, too, was a stimulant.[46]

Although most physicians and parents had accepted biological explanations and treatments for hyperactivity by the early 1970s, worries about Ritalin and dissatisfaction with conventional understanding of the disorder encouraged some parents and physicians to consider alternative theories and solutions. Among the culprits blamed for the hyperactivity epidemic were lead exposure, fluorescent lighting, television and pesticides, but the theory that attracted the most attention and controversy was that of Ben Feingold, a San Francisco allergist who believed that food additives were responsible for the phenomenon.[47] Feingold's hypothesis, which he first presented to the American Medical Association in 1973, was controversial for many reasons, not least of which was that it threatened the prevailing biological approaches to and treatment of hyperactivity. According to critic John Werry:

the most chilling aspect of Feingold's work lies in the enthusiasm with which it has been embraced by the anti-medication, anti-psychiatry section of the American public and used as a cudgel to try to close down paediatric psychopharmacological research in that country.[48]

Concerned that media interest in the Feingold diet was overshadowing scientific evidence, physicians designed dozens of trials to test Feingold's hypothesis. Although the results were inconclusive, and despite the fact many of the trials were poorly designed, most physicians believed that they proved that the Feingold diet did not work, and following Feingold's death in 1982, most of the medical and media interest in his idea faded away. Nevertheless, many parents found that the Feingold diet worked and, through the work of the Feingold Association of the United States (FAUS), parents have continued to turn to Feingold's hypothesis. Responding to parents' calls to reconsider the link between food additives and hyperactivity, recent British research funded by the Food Standards Agency has provided compelling evidence in support of Feingold's idea, re-opening the debate once more.[49] In response to the British findings, the American Academy of Pediatrics, who condemned Feingold's theory in the 1970s, have admitted that they might have been wrong.[50] Although the debates continue, if it had not been for parents finding success with the Feingold diet and working with organizations such as FAUS to promote it, it is likely that the link between food additives and hyperactivity, which raises questions about the effects of other food chemicals on health, would have been forgotten. Parents, therefore, have been instrumental not only in advocating for the legitimacy of hyperactivity and the efficacy of stimulant treatment, but also promoting radically different approaches to the disorder.

Conclusion

So what, then, is hyperactivity? A genetic, neurological disability? A paranoid response to educational failure? A disorder manufactured to boost pharmaceutical profits? An explanation for childhood behaviour that has salved the consciences of parents and aided the professional ambitions of psychiatrists? A condition caused by food additives? Or is hyperactivity merely a personality quirk that has always been present in human populations and deemed to be beneficial or detrimental according to circumstance?[51] The history of hyperactivity suggests that it has been all of these things, and more, to differing degrees and at different times and places. What can be learned from the history of hyperactivity, therefore, is a lesson about the contexts in which certain behaviours become perceived as being disabling.

The history of hyperactivity is also a particularly American story, not least because the disorder emerged and became widespread in the United States long before other countries, including the United Kingdom.[52] Through the lens of hyperactivity it is possible to chart key developments, not only in American disability history, but also in many other areas of American history. Although I have focused here on the histories of American education, psychiatry and patient/parent activism, it is also useful to use the history of hyperactivity to explore the history of childhood, the pharmaceutical industry, family life, career trends, and many other facets of American social and cultural history. In many ways, hyperactivity and the controversy that has surrounded it highlight many of the tensions that have characterized American history. While some have seen hyperactivity diagnoses as an ideal means by which to help individuals reach their potential and, thus, improve the intellectual strength of the nation, others have seen them as an example of how society controls children at the expense of self-expression. Hyperactivity drugs have been perceived as magic bullets by some, but they have also been seen as an example of where pharmaceutical companies, and in particular their marketing departments, have gone too far in their efforts to convince teachers, parents and physicians that millions of children are in need of their products. Hyperactivity remains divisive in large part because it reflects many of the key and ongoing ideological debates in American society.

It is crucial to understand these contexts if physicians, parents and policy-makers are to make sensible decisions about controversial issues such as hyperactivity. Ritalin might prove to be a godsend for some parents dealing with a hyperactive child. But so too might the Feingold diet, or a different approach to their child's education, or more physical activity, or less television and computer games, or the painful realization that there are parenting problems and/or family tensions, or all of these things at once. Despite what conventional medical opinion might suggest, there are choices when it comes to hyperactivity and there always have been, choices that can lead to better health outcomes for both parents and their children. The history of hyperactivity, when focused in the right areas, can help in this process of empowerment.

NOTES

Borsay and Dale, 'Introduction'

1.   H. Hendrick, *Children, Childhood and English Society, 1880–1990* (Cambridge: Cambridge University Press, 1997), p. 10.
2.   Modern histories of childhood begin with P. Ariès, *Centuries of Childhood*, trans. R. Baldick (London: Cape, 1962). Another landmark text was D. G. Pritchard, *Education and the Handicapped 1760–1960* (London: Routledge and Kegan Paul, 1963). Disability history came later, and from the 1980s was closely linked with the disability rights movement.
3.   P. N. Stearns, *Childhood in World History*, 2nd edn (London: Routledge, 2010); A. Borsay, *Disability and Social Policy in Britain since 1750: A History of Exclusion* (Basingstoke: Palgrave Macmillan, 2005), pp. 10–13.
4.   H. Newton, 'Children's Physic: Medical Perceptions and Treatment of Sick Children in Early Modern England, *c.* 1580–1720', *Social History of Medicine*, 23:3 (2010), pp. 456–74; M. Pelling, 'Child Health as a Social Value in Early Modern England', *Social History of Medicine*, 1:2 (1988), pp. 135–64.
5.   J. Walmsley, 'Ideology, Ideas and Care in the Community, 1971–2001', in J. Welshman and J. Walmsley (eds), *Community Care in Perspective: Care, Control and Citizenship* (Basingstoke: Palgrave Macmillan, 2006), pp. 38–55, on p. 53.
6.   Scottish Executive, *The Same as You: A Review of Services for People with Learning Disabilities* (Edinburgh: The Stationary Office, 2000).
7.   R. Rapoport, R. N. Rapoport and Z. Strelitz with S. Kew, *Fathers, Mothers and Others: Towards New Alliances* (London: Routledge and Kegan Paul, 1977), p. 171, quoting Fraiberg, 1974.
8.   S. Blume, *The Artificial Ear: Cochlear Implants and the Culture of Deafness* (London: Rutgers University Press, 2010).
9.   J. Mepsted, *Your Child Needs You: A Positive Approach to Down's Syndrome* (Plymouth: Northcote House, 1988).
10.   Books aimed at parents do address these points, for example, R. Wyman, *Multiply Handicapped Children* (London: Souvenir Press, 1986), pp. 11–31.
11.   Clara Claiborne Park summarizes some of the early studies by Bruno Bettelheim, Beata Rank and Leo Kanner. C. C. Park, *The Siege: The Battle for Communication with an Autistic Child* (1967; Harmondsworth: Pelican Books, 1972).
12.   D. Atkinson, M. Jackson and J. Walmsley (eds), *Forgotten Lives: Exploring the History of Learning Disability* (Plymouth: BILD, 1997); D. Mitchell et al. (eds) *Exploring Experi-*

        ences of *Advocacy by People with Learning Disabilities: Testimonies of Resistance* (London:
        Jessica Kingsley, 2006); M. T. Fray, *Caring for Kathleen: A Sister's Story about Down's
        Syndrome and Dementia* (Plymouth: BILD, 2000).

13. Park, *The Siege*, p. 20.

14. C. Moore, *George and Sam* (London: Viking Books, 2004); M. Green, *Elizabeth: A
     Mentally Handicapped Daughter* (London: Hodder and Stoughton, 1966); J. Wilks and
     E. Wilks, *Bernard: Bringing up our Mongol Son* (London: Routledge and Kegan Paul,
     1974).

15. M. Jefferys, 'The Uncertain Health Visitor: A Detailed Study of Buckinghamshire's
     Social Services Shows that the Health Visitor has to Face Special Difficulties of Role and
     Confidence', *New Society*, 6:161 (1965), pp. 16–18.

16. A. T. Sutherland and P. Soames, *Adventure Play with Handicapped Children* (London:
     Souvenir Press, 1984).

17. F. Armstrong, 'Writing History: Education and the Experience of Disabled Children',
     presentation to ESRC seminar series Social Change in the History of Education, 10
     March 2006. This was developed as F. Armstrong, 'Disability, Education and Social
     Change since 1960', in J. Goodman, G. McCulloch and W. Richardson (eds), *Social
     Change in the History of Education: The British Experience in International Context* (Lon-
     don: Routledge, 2009).

18. These points, and the key text *Mind-forg'd Manacles* by Roy Porter, are introduced in J.
     Melling, B. Forsythe and R. Adair, 'Families, Communities and the Legal Regulation of
     Lunacy in Victorian England: Assessments of Crime, Violence and Welfare in Admis-
     sions to the Devon Asylum, 1845–1914', in P. Bartlett and D. Wright (eds), *Outside
     the Walls of the Asylum: The History of Care in the Community 1750–2000* (London:
     Athlone Press, 1999), pp. 153–80, on p. 156.

19. L. Tilley, 'The Voluntary Sector', in Welshman and Walmsley (eds), *Community Care in
     Perspective*, pp. 219–32.

20. The chapters in this volume use the terminology deployed by contemporary actors,
     although many of these words are now treated as obsolete and even discriminatory. We
     regret any offence this may inadvertently cause.

21. R. Cooter (ed.), *In the Name of the Child: Health and Welfare, 1880–1940* (London:
     Routledge, 1992).

22. S. Pooley, '"All We Parents Want is that Our Children's Health and Lives Should Be
     Regarded": Child Health and Parental Concern in England, *c.* 1860–1910', *Social His-
     tory of Medicine*, 23:3 (2010), pp. 528–48.

23. M. Thomson, *The Problem of Mental Deficiency: Eugenics, Democracy and Social Policy in
     Britain c. 1870–1959* (Oxford: Clarendon Press, 1998), pp. 1–35.

24. Since the 1970s housing policy in the UK has tended to concentrate disabled people
     in poorer neighbourhoods through the supply of, and demand for, social housing. M.
     Oliver and C. Barnes (eds), *Disabled People and Social Policy: From Exclusion to Inclusion*
     (London: Longman, 1998), pp. 45–6.

25. An Edwardian case study that introduces the notion of domestic violence as a cause of
     childhood disabilities is provided by 'Thomas Morgan', in T. Thompson, *Edwardian
     Childhoods* (London: Routledge and Kegan Paul, 1981), pp. 9–35. This oral history
     project was published at a time when medical discussion about 'battered babies' was
     becoming a wider debate about child abuse, see N. Parton, *The Politics of Child Abuse*
     (Basingstoke: Macmillan, 1985).

26. Privately funded care of the mentally ill has been evaluated as different but not clearly superior to that offered to clients of public services. C. MacKenzie, *Psychiatry for the Rich: A History of Ticehurst Private Asylum, 1792–1917* (London: Routledge, 1992).

27. Studies of Presidents George and George W. Bush sometimes discuss Barbara Bush's unhappiness with the fact that her family's affluence and influential connections encouraged them to pursue aggressive and ultimately heartbreaking treatment options for one of her daughters.

28. Here the British Royal family serves as an exemplar with recent media interest in the care of Prince John (youngest son of George V) in a separate household and the institutionalization of relatives of Queen Elizabeth (wife of George VI). W. Shawcross, *Queen Elizabeth. The Queen Mother. The Official Biography* (Basingstoke: Macmillan, 2009), p. 313n.

29. Claire Rayner believed that it was her mother rather than her childhood self who had problems. She was therefore extremely sceptical about the value of her attendance at a child guidance clinic that was financed by concerned relatives. C. Rayner, *How Did I Get Here From There?* (London: Virago, 2003), pp. 24–6.

30. There is some discussion about these issues, especially in relation to the quest for beauty and successful marriage, in (auto)biographical work by debutantes. Vivian Winch noted many American friends had orthodontic braces (then largely unknown amongst her contemporaries in the UK) in the 1920s. V. Winch, *A Mirror for Mama* (London: Macdonald, 1965), p. 124. While Edwina Mountbatten was regularly prescribed spectacles she wouldn't wear. J. Morgan, *Edwina Mountbatten: A Life of her own* (London: Fontana, 1992), p. 61.

31. Janet Aitken had a privileged childhood but nonetheless required a series of medical procedures to treat a tubercular neck gland and plastic surgery to her face following a car accident. J. Aitken Kidd, *The Beaverbrook Girl: An Autobiography* (London: Collins, 1987), pp. 24–5 and p. 56.

32. M. Jackson (ed.), *Health and the Modern Home* (London: Routledge, 2007).

33. D. Hirst, 'The Early School Medical Service in Wales: Public Care or Private Responsibility?', in A. Borsay (ed.), *Medicine in Wales c. 1800–2000: Public Service or Private Commodity?* (Cardiff: University of Wales Press, 2003), pp. 65–85.

34. M. A. Crowther, *The Workhouse System, 1834–1929: The History of an English Social Institution* (Athens, GA: University of Georgia Press, 1982); L. H. Lees, *The Solidarities of Strangers: The English Poor Laws and the People 1700–1948* (Cambridge: Cambridge University Press, 1998).

35. For literature review, see Borsay, *Disability and Social Policy*, pp. 94–116.

36. *History of Education, Special Issue, Disability and Education: Historical Perspectives from Europe*, 34:2 (2005).

37. H. Hendrick, *Child Welfare: England 1872–1989* (London: Routledge, 1994), pp. 1–15.

38. H. Hendrick, 'Optimism and Hope Versus Anxiety and Narcissism: Some Thoughts on Children's Welfare Yesterday and Today', *History of Education*, 36:6 (2007), pp. 747–68.

39. L. Purves, 'The Moral Is: Question Your Motives, Parents – Callous Neglect, "Mercy Killing" and Sickness-faking – Three Extreme Cases Reveal Some Awkward Truths About Parenting', *The Times*, 25 January 2010, p. 25.

40. Walmsley, 'Ideology, Ideas and Care', pp. 49–51.

41. A problem compounded by a lack of differentiation between children whose special educational needs require additional support (such as Braille books) and children whose medical condition precludes ordinary schooling.

42. A useful survey of issues is provided by R. Viner and J. Golden, 'Children's Experiences of Illness', in R. Cooter and J. Pickstone (eds), *Medicine in the Twentieth Century* (Harwood Academic Publishers, Amsterdam, 2000), pp. 575–87.

43. For example, A. Shaw and C. Reeves, *The Children of Craig-y-nos: Life in a Welsh TB Sanatorium, 1922–1959* (London: Wellcome Trust Centre for the History of Medicine at UCL, 2009).

44. This helps explain the contentious, but unresolved, debate about the merits of educating disabled children in mainstream or special schools in the UK.

45. H. Hendrick, *Child Welfare: Historical Dimensions, Contemporary Debates* (Bristol: Policy Press, 2003), pp. 205–53.

46. W. S. Paine (ed.), *Job Stress and Burnout: Research, Theory and Intervention Perspectives* (Beverly Hills, CA: Sage Publications, 1982).

47. The Camden Society, *I Want What You Have: Five Decades of Making it Happen. The Story of the Camden Society* (London: The Camden Society, 2010).

48. This was associated with recognition of the special burden placed on the mother. P. Abbot and R. Sapsford, *Community Care for Mentally Handicapped Children* (Milton Keynes: Open University Press, 1987).

49. J. Twigg and K. Atkin, *Carers Perceived: Policy and Practice in Informal Care* (Buckingham: Open University Press, 1994).

50. G. Hendey, 'Disability and Transition to Adulthood: The Politics of Parenting', *Critical Social Policy*, 24:2 (2004), pp. 165–86.

51. This is not to decry the significant ongoing efforts of long-established charities working with veterans but to suggest that charities like Help for Heroes mark something of a new departure. In other countries, most notably the USA, provision for veterans has traditionally had an even greater influence on statutory responses to disability issues and welfare policy more generally. B. Linker, '"Feet for Fighting": Locating Disability and Social Medicine in First World War America', *Social History of Medicine*, 20:1 (2007), pp. 91–107.

52. The way new categories of need/demands for services are problematically created by adult activists dissatisfied with existing categories of illness/disability has been usefully explored using the example of breast cancer survivors. E. Abel and S. Subramanian, *After the Cure: The Untold Stories of Breast Cancer Survivors* (New York: New York University Press, 2008).

53. Hendrick, 'Optimism and Hope'.

1 Starkey, 'Club Feet and Charity'

1. One of its members was William Ewart Gladstone, who was instrumental in setting up the House and, during its early days, an active member of its Council. Gladstone (1809–98), was Prime Minister four times. He and his wife Catherine were active supporters of the House of Charity (hereafter HoC).

2. The House of Charity Prospectus, 11 June 1846, Flintshire Record Office, Hawarden. Deeside, Glynne-Gladstone MSS 1668.

3. P. Starkey, '"Temporary Relief for Specially Recommended or Selected Deserving Persons". The Mission of the House of Charity, Soho 1846–1914', *Urban History*, 35:1 (2008), pp. 96–115; HoC Minute Books, 4 December 1874 and 11 December 1874, Westminster Archive Centre (hereafter WAC), ACC2091.

4. HoC Minute Books, 3 August 1866. On that occasion, it was agreed that fifteen children should be admitted, although this was a number that was greatly exceeded.

5. R. Cooter, *Surgery and Society in Peace and War: Orthopaedics and the Organization of Modern Medicine, 1880–1948* (Manchester: Manchester University Press, 1993), p. 64.
6. In the twenty-first century the National Health Service operates not dissimilar schemes for certain cancer patients.
7. HoC Case Books (hereafter HoC CB), 1 April 1869, WAC, ACC2091.
8. HoC CB, 18 January 1878.
9. HoC CB, 31 May 1889.
10. When the House of Charity outgrew its premises in Rose Street in Soho and moved to 1 Greek Street in 1860, the Sisters took over the original premises for a House of Mercy as well as beginning to manage the housekeeping at the House of Charity. HoC, Fifteenth Annual Report, 26 June 1861, WAC, ACC2091.
11. V. Bonham, *A Place in Life: The Clewer House of Mercy 1849–83* (Reading: Thameslink, 1992), pp. 173–4.
12. HoC CB, 11 October 1872.
13. J. A. Cholmeley, *History of the Royal National Orthopaedic Hospital* (hereafter RNOH) (London: Chapman and Hall, 1985), pp. 4–6 and p. 10.
14. Cooter, *Surgery and Society*, p. 15.
15. Cholmeley, *History of the RNOH*, p. 15.
16. Ibid., p. 15 and p. 52.
17. Ibid., p. 46 and p. 72. The three hospitals eventually united as the RNOH in 1903.
18. See D. LeVay, *The History of Orthopaedics: An Account of the Study and Practice of Orthopaedics from the Earliest Times to the Modern Era* (Carnforth and Park Ridge: Parthenon, 1990), p. 63.
19. Cholmeley, *History of the RNOH*, p. 32. See also, F. Prochaska, *Royal Bounty. The Making of a Welfare Monarchy* (New Haven, CT: Yale University Press, 1995), p. 100.
20. Cholmeley, *History of the RNOH*, p. 10, and p. 32.
21. HoC CB, 2 October 1855.
22. HoC CB, 20 August 1861.
23. HoC CB, 26 November 1890.
24. LeVay, *History of Orthopaedics*, pp. 489–93.
25. 'Little, William John (1810–1894), orthopaedic surgeon', in *ODNB*.
26. J. D. Brown, *Remarks on the Operation for the Cure of Club Foot, With Cases, also Letters to John C Warren MD on Curvature of the Spine*, republished from the *Boston Medical and Surgical Journal* (Boston, MA: D. Clapp Jnr, 1839), p. 7; Cholmeley, *History of the RNOH*, p. 3; Cooter, *Surgery and Society*, p. 14; LeVay, *History of Orthopaedics*, pp. 492–501; A. Rocyn Jones, 'The British Orthopaedic Association', *The Journal of Bone and Joint Surgery*, 51B (1969), pp. 2–3.
27. LeVay, *History of Orthopaedics*, p. 70.
28. Cholmeley, *History of the RNOH,* p. 15.
29. HoC CB, 23 June 1868 and 10 February 1874.
30. HoC CB, 25 October and 8 December 1879.
31. HoC CB, 2 October 1855 and 23 June 1868.
32. Cholmeley, *History of the RNOH*, p. 19 and p. 22.
33. Ibid., p. 31 and p. 37.
34. G. Roberts, 'The London Hospital', in R. B. D. Acland (ed.), *Hospital Saturday and the Medical Charities* (London, 1898), p. 15.
35. Cholmeley, *History of the RNOH*, p. 66.
36. Brown, *Remarks on the Operation*, pp. 13–15.

37. Ibid., pp. 19–20.
38. LeVay, *History of Orthopaedics*, p. 127.
39. HoC CB, 9 July 1870 and 27 November 1872.
40. HoC CB, 18 July 1872.
41. HoC CB, 24 November 1854 and 19 January 1855.
42. HoC CB, 3 May 1863.
43. O. Temkin, *The Falling Sickness. A History of Epilepsy from the Greeks to the Beginnings of Modern Neurology*, 2nd edn (1945; Baltimore, MD and London: Johns Hopkins Press, 1971), p. 256.
44. J. Maley, 'On Epilepsy', *Journal of Mental Science*, 4 (1858), pp. 245–8.
45. Temkin, *The Falling Sickness*, p. 293 and pp. 298–9; Also see, 'Correspondence', *Lancet*, II (1852), pp. 337–8; M. Ward, 'Clinical Notes', *Lancet*, II (1852), pp. 374–5; C. B. Radcliffe, 'On the Pathology of Affections Allied to Epilepsy', *Lancet*, I (1853), pp. 264–6; J. Williams, 'Practical Observations on the Cure of Epilepsy', *Lancet*, I (1854), pp. 128–30.
46. 'Jackson, John Hughlings (1835–1911) Physician', *ODNB*.
47. HoC CB, 14 October 1853.
48. HoC CB, 12 January 1853.
49. HoC CB, 4 February 1859.
50. HoC CB, 29 April 1862.
51. HoC CB, 18 January 1867.
52. HoC CB, 8 February 1866.
53. HoC CB, 9 August 1872.
54. HoC CB, 4 June 1855.
55. HoC Annual Report 1856.
56. HoC CB, 20 May 1881.
57. HoC CB, 17 March 1921.
58. HoC CB, 29 April, 1862 and 4 April 1854.
59. HoC CB, 7 April 1854.
60. HoC CB, 25 June 1866.
61. HoC CB, 26 November 1890.
62. Cooter, *Surgery and Society*, pp. 53–5.
63. Temkin, *The Falling Sickness*, p. 303.
64. For discussion of London hospital finances see K. Waddington, *Charity and the London Hospitals, 1850–1898* (Woodbridge: Royal Historical Society, Boydell Press, 2000), p. 21.

2 Rosenthal, 'Insanity, Family and Community in Late-Victorian Britain'

1. W. Bernard, 'Infantile Insanity', *Transactions of the Royal Academy of Medicine in Ireland*, 7 (1899–1900), pp. 416–20, on p. 418.
2. A rare exception is J. Melling, R. Adair and B. Forsythe, '"A Proper Lunatic for Two Years": Pauper Lunatic Children in Victorian and Edwardian England. Child Admissions to the Devon County Asylum, 1845–1914', *Journal of Social History*, 31:2 (1997), pp. 371–405.
3. J. Walton, 'Casting Out and Bringing Back in Victorian England: Pauper Lunatics 1840–1870', in W. F. Bynum, R. Porter, and M. Shepherd (eds) *The Anatomy of Madness: Essays in the History of Psychiatry. Volume II: Institutions and Society* (London: Tavistock, 1985), pp. 132–46.

4. Wealthier families could seek private medical advice about the care of insane relatives who might be looked after at home or admitted to private asylums at this time.
5. W. Ireland, *The Mental Affections of Children: Idiocy, Imbecility and Insanity*, 2nd edn (London: J. and A. Churchill, 1900), p. 272.
6. H. Maudsley, *The Pathology of the Mind: A Study of Its Distempers, Deformities, and Disorders* (London: J. Friedmann, 1979 reprint, 1895), p. 364.
7. Patients admitted to Victorian idiot asylums were typically younger than those admitted to lunatic asylums. D. Wright, *Mental Disability in Victorian England: The Earlswood Asylum, 1847–1901* (Oxford: Oxford University Press, 2001), p. 90.
8. Melling et al., 'A Proper Lunatic', p. 372.
9. A formal diagnosis of moral insanity was however rarely applied to children.
10. H. Cunningham, *Children and Childhood in Western Society since 1500* (London: Longman, 1995), p. 61.
11. Ibid., pp. 74–5.
12. R. Cooter (ed.), *In the Name of the Child: Health and Welfare, 1880–1940* (London: Routledge, 1992).
13. J. Walvin, *A Child's World: A Social History of English Childhood, 1800–1914* (New York: Penguin Books, 1982), p. 15.
14. F. Davenport Hill, *Children of the State*, 2nd edn, ed. F. Fowke (London: Macmillan, 1889), p. 22.
15. Maudsley, *Pathology of the Mind*, p. 380.
16. M. Thomson, *The Problem of Mental Deficiency: Eugenics, Democracy and Social Policy in Britain c. 1870–1959* (Oxford: Clarendon Press, 1998).
17. Anon., 'Lunatics at Home', *British Medical Journal*, 1:491 (1870), pp. 552–3, on p. 552.
18. Maudsley, *Pathology of the Mind*, p. 383.
19. Ibid., pp. 383–4.
20. M. Brierre de Boismont, 'On the Insanity of Early Life', *Journal of Psychiatric Medicine*, 10 (1875), pp. 622–38, on p. 630.
21. Ibid., p. 629.
22. J. Crichton-Browne, 'Psychical Diseases of Early Life', *Journal of Mental Science*, 6 (1859–60), pp. 284–320, on p. 289.
23. Ibid., p. 290.
24. Cunningham, *Children and Childhood*, p. 62.
25. 'Children's Faults: A Few Hints for Mothers', *Bow Bells* (26 May 1869), pp. 429–30, on p. 429.
26. Ibid., p. 429.
27. 'Early Training', *Bow Bells* (February 1867), p. 45.
28. 'Our Young Servants', *Longman's Magazine* (April 1895), pp. 631–44, on p. 631.
29. H. Hendrick, *Children, Childhood and English Society, 1880–1990* (Cambridge: Cambridge University Press, 1997), p. 10.
30. Ibid., pp. 11–12.
31. Biographical details for Florence Davenport Hill (1828–1919) are included in the ODNB entry for her sister Rosamond. 'Hill, Rosamond Davenport (1825–1902)', *ODNB*.
32. Davenport Hill, *Children of the State*, p. 2.
33. Cunningham, *Children and Childhood*, p. 152.
34. Ibid., p. 153.
35. Melling et al., 'A Proper Lunatic', p. 371.
36. Anon., 'Lunatics at Home', *British Medical Journal*, 2:312 (22 December 1866), pp. 700–1, on p. 701.

37. Davenport Hill, *Children of the State*, p. 2.
38. The *Oxford English Dictionary* suggests that 'vicious' referred to parents who had bad or immoral habits and practices.
39. Walvin, *A Child's World*, pp. 14–15.
40. Melling et al., 'A Proper Lunatic', p. 372.
41. Ibid.
42. R. Hunter and I. Macalpine, *Psychiatry for the Poor: 1851 Colney Hatch Asylum-Friern Hospital 1973: A Medical and Social History* (Folkestone: Dawsons of Pall Mall, 1974), p. 13.
43. D. Wright, 'Getting out of the Asylum: Understanding the Confinement of the Insane in the Nineteenth Century', *Social History of Medicine*, 10:1 (1997), pp. 137–55, on p. 138.
44. The general trend was towards greater therapeutic pessimism and a corresponding emphasis on long-term care/control rather than cure.
45. A. Roberts, Index of English and Welsh Lunatic Asylums and Mental Hospitals, http://studymore.org.uk/4_13_ta.htm [accessed 15 April 2011].
46. R. Allen, 'History of a Hospital: St. Augustine's Hospital, Chartham', *Bygone Kent*, 2:12 (1990), pp. 698–704, on p. 699.
47. Roberts, Index of English and Welsh Lunatic Asylums.
48. Allen, 'History of a Hospital', p. 699.
49. Ibid., p. 701.
50. A. Roberts, 'The Lunacy Commission: A Study of its Origins, Emergence and Character', http://studymore.org.uk/01.htm [accessed 16 March 2011].
51. D. Wright, '"Childlike in his Innocence": Lay Attitudes to "Idiots" and "Imbeciles" in Victorian England', in D. Wright and A. Digby (eds), *From Idiocy to Mental Deficiency: Historical Perspectives on People with Learning Disabilities* (London: Routledge, 1996), pp. 118–33, on p. 119.
52. P. Bartlett, 'The Asylum and the Poor Law: The Productive Alliance', in J. Melling and B. Forsythe (eds), *Insanity, Institutions and Society, 1880–1914: A Social History of Madness in Comparative Perspective* (London: Routledge, 1999), pp. 48–67, on p. 51.
53. Ibid.
54. Wright, *Mental Disability in Victorian England*, p. 13.
55. Wright, 'Childlike in his Innocence', p. 120.
56. The continuing importance of the legal age of majority meant that legislation (such as the 1913 Mental Deficiency Act) dictated that certain cases had to be reviewed when a person attained twenty-one years. The changing official school leaving age also impacted on care arrangements.
57. East Kent Lunatic Asylum/St. Augustine's Hospital (hereafter EKLA), 'Case Book B', 1877–81, East Kent Archive Centre, Dover, Kent (hereafter EKAC), p. 368.
58. EKLA, 'Case Book B', p. 368.
59. Ibid.
60. Ibid.
61. EKLA, 'Case Book C', 1881–5, p. 187.
62. Ibid.
63. Ibid. Ann E. was discharged on 31 August 1883.
64. Melling et al., 'A Proper Lunatic', p. 386.
65. EKLA, 'Case Book C', p. 77.
66. Ibid.
67. Ibid., p. 81.

68. Ibid.
69. Ibid.
70. Ibid.
71. EKLA, 'Case Book D', 1885–9, p. 166. Asylum records give conflicting information about the type of disorder Matilda B. suffered from. While the register of admissions indicates imbecility, her casebook record does not record the form of disorder at all. EKLA, 'Register of Pauper Admissions', 1880–7, EKAC, entry 2243.
72. EKLA, 'Case Book D', p. 166.
73. EKLA, 'Case Book I', p. 151.
74. EKLA, 'Case Book J', p. 57.
75. 'The Cry of the Parents (by One of Them)', *Macmillan's Magazine* (May/October 1890), pp. 55–8, on p. 55.
76. H. Hendrick, *Child Welfare: England 1872–1989* (London: Routledge, 1994), p. 127.

3 Thompson, 'The Mixed Economy of Welfare and the Care of Sick and Disabled Children in the South Wales Coalfield'

1.   The importance and utility of the concept is explored in M. Katz and C. Sachße (eds), *The Mixed Economy of Social Welfare: Public/Private Relations in England, Germany and the United States, the 1870s to the 1930s* (Baden Baden: Nomos, 1996); N. Johnson, *Mixed Economies of Welfare: A Comparative Perspective* (Hemel Hempstead: Prentice Hall, 1999); B. Harris and P. Bridgen (eds), *Charity and Mutual Aid in Europe and North America since 1800* (London: Routledge, 2007); M. Powell (ed.), *Understanding the Mixed Economy of Welfare* (Bristol: Policy, 2007). Crucial to the development of this approach is G. Finlayson, *Citizen, State and Social Welfare in Britain, 1830–1990* (Oxford: Oxford University Press, 1994) and G. Finlayson, 'A Moving Frontier: Voluntarism and the State in British Social Welfare 1911–1949', *Twentieth Century British History*, 1:2 (1990), pp. 183–206.
2.   Devolution has focused some attention on the particular national trajectories of welfare development in the devolved countries. C. Webster, 'Devolution and the Health Service in Wales, 1919–1969', in P. Michael and C. Webster (eds), *Health and Society in Twentieth-Century Wales* (Cardiff: University of Wales Press, 2006), pp. 240–69; J. Stewart, 'The National Health Service in Scotland, 1947–74: Scottish or British?', *Historical Research*, 76:193 (2003), pp. 389–410; C. Nottingham (ed.), *The N.H.S. in Scotland: The Legacy of the Past and the Prospect of the Future* (Aldershot: Ashgate, 2000).
3.   S. Thompson, 'A Proletarian Public Sphere: Working-class Self-provision of Medical Services and Care in South Wales, c. 1900–1948', in A. Borsay (ed.), *Medicine in Wales, c. 1800–2000: Public Service or Private Commodity?* (Cardiff: University of Wales Press, 2003), pp. 86–107.
4.   J. Ginswick (ed.), *Labour and the Poor in England and Wales 1849–1851: The Letters to the Morning Chronicle. Vol. III: The Mining and Manufacturing Districts of South Wales and North Wales* (London: Cass, 1983), p. 144; *Report from the Select Committee on Payment of Wages* (471), 1842, ix, pp. 67–8; O. Jones, *The Early Days of Sirhowy and Tredegar* (Newport: Tredegar Local History Society, 1969), p. 70.
5.   L. W. Evans, *Education in Industrial Wales 1700–1900: A Study of the Works Schools System* (Cardiff: Avalon Books, 1971).

6. J. Williams, *Digest of Welsh Historical Statistics: vol. 1* (Cardiff: Welsh Office, 1985), p. 63; Ginswick, *Labour and the Poor in England and Wales*, p. 74.
7. T. Thomas, *Poor Relief in Merthyr Tydfil Union in Victorian Times* (Cardiff: Glamorgan Archive Service, 1992), p. 108.
8. Evidence for the Cardiff and Carmarthen workhouses in the late 1860s suggests that sick children were accommodated in the female wards. *Report of Dr. E. Smith, Medical Officer to Poor Law Board, on Sufficiency of Arrangements for Care and Treatment of Sick Poor in Forty-eight Provincial Workhouses in England and Wales*, 1867–8, lx, pp. 55–9.
9. Quoted in S. King and J. Stewart, 'Death in Llantrisant: Henry Williams and the New Poor Law in Wales', *Rural History*, 15:1 (2004), p. 81.
10. For an early articulation of this belief, see Col. Thomas Wood to John Jones, 22 January 1822, National Library of Wales, Maybery (3), 6589; for a broader treatment of this matter, see P. Michael, *Care and Treatment of the Mentally Ill in North Wales 1800–2000* (Cardiff: University of Wales Press, 2003).
11. Resolutions passed by a public meeting of the Dowlais workmen protesting against the treatment of the sick and dead members of their families, 1866, Glamorgan Record Office (hereafter GlamRO), Cardiff, Dowlais Iron Company Collection, DG/C/5/43.
12. King and Stewart, 'Death in Llantrisant', p. 73 and p. 79; A. Hardy, *Health and Society in Britain since 1860* (Basingstoke: Macmillan, 2001), p. 20.
13. Williams, *Digest of Welsh Historical Statistics*, p. 17 and p. 20.
14. *Western Mail*, 12 March 1879, p. 4; such was the nature of the economy in the town at this time that accident cases among children from the local industries were brought to the hospital. See, for example, *Merthyr Express*, 30 June 1883, p. 5. The hospital was eventually subsumed into the larger General Hospital opened in 1888.
15. *Aberdare Times*, 26 March 1881, p. 4.
16. See for example Local Government Board (hereafter LGB), *Twentieth Annual Report* [C.6460], 1890–91, xxxiii, p. 257; *Western Mail*, 2 September 1874, p. 5; *Western Mail*, 12 June 1883, p. 2; *Merthyr Express*, 26 February 1881, p. 5; *Merthyr Express*, 24 July 1886, p. 3, and pp. 4–5.
17. For examples of such additional payments see Park Slip Fund committee minutes, 29 March 1897, GlamRO, D/D NCB 22/1.
18. Llanerch Colliery Explosion Fund (hereafter Llanerch CEF), Executive Committee Minute Book (hereafter ECMB), 25 January 1895, Gwent Record Office (hereafter Gwent RO), Cwmbran; Senghenydd Relief Fund minute book, 27 January 1916, South Wales Coalfield Collection (hereafter SWCC), MNA/NUM/3/7/6; Senghenydd Relief Fund minute book, 21 July 1916.
19. Llanerch CEF, ECMB, Local committee, 24 April 1899; Abercarn Colliery Explosion Trust Fund, Minute Book of the Distribution Committee, 28 July 1881, Gwent RO, D.184.0004; Park Slip Fund committee minutes, 29 March 1897.
20. Llanerch CEF, ECMB, 24 April 1899 and 29 October 1900.
21. Park Slip Fund committee minutes, 29 March 1897; 2 October 1899; 17 October 1899; 18 January 1900; 4 April 1901; 7 November 1901.
22. Royal Commission on the Blind, the Deaf and Dumb of the United Kingdom (hereafter Royal Commission, 1889), Appendices [C.5781–I], xix, 1889, Appendix 2, pp. 27–9; also, Education Department, *Reports on Education of Deaf and Dumb Children in Metropolitan, Manchester and Swansea Districts by H. M. Inspectors* [C.4639], 1886, xxv, pp. 6–7.

23. Pontardawe Board of Guardians minutes, 3 August 1876, West Glamorgan Archive Service (hereafter WGAS), U/Pd 1/1; Pontardawe Board of Guardian minutes, 1 March 1877.

24. Royal Commission, 1889, xix, Appendix 2, p. 152; Neath Union Board of Guardians minutes, 16 February 1897, WGAS, U/N 1/8.

25. Education Department, *Report of the Committee of Council of Education on Schools for the Blind and Deaf, with Appendices, 1896–97* [C.8608], 1897, xxvii, pp. 24, 29.

26. See for example LGB, *Twentieth Annual Report, 1890–91* [C.6460], 1890–1, xxxiii, pp. 256–8; LGB, *Twenty-First Annual Report, 1891–92* [C.6745], 1892, xxxviii, pp. 174–6; LGB, *Twenty-Fifth Annual Report, 1895–96* [C.8212], 1896, xxxvi, p. 221.

27. LGB, *Twenty-First Annual Report*, pp. 174–6.

28. LGB, *Twenty-Ninth Annual Report, 1899–1900* [Cd.292], 1900, xxxiii, p. 152.

29. *Western Mail*, 15 November 1883, p. 3.

30. *Western Mail*, 25 March 1897, p. 3.

31. *Western Mail*, 29 January 1897, p. 3.

32. *The Welsh Housing and Development Year Book* (1920), pp. 105–7.

33. See for example C. Williams, 'Labour and the Challenge of Local Government, 1919–1939', in D. Tanner, C. Williams and D. Hopkin (eds), *The Labour Party in Wales 1900–2000* (Cardiff: University of Wales Press, 2000), pp. 140–56; as an example of the greater focus on children in local and national politics see Election handbill: 'Vote for Labour and Give the Children a Chance', *c.* 1910, GlamRO, D/D Vau 24/11.

34. See the clipping from *The Labour Woman* (1920), p. 157, GlamRO, Alderman Rose Davies' Papers; see also Pontypridd Board of Guardians By-Election, Handbill of Labour Party candidate, Catherine Jenkins, 1925, SWCC, MNA/NUM/PP/52/1; West Wales Labour Women's Advisory Council, minute books, 1937–57, especially 23 April 1938 and 27 March 1944, WGAS.

35. LGB, *Twenty-Fifth Annual Report, 1895–96*, p. 221; see also J. Prowle, 'Poor Law Administration of Merthyr Parish', in *The Democrat's Handbook to Merthyr, Published for the Twentieth Annual Conference of the ILP* (Merthyr: The Educational Publishing Co., 1912), pp. 84–9.

36. LGB, *Thirty-ninth Annual Report, 1909–10*, [Cd.5260, 5275], 1910, xxxviii, pp. 95–6.

37. Cardiff Poor Cripples Aid Society (hereafter Cardiff PCAS) minutes, 1908–49, passim, GlamRO, DPC/1/1–2.

38. For examples, see Cardiff PCAS minutes, 16 December 1912, 8 February 1917, 4 May 1925 and 7 September 1925.

39. There were also instances in which the Society arranged for surgical appliances and equipment to be provided but where the cost was borne by the Royal Surgical Aid Society, a national body founded in 1862 to assist disabled people. Cardiff PCAS minutes, 4 May 1925 and 27 August 1930.

40. Cardiff PCAS minutes, 4 May 1925, 8 June 1925, 30 January 1929. The Cardiff Guardians donated £20 a year in the 1910s; see Cardiff PCAS minutes, 21 February 1916.

41. Cardiff PCAS minutes, 20 October 1927 and 20 September 1928.

42. Cardiff PCAS minutes, 7 January 1931.

43. See the column of John Morgan in *Pontypridd Observer*, 28 March 1908, supplement; *Pontypridd Observer*, 11 April 1908, p. 1.

44. A. E. Remmett Weaver, 'The Abertillery School Clinic', *Public Health*, 24 (July 1911), pp. 388–93; see also *The Hospital*, 13 April 1912, pp. 39–40.

45. Abertillery Urban District Council (hereafter UDC), *Report of the Medical Officer of Health and School Medical Officer* (1909), p. 100.
46. Ibid. (1927), p. 110, and (1928–34), *passim*.
47. The surgical registrar at the National Hospital, Arthur Rocyn Jones, was brother to David Rocyn Jones, the County Medical Officer and School Medical Officer.
48. Monmouthshire County Council (hereafter CC), Annual Report of the Medical Inspection Department to the Education Committee (hereafter AR MID) (1914), p. 58.
49. Ibid., (1938), pp. 24–5.
50. Ibid., (1908–38), *passim*.
51. Ibid., (1932) p. 43.
52. Aberdare Open Air School Log Book, 1914–50, *passim*, GlamRO, EA/5/1; M. Thomas, *Aberdare Open-Air Schools* (Aberdare, 1931). See also *Labour Woman*, 1 February 1927, p. 18; K. Freeman, *If Any Man Build. The History of the Save the Children Fund* (London: Hodder & Stoughton, 1965), p. 50; D. Hughes, 'Just a Breath of Fresh Air in an Industrial Landscape? The Preston Open Air School in 1926: A School Medical Insight', *Social History of Medicine*, 17:3 (2004), pp. 443–61.
53. Rhondda UDC, Annual Report of the Medical Officer of Health and School Medical Officer (hereafter AR MOH) (1912), pp. 199–200.
54. Ibid. (1919), p. xxii.
55. Ibid. (1927), p. xxix.
56. Ibid. (1928), p. xxxiv.
57. Ibid. (1927), p. xxxvi.
58. *Third Annual Report of the Ministry of Health, 1921–1922* [Cmd.1713], 1922, viii, p. 15; see also, M. Rooff, *Voluntary Societies and Social Policy* (London: Routledge and Kegan Paul, 1957), p. 52.
59. Rhondda UDC, AR MOH (1927), p. vii.
60. Ibid., pp. vii, xxxii, pp. xxxvi–xxxvii; (1928), p. vi; (1939), pp. xxx–xxxi.
61. Ibid. (1937), p. vi.
62. Ibid., pp. vi and xxiv–xxv.
63. Ibid., p. vii.
64. LGB, *Twenty-Eighth Annual Report, 1898–99* [C.9444], 1899, xxxvii, p. 179.
65. Election handbill of Morgan Williams, April 1913, Aberdare Central Library.
66. *List of Certified Schools for Blind, Deaf, Defective, and Epileptic Children in England and Wales in 1914* [Cd.7724], 1914–16, l, p. 36.
67. J. H. L. Mabbitt, *The Health Services of Glamorgan* (Cowbridge: D. Brown, 1973), pp. 16–26.
68. Rhondda UDC, AR MOH (1932), pp. xlvii–xlix; (1933), p. xlii.
69. Monmouthshire CC, AR MID (1909), pp. v–vii.
70. These changes can be followed in ibid., (1910–15).
71. Ibid., (1930), p. 53; (1932), pp. 57–60.
72. For example, see Nine Mile Point Lodge, Committee Meeting minutes, 2 February 1925, SWCC, MNA/NUM/L/57/A/1; on donations to Barnardo's Homes see, for example, Blaenavon Lodge, General and Committee Meetings minutes, 19 June 1916, SWCC, MNA/NUM/L/11/4.
73. See, for example, Caerau Lodge, Annual, General and Committee Meetings minutes, 1906–33, SWCC, MNA/NUM/L/19/1–12, lists of recipients of tickets can be found at the back of each minute book; see, in particular, the lists for 1918, 1923 and 1924.

74. S. Thompson, "'Brodyr trwyadl mewn tywydd garw'": Welfare Provision and the Social Centrality of the South Wales Miners' Federation', *Welsh History Review*, 24:4 (2009), pp. 141–67.

75. Aberdare District Council Election Handbill, Thomas Bowen, Labour Party, 1908, Aberdare Central Library, Aberdare.

76. Ministry of Health, *First Report of the Welsh Consultative Council on Medical and Allied Services in Wales* [Cmd.703], 1920, xvii, pp. 5–6; the Welsh Hospital Survey found that the region only possessed one children's hospital (an institution of 25 beds provided by Cardiff County Borough) and one paediatrician, who was employed jointly by the Welsh National School of Medicine, Cardiff Royal Infirmary and Cardiff CBC; A. Trevor Jones, J. A. Nixon and R. M. F. Picken, *Hospital Survey: The Hospital Services of South Wales and Monmouthshire* (London: HMSO, 1945), p. 24 and p. 27.

4 Mantin, 'The Question of Oralism and the Experiences of Deaf Children'

1. P. Ladd, *Understanding Deaf Culture: In Search of Deafhood* (Clevedon: Multilingual Matters, 2003), p. 121; J. Rée, *I See a Voice: A Philosophical History of Language, Deafness and the Senses* (London: Harper Collins, 1999), p. 228; A. F. Dimmock, *Cruel Legacy: An Introduction to the Record of Deaf People in History* (Edinburgh: Scottish Workshop Publications, 1993), p. 32.

2. Second International Congress on Education of the Deaf (1880) cited in H. G. Lang, 'Perspectives on the History of Deaf Education', in M. Marschark and P. E. Spencer (eds), *Oxford Handbook of Deaf Studies, Language and Education* (Oxford: Oxford University Press, 2003), pp. 9–20, on p. 15.

3. R. Elliott, 'The Milan Congress and the Future of the Education of the Deaf and Dumb', in *Proceedings of the Conference of Head Masters of Institutions and of Other Workers for the Education of the Deaf and Dumb, 22–24 June, 1881* (London: W. H. Allen, 1882), pp. 7–18, on p. 18.

4. K. W. Hodgson, *The Deaf and their Problems: A Study in Special Education* (London: Watts & Co., 1953).

5. D. G. Pritchard, *Education and the Handicapped 1760–1960* (London: Routledge, 1963), p. 27.

6. See J. Vickrey Van Cleve, 'Preface', in J. Vickrey Van Cleve (ed.), *Deaf History Unveiled: Interpretations from the New Scholarship* (Washington, DC: Gallaudet University Press, 2000), pp. ix–x. Some use the capitalization of Deaf to refer to those who belonged to the deaf community.

7. Ladd, *Understanding*, p.4.

8. J. Branson and D. Miller, *Damned for their Difference: The Cultural Construction of Deaf People as Disabled* (Washington, DC: Gallaudet University Press, 2002); Ladd, *Understanding*; H. Lane, *The Mask of Benevolence: Disabling the Deaf Community* (New York: Knopf, 1993); O. Sacks, *Seeing Voices: A Journey into the World of the Deaf* (Berkeley, CA: University of California Press, 1989).

9. C. J. Kudlick, 'Disability History: Why We Need Another "Other"', *American Historical Review*, 108:3 (2003), pp. 763–93, on p. 781.

10. R. M. Buchanan, *Illusions of Equality: Deaf Americans in School and Factory 1850–1950* (Washington, DC: Gallaudet University Press, 1999), pp. 20–36.

11. Ibid., p. xiv.
12. F. Buton, 'Making Deaf Children Talk: Changes in Educational Policy towards the Deaf in the French Third Republic', in D. M. Turner and K. Stagg (eds.), *Social Histories of Disability and Deformity* (London: Routledge, 2006), pp. 117–25, on p. 119.
13. P. Beaver, *A Tower of Strength: Two Hundred Years of the Royal School for Deaf Children Margate* (Brighton: Book Guild, 1992), p. 29; Lang, 'Perspectives', p. 13; M. G. McLoughlin, *A History of the Education of the Deaf in England* (Liverpool: G. M. McLoughlin, 1987), p. 24.
14. Branson and Miller, *Damned for their Difference*, p. 123; I. Hutchison, 'Oralism: A Sign of the Times? The Contest for Deaf Communication in Nineteenth-century Scotland', *European Review of History*, 14:4 (2007), pp. 481–501, on p. 483.
15. P. Jackson, *A Pictorial History of Deaf Britain* (Winsford: Deafprint, 2001), p. 52.
16. Beaver, *A Tower of Strength*, p. 32.
17. Pritchard, *Education and the Handicapped*, p. 26.
18. J. S. Hurt, *Outside the Mainstream: A History of Special Education* (London: Batsford, 1988), p. 100.
19. Pritchard, *Education and the Handicapped*, p. 76; S. Tomlinson, *A Sociology of Special Education* (London: Routledge, 1982), p. 26.
20. P. H. Butterfield, 'The First Training Colleges for Teachers of the Deaf', *British Journal of Educational Studies*, 19:1 (1971), pp. 51–69, on p. 55.
21. *Proceedings of the Conference of Head Masters of Institutions and of Other Workers for the Education of the Deaf and Dumb, 24–26 July, 1877* (London: G. Hill, 1877), p. 18.
22. *British Medical Journal* (12 April 1884), p. 743.
23. Pritchard, *Education and the Handicapped*, p. 77; *British Medical Journal*, 1:1013 (1880), pp. 822–3.
24. *Report of the Royal Commission on the Blind, the Deaf and Dumb of the United Kingdom* (C. 5781), 1889 (hereafter Report of the RC), pp. xi–xii.
25. Ibid., pp. 406–89.
26. Ibid., p. 427.
27. Ibid., p. 298.
28. Ibid., p. 484.
29. D. C. Baynton, 'Savages and Deaf-Mutes: Evolutionary Theory and the Campaign against Sign Language in the Nineteenth Century', in J. V. Van Cleve (ed.), *Deaf History Unveiled*, pp. 92–112, on p. 99.
30. Rée, *I See*, p. 223; Ladd, *Understanding*, p. 118.
31. *Report of the RC*, p. 572. The importance of statistics in the eugenics movement is explored in R. Soloway, 'Counting the Degenerates: The Statistics of Race Deterioration in Edwardian England', *Journal of Contemporary History*, 17:1 (1982), pp. 137–64.
32. Branson and Miller, *Damned for their Difference*, p. 127.
33. *British Deaf-Mute*, 3:33 (July 1894), p. 114.
34. Other historians have pointed out the inaccuracy of reducing British deaf education to the dominance of one method. See McLoughlin, *A History of the Education of the Deaf*, p. 26; Branson and Miller, *Damned for their Difference*, p. 123.
35. Elliott, 'The Milan Congress', p. 18.
36. Hutchison, 'Oralism', p. 493.
37. Llandaff and Pontypridd had both founded deaf schools towards the end of the nineteenth century; the former created by the disillusioned ex-principal of the Cambrian Institution, in protest at the religious makeup of the committee. For more details about

Welsh deaf institutions, see D. Woodford, *A Man and his School: The Story of the Llandaff School for the Deaf and Dumb* (Cardiff: Llandaff Society, 1996); C. J. Moon, *A Tale of Three Deaf Schools in South Wales* (Warrington: British Deaf History Society, 2010).

38. Meeting of the [Cambrian Institution] Committee (hereafter CIC) 28 November 1849, Minute Book (hereafter MB) 1847–55, West Glamorgan Archives (hereafter WGA), Swansea, E/Cam 1/1.

39. Most deaf institutions at the time would use public demonstrations to raise funds and publicize their alleged success stories and the 'miracle' of deaf education. See, A. Borsay, 'Deaf Children and Charitable Education in Britain 1790–1914', in A. Borsay and P. Shapely (eds), *Medicine, Charity and Mutual Aid: The Consumption of Health and Welfare in Britain, c. 1550–1950* (Aldershot: Ashgate, 2007), pp. 71–90.

40. *Welshman,* 5 February 1847.

41. *Ephphatha: A Monthly Magazine, Published in the Interests of the Deaf* (May 1896), p. 78.

42. *Proceedings of the Conference of Head Masters,* 1877, p. 104.

43. Ibid., 1881, pp. 138–9.

44. *Thirtieth Annual Report of the Cambrian Institution for the Deaf and Dumb, Swansea, for the year ending 30th June, 1888,* p. 16.

45. B. H. Payne to Joseph Hall, 23 February 1879, Principal's Letter Book (hereafter PLB), 1876–1880, WGA, E/Cam 5/1.

46. Payne to Joseph Hall, 23 February 1879, PLB.

47. Payne to D. Buxton, 20 April 1880, PLB.

48. CIC, 15 October 1883, MB 1867–1887, WGA, E/Cam 1/3.

49. Payne to Mr John Davies, 5 April 1878, PLB.

50. Payne to Miss Maclaran, 10 January 1879, PLB.

51. *Annual Report 1888,* p. 18. This information was repeated in every Annual Report hereafter.

52. *Proceedings of the Conference of Head Masters of Institutions and of Other Workers for the Education of the Deaf and Dumb, 1–3 July, 1885* (Margate: W. H. Allen, 1886), p. 90.

53. H. Hendrick, 'The Child as Social Actor in Historical Sources: Problems of Identification and Interpretation', in P. Christensen and A. James (eds), *Research with Children: Perspectives and Practices* (London: Falmer, 2000), pp. 36–61, on p. 38. Davis and Watson also approach this question from a modern sociological perspective. See, J. M. Davis and N. Watson, 'Where Are the Children's Experiences? Analysing Social and Cultural Exclusion in "Special" and "Mainstream" Schools', *Disability & Society,* 16:5 (2001), pp. 671–87.

54. F. Armstrong, 'The Historical Development of Special Education: Humanitarian Rationality or "Wild Profusion of Entangled Events"?', *History of Education,* 31:5 (2002), pp. 437–56, on p. 438.

55. Hendrick, 'Child as Social Actor', p. 42.

56. J. Read and J. Walmsley, 'Historical Perspectives on Special Education, 1890–1970', *Disability & Society,* 21:5 (2006), pp. 455–69, on p. 457.

57. Payne to John Davies, 26 April 1879, PLB.

58. Payne to John Davies, 11 and 13 April 1878, PLB.

59. Payne to Miss Phillips, 15 July 1891, PLB, 1889–1893, WGA, E/Cam/5/2.

60. Payne to George Taylor, 25 June 1891, PLB, 1889–1893.

61. The British and international deaf community's challenge to oralism is summarized in Ladd, *Understanding,* pp. 124–8.

62. B. Grant, *The Deaf Advance: A History of the British Deaf Association* (Edinburgh: Pentland Press, 1990), p. 11.

63. Ladd, *Understanding*, p. 128.

64. M. Atherton, 'Reading Between the Lines: The Value of Deaf Newspapers as Research Resources', *Deaf Worlds*, 19:3 (2003), pp. 82–93, on p. 82. This is so far the only dedicated study of deaf newspapers in Britain, but this topic is explored further in Atherton's book on deaf leisure. M. Atherton *Deafness, Community and Culture in Britain: Leisure and Cohesion, 1945–1995* (Manchester: Manchester University Press, 2011). See also Jackson, *A Pictorial History*, p. 231; Ladd, *Understanding*, p. 52.

65. Atherton, 'Reading Between the Lines', p. 83; Jackson, *A Pictorial History*, p. 231.

66. *British Deaf-Mute*, 3:33 (July 1894), pp. 113–4.

67. Ibid., 3.34 (August 1894), p. 137.

68. *Our Monthly Church Messenger to the Deaf*, 2 (no date), p. 120. It is unclear how realistic the orally educated, elitist deaf people portrayed here would have been, but it has been noted by Rée that signs began to be a symbol of embarrassment to 'more respectable members of the deaf community'. Rée, *I See*, p. 236.

69. *Our Monthly Church Messenger to the Deaf*, 2, p. 148.

70. Rée, *I See*, p. 231.

71. *British Deaf-Mute*, 4:40 (February 1895), p. 57.

72. Ibid., 3:35 (September 1894), p. 150.

73. Ibid., 3:36 (October 1894), p. 175.

74. See Sacks, *Seeing Voices*, p. 28.

5 Monk and Manning, 'Exploring Patient Experience in an Australian Institution for Children with Learning Disabilities'

1. No title, *Argus* (Melbourne), 5 January 1887, p. 5.

2. D. Wright, *Mental Disability in Victorian England: The Earlswood Asylum, 1847–1901* (Oxford: Oxford University Press, 2001), p. 97.

3. D. Atkinson and J. Walmsley, 'Using Autobiographical Approaches with People with Learning Difficulties', *Disability and Society*, 14:2 (1999), pp. 203–16.

4. For example, M. Potts and R. Fido, *'A Fit Person to be Removed': Personal Accounts of Life in a Mental Deficiency Institution* (Plymouth: Northcote House, 1991); 'Mabel Cooper's Life Story', in D. Atkinson, M. Jackson, and J. Walmsley (eds), *Forgotten Lives: Exploring the History of Learning Disability* (Kidderminster: BILD Publications, 1997), pp. 21–34.

5. J. Walmsley, 'Institutionalization: A Historical Perspective', in K. Johnson and R. Traustadóttir (eds), *Deinstitutionalization and People with Intellectual Disabilities: In and Out of Institutions* (London: Jessica Kingsley, 2005), pp. 50–65, on pp. 52–3.

6. C. Fox, '"Forehead Low, Aspect Idiotic": Intellectual Disability in Victorian Asylums, 1870–1887', in C. Coleborne and D. MacKinnon (eds), *'Madness' in Australia: Histories, Heritage and the Asylum* (St Lucia: University of Queensland Press, 2003), pp. 145–56, on p. 153.

7. *Lunacy Statute 1867*, s. 21; *Lunacy Act 1890*, s. 31; *Lunacy Act 1903*, s. 37.

8. J. Andrews, 'Case Notes, Case Histories and the Patient's Experience of Insanity at Gartnavel Royal Asylum, Glasgow, in the Nineteenth Century', *Social History of Medicine*, 11:2 (1998), pp. 255–81, on pp. 264–6.

9. G. Reaume, "'Keep Your Labels Off My Mind"! Or "Now I Am Going to Pretend I Am Craze but Don't Be A Bit Alarmed": Psychiatric History from the Patients' Perspectives', *Canadian Bulletin of Medical History*, 11:2 (1994), pp. 397–424, on p. 401; K. Johnson, *Deinstitutionalising Women: An Ethnographic Study of Institutional Closure* (Cambridge: Cambridge University Press, 1998), p. 57.

10. Fox, 'Forehead Low', p. 147.

11. Public Record Office Victoria (hereafter PROV), VPRS 7420/P1, Unit 3, p. 54.

12. Reaume, 'Keep Your Labels', p. 399 and p. 402.

13. Ibid., p. 397 and p. 399; G. Reaume, 'Portraits of People with Mental Disorders in English Canadian History', *Canadian Bulletin of Medical History*, 17:1 and 17:2 (2000), pp. 93–125, on pp. 99–100.

14. J. Ryan with F. Thomas, *The Politics of Mental Handicap* (London: Free Association Books, 1987).

15. R. Traustadóttir and K. Johnson, 'Introduction: In and Out of Institutions', in Traustadóttir and Johnson (eds), *Deinstitutionalization*, pp. 13–29, on pp. 18–19.

16. Wright, *Mental Disability*, pp. 25–6, and p. 137; D. Gladstone, 'The Changing Dynamic of Institutional Care: The Western Counties Idiot Asylum, 1864–1914', in D. Wright and A. Digby (eds), *From Idiocy to Mental Deficiency: Historical Perspectives on People with Learning Disabilities* (London: Routledge, 1996), pp. 134–60, on p. 138.

17. Wright, *Mental Disability*, pp. 26–36.

18. Ibid., p. 138.

19. Ibid.

20. Gladstone, 'The Changing Dynamic', pp. 137–8.

21. Wright, *Mental Disability*, pp. 41, 138, 144–9, 153; Gladstone, 'The Changing Dynamic', pp. 151–4.

22. Report of the Inspector of Lunatic Asylums on the Hospitals for the Insane, 1875, *Victorian Parliamentary Papers* (hereafter *VPP*), 1876, vol. 2, p. 12.

23. Report of the Inspector of Lunatic Asylums, 1875, p. 12.

24. Royal Commission on Asylums for the Insane and Inebriate, *VPP*, vol. 2, 1886 (hereafter Royal Commission), Minutes of Evidence (hereafter ME), Q.9180–3, p. 380; Q.9627–31, pp. 405–6; Q.10323–7, p. 436; Q.12942–7, p. 550.

25. Royal Commission, ME, Q.9383, p. 394.

26. Royal Commission, ME, Q.8677–80, p. 349; Q.9310–11, p. 300; Q.9383–6, p. 394; Q.9625, p. 405; Q.10322–5, p. 436; Q.11027–9, p. 477; Q. 12345, p. 529; Q.12949–50, p. 550.

27. Report of the Inspector of Lunatic Asylums, 1875, p. 12.

28. Royal Commission, ME, Q.9310, p. 390; Q.9383, p. 394; Fox, 'Forehead Low', pp. 153–4.

29. Royal Commission, ME, Q.9625, p. 405.

30. Inspector to the Chief Secretary, PROV, VPRS 3992/P, Unit 176, File 87/J3370; Report of Inspector of Asylums on the Hospitals for the Insane, 1887, *VPP*, 1888, vol. III, p. 5.

31. Report of the Inspector-General of the Insane (hereafter Report of IGI), 1907, *VPP*, 1908, vol. I, p. 3.

32. J. V. McCreery, 'Idiocy and Juvenile Insanity in Victoria', *Intercolonial Medical Congress of Australasia* (Sydney: Charles Potter, 1893), pp. 665–8, on pp. 665–6.

33. PROV, VPRS 7419/P1, Units 1 and 2; VPRS 7420/P1, Unit 1.

34. Royal Commission, ME, Q.11023–6, p. 477.

35. Ryan, *Politics of Mental Handicap*, pp. 104–8; Wright, *Mental Disability*, pp. 188–91; M. Jackson, 'Institutional Provision for the Feeble-Minded in Edwardian England: Sandlebridge and the Scientific Morality of Permanent Care', in Wright and Digby (eds), *From Idiocy to Mental Deficiency*, pp. 161–83, on pp. 168–72.
36. R. Jones, 'The Master Potter and the Rejected Pots: Eugenic Legislation in Victoria, 1918–1939', *Australian Historical Studies*, 30:113 (October 1999), pp. 319–42, p. 324.
37. 'The Mentally Infirm', *Argus*, 12 March 1913, p. 12.
38. Report of IGI, 1912, *VPP*, vol. II, 1913, pp. 60–1; 'Feeble-Minded Children', *Argus*, 13 February 1913, p. 12; 'Feeble-Minded Children: "Danger to Community"', *Argus*, 5 April 1913, p. 9.
39. J. Lewis, 'Removing the Grit: The Development of Special Education in Victoria, 1887–1947' (PhD dissertation, La Trobe University, 1989).
40. Report of IGI, 1912, p. 61.
41. Ibid., 1907, *VPP*, vol. I, 1908, p. 3; 1925, *VPP*, vol. 2, 1927, p. 4.
42. McCreery, 'Idiocy', pp. 665–7; PROV, VPRS 7420/P1, Unit 1, p. 25, p. 145, p. 173, p. 251, p. 271, p. 288, p. 303, p. 345, p. 351; Unit 2, p. 19, p. 29, p. 33; VPRS 7419/P1, Unit 1, p. 26, p. 70, pp. 101–2, p. 121, p. 176, p. 211, p. 226, pp. 228–9, p. 242, p. 256 and p. 286.
43. A. Henry, 'Teaching the Unteachable', *Argus*, 8 January 1898, p. 14.
44. PROV, VPRS 7420/P1, Unit 1, p. 1 and p. 57.
45. Report of IGI, 1907, p. 28 and p. 31.
46. Ibid., 1909, *VPP*, vol. 2, 1910, p. 47.
47. For example Jones to the Chief Secretary, 4 October 1911, PROV, VPRS 3992/P, Unit 1334, File 1914/P4037; PROV, Jones to the Under Secretary, 15 July 1916, VPRS 3992/P, Unit 1420, File 1916/U8760; VPRS 892/P, Unit 89, File 1113 and Unit 102, File 1196, *passim*.
48. Lewis, 'Removing the Grit', p. 309.
49. Appendix A, Draft of Suggested Recommendations for the Minister, 6 February 1911, PROV, VPRS 892/P, Unit 89, File 1113.
50. 'Lunatic Asylums: Shocking Neglect', *Argus*, 7 February 1922, p. 7; 'Neglected Asylums', *Argus*, 8 February 1922, p. 11; 'Kew Asylum Buildings', *Argus*, 9 February 1922, p. 7; 'Kew Asylum Buildings', *Argus*, 11 February 1922, p. 21.
51. 'Kew Asylum Administration', *Argus*, 27 November 1924, p. 13.
52. Visitors Book, 26 March 1923, PROV, VPRS 7468/P1, Unit 2, p. 97.
53. Ibid., 31 October 1922, pp. 91–2.
54. Wright, *Mental Disability*, pp. 137–8.
55. Henry, 'Teaching the Unteachable', p. 14.
56. Ryan, *Politics of Mental Handicap*, pp. 92–3; A. Borsay, *Disability and Social Policy in Britain since 1750: A History of Exclusion* (Basingstoke: Palgrave Macmillan, 2005), p. 101.
57. McCreery, 'Idiocy', p. 666.
58. PROV, VPRS 7419/P1, Unit 1, p. 110 and p. 200.
59. D. O'Driscoll and J. Walmsley, 'Absconding from Hospitals: A Means of Resistance?', *British Journal of Learning Disabilities*, 38:2 (2010), pp. 97–102, on p. 101.
60. PROV, VPRS 7420/P1, Unit 1, p. 35, p. 107, p. 129, p. 143, p. 153, p. 157, p. 169, p. 325; Unit 3, p. 52, p. 60, p. 93, p. 96, p. 98; VPRS 7419/P1, Unit 1, p. 88, p. 110, p. 182, p. 229, p. 310, p. 328; Unit 2, p. 71; Department of Health Services Archives (hereafter

DHSA), 92/184, Unit 2, File Dennis H. and Unit 3, File Francis M.; Fox, 'Forehead Low', p. 153.

61. Wright, *Mental Disability*, p. 97.
62. PROV, VPRS 7419/P1, Unit 1, p. 229.
63. PROV, VPRS 7448/P1, Unit 1, File 57; also VPRS 7420/P1, Unit 3, p. 54 and p. 98; VPRS 7419/P1, Unit 1, p. 229.
64. PROV, VPRS 7420/P1, Unit 3, p. 34; 'Boy's Body in the Yarra', *Argus*, 19 February 1910, p. 20.
65. Compare O'Driscoll and Walmsley, 'Absconding', pp. 101–2.
66. Wright, *Mental Disability*, pp. 142–3.
67. Henry, 'Teaching the Unteachable', p. 14.
68. McCreery, 'Idiocy', p. 667; Memo, Superintendent McCreery to the Inspector of Asylums, 20 March 1890, PROV, VPRS 3992/P, Box 341, File 90/P3520.
69. L. Monk, '"Made Enquiries, Can Elicit No History of Injury": Researching the History of Institutional Abuse in the Archives', *Provenance* (September 2007), at www.prov.vic.gov.au/provenance/no6/MadeEnquiries1.asp [accessed 15 April 2011].
70. PROV, VPRS 7419/P1, Unit 1, 10 January 1906, p. 42.
71. PROV, VPRS 7420/P1, Unit 1, 14 June 1906, p. 168.
72. PROV, VPRS 4723/P, Unit 493, 1917/W4997.
73. PROV, VPRS 7420/P1, Units 1 and 2 and VPRS 7419/P1, Unit 1.
74. For example, PROV, VPRS 7420/P1, Unit 1, p. 75, p. 153, p. 229.
75. PROV, VPRS 7420/P1, Units 1 and 2 and VPRS 7419/P1, Unit 1. The 'destination' of the remaining proportion of patients for these years is unknown.
76. PROV, VPRS 7420/P1, Unit 3, VPRS 7449/P1, Unit 1; DHSA, 92/184, Units 1–4; PROV VPRS 7419/P1 Unit 2 and VPRS 7448/P1, Unit 1.
77. Kew Cottages History Project www.latrobe.edu.au/history/kew_project.html [accessed 15 April 2011].
78. C. Manning, '"My Memory's Back!" Inclusive Learning Disability Research using Ethics, Oral History and Digital Storytelling', *British Journal of Learning Disabilities*, 38:3 (2010), pp. 160–7; C. Manning, *Bye-Bye Charlie: Stories from the Vanishing World of Kew Cottages* (Sydney: UNSW Press, 2008).
79. 'Kew Asylum Inspected', *Argus*, 17 March 1922, p. 8; Visitors Book, PROV, VPRS 7468/P1, Unit 2, pp. 87–97, *passim*.
80. 'Kew Idiot Asylum Improvements', *Argus*, 17 December 1924, p. 22.
81. Report of IGI, 1928, *VPP*, vol. 1, 1930, p. 23.
82. E. Rowe, Interview with C. Manning, Kew Cottages History Project Archive, Melbourne, La Trobe University, 20 April 2006 (hereafter Rowe Interview).
83. Visitors Book, 29 September 1926, PROV, VPRS 7468/P1, Unit 2, p. 139.
84. Rowe Interview.
85. 30 June 1931, Visitors Book, PROV, VPRS 7468/P1, Unit 2, p. 187.
86. L. Monk, 'Exploiting Patient Labour at Kew Cottages, Australia, 1887–1950', *British Journal of Learning Disabilities*, 38:2 (2010), pp. 86–94, on p. 91; Manning, *Bye-Bye Charlie*, pp. 156–9.
87. PROV, VPRS 7420/P1, Unit 3, p. 36.
88. We would like to acknowledge Ms Kerrie Soraghan for first suggesting this to us.
89. S. D. Porteus, *A Psychologist of Sorts: The Autobiography and Publications of the Inventor of the Porteus Maze Tests* (California: Pacific Books, 1969), pp. 37–8.
90. Rowe Interview.

91. Ibid.
92. Ibid.
93. PROV, VPRS 7420/P1, Unit 3, p. 98.
94. For example, ibid., p. 18, p. 22, p. 48, p. 50 and p. 96.
95. P. Carpenter, 'Resistance and Control: Mutinies at Brentry', in D. Mitchell et al. (eds), *Exploring Experiences of Advocacy by People with Learning Disabilities: Testimonies of Resistance* (London and Philadelphia, PA: Jessica Kingsley, 2006), pp. 172–8.
96. Rowe Interview.
97. Ibid.; Report of IGI, 1928, p. 26; Inspector-General to the Director of Education, 18 September 1916, PROV, VPRS 892/P0, Unit 102, File 1196.
98. Jones, 'The Master Potter', p. 325.
99. Ibid., pp. 319–42.
100. Report of IGI, 1926, *VPP*, vol. 2, 1927, p. 39.
101. M. L. Jones, *Colony to Community: The Janefield and Kingsbury Training Centres* (Kew: Janefield and Kingsbury Redevelopment Project with Australian Scholarly Publishing, 1997), p. 40.
102. Report of IGI, 1926, p. 39.
103. Ibid., 1935, *VPP*, vol. 1, 1934, p. 24.
104. Ibid., 1933, p. 24.
105. Rowe Interview; Report of IGI, 1932, *VPP*, vol. 1, 1933, p. 27.
106. Rowe Interview; Manning, *Bye-Bye Charlie*, pp. 118–19.

6 Borsay, 'From Representation to Experience'

1. V. Long and H. Marland, 'From Danger and Motherhood to Health and Beauty: Health Advice for the Factory Girl in Early Twentieth-Century Britain', *Twentieth-Century British History*, 20:4 (2009), pp. 454–81, on pp. 454–5.
2. E. Pritchard, *The New-Born Baby: A Manual for the Use of Mid-wives and Maternity Nurses* (London: Henry Kimpton, 1934).
3. F. Horspool, *Mothercraft for Schoolgirls* (London: Macmillan, 1914).
4. C. Urwin and C. Sharland, 'From Bodies to Minds in Childcare Literature: Advice to Parents in Inter-War Britain', in R. Cooter (ed.), *In the Name of the Child: Health and Welfare, 1880–1940* (London: Routledge, 1992), pp. 174–99.
5. *Mother and Child: The Official Organ of the National Council for Maternity and Child Welfare*, 1:1 (1930).
6. *Motherhood: A Guide for Mothers*, 8th edn (Guildford: Cow and Gate, no date).
7. *A Moving Sight* (London: Scope, 1964).
8. H. Graham, 'Images of Pregnancy in Antenatal Literature', in R. Dingwall, C. Heath, M. Reid and M. Stacey (eds), *Health Care and Health Knowledge* (London: Croom Helm, 1977), pp. 15–37, on p. 21.
9. Urwin and Sharland, 'From Bodies', p. 177.
10. F. Truby King, *Feeding and Care of Baby* (London: Macmillan, 1913), p. 36.
11. D. King, *In the Name of Liberalism: Illiberal Social Policy in the United States and Britain* (Oxford: Oxford University Press, 1999), pp. 51–7.
12. Infant mortality is defined as the death of children before their first birthday.
13. A. Oakley, *The Captured Womb: A History of the Medical Care of Pregnant Women* (Oxford: Blackwell, 1984), pp. 12–4, 37.

14. J. Lewis, *The Politics of Motherhood: Child and Maternal Welfare in England, 1900–1939* (London: Croom Helm, 1980), pp. 89–113.
15. G. Tucker, *Mother, Baby, and Nursery: A Manual for Mothers* (London: T. Fisher Unwin, 1900), pp. xiii–xiv.
16. J. S. Fairbairn, 'Introduction', in M. Liddiard, *The Mothercraft Manual* (London: J. and A. Churchill, 1924), p. xii.
17. A. R. Dafoe, *Baby-Guide for Mothers* (London: Constable, 1936), 'Foreword'.
18. J. B. Dawson, *The Young Mother* (London: Ewart, Seymour and Co., 1912); J. B. Dawson, *Babyhood* (London: Ewart, Seymour and Co., 1912).
19. L. E. Ashby and K. Atherton Earp, *The Coming of Baby* (London: Scientific Press, 1925), p. 11.
20. A. M. Hewer, 'Introduction', in J. L. Hewer, *Our Baby: For Mothers and Nurses*, 12th edn (1891; Bristol: John Wright and Sons Ltd, 1910), p. v.
21. E. A. Cocker, *What does my Baby Want? Health Requirements from before Birth to One Year: Practical Talks on Infant Care by a Mother to Mothers* (London: Lutterworth's Ltd, 1926), 'Preface', p. 42.
22. A. Borsay, 'Disciplining Disabled Bodies: The Development of Orthopaedic Medicine in Britain, *c.* 1800–1939', in D. M. Turner and K. Stagg (eds), *Social Histories of Disability and Deformity* (London: Routledge, 2006), pp. 97–116, on p. 101.
23. Tucker, *Mother*, p. 7.
24. *Report of the Inter-Departmental Committee on Physical Deterioration*, Cd. 2175 (London: HMSO, 1904), pp. 13–14.
25. Dawson, *Young Mother*, p. 2 and p. 37.
26. Tucker, *Mother*, p. 1, p. 2, p. 4, p. 7, p. 8, p. 16.
27. E. Pantin, *Preparing for Motherhood and Training in Infancy and Childhood* (London and Hereford: Hereford Times, 1932), p. 5.
28. Tucker, *Mother*, p. 17, p. 19, and p. 21.
29. Hewer, *Our Baby* (1910), p. 19.
30. Cocker, *What does my Baby Want?*, p. 58.
31. King, *Feeding*, p. 11.
32. Tucker, *Mother*, p. 94.
33. Dafoe, *Baby-Guide*, p. 83, and p. 231; Dawson, *Babyhood*, p. 66; *Every Woman's Doctor Book* (London: Amalgamated Press, 1934), p. 141, and p. 145; Hewer, *Our Baby* (1910), p. 139, p. 140, and p. 151.
34. Dawson, *Babyhood*, p. 67.
35. Cocker, *What does my Baby Want?* p. 59; *Every Woman's Doctor Book*, pp. 138–9, p. 142, and p. 145.
36. Hewer, *Our Baby* (1891), pp. 6–12.
37. Hewer, *Our Baby* (1910), pp. 114–16.
38. W. Ernst, 'The Normal and the Abnormal: Reflections on Norms and Normativity', in W. Ernst (ed.), *Histories of the Normal and the Abnormal: Social and Cultural Histories of Norms and Normativity* (London: Routledge, 2006), pp. 1–25, on pp. 2–3.
39. Hewer, *Our Baby* (1891), pp. 86–7.
40. Tucker, *Mother*, p. 48, p. 51, and p. 52; Hewer, *Our Baby* (1910), p. 49, pp. 51–5, and p. 87; Dawson, *Babyhood*, p. 6.
41. D. Armstrong, *Political Anatomy of the Body: Medical Knowledge in Britain in the Twentieth Century* (Cambridge: Cambridge University Press, 1983), pp. 9, 11, 42, 51, 64, 66–7, and 86–7.

42. Hewer, *Our Baby* (1891), p. 11; Hewer, *Our Baby* (1910), p. 51, and p. 116.
43. Dawson, *Babyhood*, p. 60.
44. Hewer, *Our Baby* (1891), pp. 113–15; Hewer, *Our Baby* (1910), pp. 149–50.
45. T. Dormandy, *The White Death: A History of Tuberculosis* (London and New York: Hambledon, 1999), pp. 161–75.
46. Hewer, *Our* Baby (1891), pp. 7–9; Hewer, *Our Baby* (1910), p. 115, p. 151, and pp. 156–7; Dawson, *Babyhood*, pp. 66–7.
47. R. Cooter, *Surgery and Society in Peace and War: Orthopaedics and the Organization of Modern Medicine, 1880–1948* (Basingstoke: Macmillan, 1993), pp. 152–79.
48. Hewer, *Our Baby* (1910), p. 115, and pp. 156–7.
49. Ibid., p. 116, and pp. 151–2.
50. J. Mechling, 'Advice to Historians on Advice to Mothers', *Journal of Social History*, 9:1 (1975), pp. 44–63, on p. 44.
51. Urwin and Sharland, 'From Bodies', pp. 186–8, and pp. 191–4.
52. B. Spock, *The Common Sense Book of Baby and Child Care* (New York: Duell, Sloan and Pearce, 1945), pp. 3–4.
53. D. M. Taylor, 'Introduction', in M. Liddiard, *The Mothercraft Manual*, 11th edn (London: J. and A. Churchill, 1948), pp. xii–xiii.
54. A. Cuthbert, *Housewife Baby Book: A Guide to the Welfare of the Young Family* (London: Hulton Press, 1948), pp. 7–8.
55. C. Beels, *The Childbirth Book* (London: Granada, 1980).
56. J. Gibbens, *The Care of Young Babies*, 3rd edn (London: J. and A. Churchill, 1953), p. 191, Appendix 1.
57. S. Kitzinger, *Pregnancy and Childbirth* (Harmondsworth: Penguin, 1980), p. 136.
58. G. Bourne, *Pregnancy* (1972; London: Cassell, 1979), p. 21.
59. P. Leach, *Baby and Child: From Birth to Age Five* (Harmondsworth: Penguin Books, 1977), p. 24, and p. 472.
60. H. Jolly, *Book of Child Care: The Complete Guide for Today's Parents* (London: George Allen and Unwin, 1975), pp. 388–97, pp. 432–7, pp. 477–89, and pp. 514–60.
61. Bourne, *Pregnancy*, pp. 503–4.
62. Good Housekeeping Family Centre, *Good Housekeeping's Mothercraft* (London: National Magazine Co. Ltd, 1959), pp. 235–42.
63. Jolly, *Book of Child Care*, pp. 389–90, pp. 395–6, and pp. 545–8; E. Rudinger (ed.), *The Newborn Baby* (London: Consumers' Association, 1972), pp. 55–6, and p. 67.
64. Jolly, *Book of Child Care*, pp. 254–5, and p. 485; Leach, *Baby and Child*, p. 475.
65. Gibbens, *The Care of Young Babies*, p. v.
66. G. Chamberlain, *The Safety of the Unborn Child* (Harmondsworth: Penguin, 1969), p. 126; Jolly, *Book of Child Care*, p. 388.
67. Bourne, *Pregnancy*, pp. 467–8.
68. Jolly, *Book of Child Care*, p. 24; Kitzinger, *Pregnancy*, pp. 44–52.
69. Oakley, *Captured Womb*, p. 89.
70. S. Pitt, 'Private Lives and Public Bodies: Childbirth in Post-War Swansea', in A. Borsay (ed.), *Public Service or Private Commodity? Medicine in Wales, c. 1800–2000* (Cardiff: University of Wales Press, 2003), pp. 154–70, on p. 166.
71. Oakley, *Captured Womb*, pp. 172–3.
72. Bourne, *Pregnancy*, pp. 504–5; Kitzinger, *Pregnancy*, pp. 183–7.
73. W. J. Gagen and J. P. Bishop, 'Ethics, Justification and the Prevention of Spina Bifida', *Journal of Medical Ethics*, 33 (2007), pp. 501–7, on p. 505.

74. Bourne, *Pregnancy*, p. 505.
75. T. Shakespeare, *Disability Rights and Wrongs* (London: Routledge, 2006), pp. 85–102.
76. Liddiard, *Mothercraft Manual* (1948), p. 3; E. Morrison, *Babies: Advice by Letter* (London: Ernest Benn, 1949), p. 17.
77. J. Peel, 'Foreword', in Chamberlain, *Safety*, p. 8.
78. Chamberlain, *Safety*, p. 91.
79. Jolly, *Book of Child Care*, p. 28.
80. Bourne, *Pregnancy*, p. 91.
81. Kitzinger, *Pregnancy*, p. 84.
82. Chamberlain, *Safety*, pp. 98–100.
83. Bourne, *Pregnancy*, p. 175.
84. Ibid., p. 176; Kitzinger, *Pregnancy*, p. 99.
85. Sunday Times Insight Team, *Suffer the Children: The Story of Thalidomide* (London: Futura Publications, 1979), p. 151.
86. Kitzinger, *Pregnancy*, pp. 94–8.
87. Bourne, *Pregnancy*, p. 179.
88. Kitzinger, *Pregnancy*, p. 94.
89. A. S. Williams, *Women and Childbirth in the Twentieth Century* (Stroud: Sutton, 1997), p. 220.
90. Good Housekeeping Family Centre, *Good Housekeeping's Mothercraft*, p. 71.
91. Bourne, *Pregnancy*, p. 167. See also Kitzinger, *Pregnancy*, p. 92.
92. Beels, *Childbirth Book*, p. 27.
93. A. Cuthbert, *Housewife Baby Book: A Guide to the General Principles of Mothercraft*, 2nd edn (London: Hulton Press, 1955), p. 11. See also National Association for the Prevention of Infant Mortality, *Mothercraft* (London: National League for Physical Education and Improvement, 1915) p. viii.
94. Cuthbert, *Housewife Baby Book* (1948), p. 95; Leach, *Baby and Child*, p. 37, p. 79, p. 126, and p. 201.
95. Jolly, *Book of Child Care*, p. 109, and p. 217.
96. Liddiard, *Mothercraft Manual* (1948), p. v.
97. Bourne, *Pregnancy*, pp. 476–96, and pp. 502–8.
98. Rudinger (ed.), *Newborn Baby*, p. 51.
99. Jolly, *Book of Child Care*, pp. 521–2.
100. Gibbens, *The Care of Young Babies*, pp. 120–1, and pp. 132–3.
101. Rudinger (ed.), *Newborn Baby*, p. 3.
102. Leach, *Baby and Child*, p. 48.
103. Gibbens, *The Care of Young Babies*, pp. 71–2.
104. Rudinger (ed.), *Newborn Baby*, p. 54.
105. Gagen and Bishop, 'Ethics', p. 504; Jolly, *Book of Child Care*, p. 396.
106. Good Housekeeping Family Centre, *Good Housekeeping's Mothercraft*, p. 115; Rudinger (ed.), *Newborn Baby*, pp. 52–3.
107. Jolly, *Book of Child Care*, p. 552; Good Housekeeping Family Centre, *Good Housekeeping's Mothercraft*, p. 64.
108. Rudinger (ed.), *Newborn Baby*, p. 67.
109. Ibid., p. 41; Jolly, *Book of Child Care*, p. 516.
110. Good Housekeeping Family Centre, *Good Housekeeping's Mothercraft*, p. 239.
111. S. Bruley, *Women in Britain since 1900* (Basingstoke: Macmillan, 1999), pp. 128–34.
112. Good Housekeeping Family Centre, *Good Housekeeping's Mothercraft*, p. 237, and p. 239.

113. Jolly, *Book of Child Care*, p. 552.
114. Good Housekeeping Family Centre, *Good Housekeeping's Mothercraft*, p. 236.
115. Ibid., p. 240.
116. Jolly, *Book of Child Care*, pp. 524–5.
117. M. Bayley, *Mental Handicap and Community Care: A Study of Mentally Handicapped People in Sheffield* (London: Routledge and Kegan Paul, 1973), pp. 208–61; C. Glendinning, *Unshared Care: Parents and their Disabled Children* (London: Routledge and Kegan Paul, 1983), pp. 41–111.
118. K. Jones, *A History of the Mental Health Services* (London: Routledge and Kegan Paul, 1972), pp. 198–215.
119. Good Housekeeping Family Centre, *Good Housekeeping's Mothercraft*, p. 241.
120. K. Jones with J. Brown, W. J. Cunningham, J. Roberts and P. Williams, *Opening the Door: A Study of New Policies for the Mentally Handicapped* (London: Routledge and Kegan Paul, 1975); M. Oswin, *The Empty Hours: A Study of the Week-End Life of Handicapped Children in Institutions* (London: Allen Lane, 1971).
121. Good Housekeeping Family Centre, *Good Housekeeping's Mothercraft*, p. 241.
122. Jolly, *Book of Child Care*, pp. 540–1.
123. E. Page, 'Obituary: Benjamin Spock, World's Pediatrician, Dies at 84' (19 March 1998), at http:// www.nytimes.com/learning/general/onthisday/bday/0502.html [accessed 15 March 2011].
124. Hewer, *Our Baby* (1910), 'Preface to the Twelfth Edition'.
125. Cuthbert, *Housewife Baby Book* (1955), p. 7.
126. Mechling, 'Advice', pp. 45–6.
127. Fairbairn, 'Introduction', p. xvi.
128. S. Pooley, '"All We Parents Want Is That Our Children's Health and Lives Should Be Regarded": Child Health and Parental Concern in England, *c.* 1860–1910', *Social History of Medicine*, 23:3 (2010), pp. 528–48, on p. 532.
129. Hewer, 'Introduction', p. iv.
130. A. Davis, '"The Ordinary Good Mother": Women's Construction of their Identity as Mothers, Oxfordshire, *c.* 1945–1970', in A. Brown (ed.), *Historical Perspectives on Social Identities* (Newcastle: Cambridge Scholars Press, 2006), pp. 114–28, on p. 121; E. Roberts, *A Woman's Place: An Oral History of Working-Class Women, 1890–1940* (Oxford: Basil Blackwell, 1984), pp. 23–4.
131. M. Young and P. Willmott, *Family and Kinship in East London* (1957; Harmondsworth: Penguin, 1962), p. 54.
132. Roberts, *A Woman's Place*, p. 177.
133. P. Willmott and M. Young, *Family and Class in a London Suburb* (1960; London: New English Library, 1976), p. 70.
134. P. M. Matthews, 'The Young Child', in P. J. Cunningham (ed.), *The Principles of Health Visiting* (London: Faber and Faber, 1967), pp. 60–81; G. Owen, 'The Development of Health Visiting as a Profession', in G. Owen (ed.), *Health Visiting* (London: Balliére Tindall, 1977), pp. 1–29.
135. J. and E. Newson, *Patterns of Infant Care in an Urban Community* (1963; Harmondsworth: Penguin, 1965), p. 24; A. Oakley, *From Here to Maternity: Becoming a Mother* (1979; Harmondsworth: Penguin, 1981), p. 278.
136. S. Humphries and P. Gordon, *Out of Sight: The Experience of Disability, 1900–1950* (Plymouth: Northcote House, 1992), p. 19.

137. C. Hannam, *Parents and Mentally Handicapped Children* (Harmondsworth: Penguin, 1975), p. 14.
138. Glendinning, *Unshared Care*, p. 30.
139. C. C. Park, *The Siege: The Battle for Communication with an Autistic Child* (1967; Harmondsworth: Penguin, 1972), p. 19, and p. 25.
140. Glendinning, *Unshared Care*, pp. 22–31; M. Brock, *Christopher: A Silent Life* (London: Bedford Square Press, 1984), p. 3; J. Copeland, *For the Love of Ann: Based on a Diary by Jack Hodges* (London: Arrow, 1973), p. 19.
141. S. Cartwright, *Why My Child?: The Grief, Shock and Anguish of Parents with Handicapped Children* (London: Rigby, 1981), p. 47.
142. A. Green, *Cultural History* (Basingstoke: Palgrave Macmillan, 2008).
143. Mechling, 'Advice', p. 55.
144. J. McLaughlin, D. Goodley, E. Clavering and P. Fisher, *Families Raising Disabled Children: Enabling Care and Social Justice* (Basingstoke: Palgrave Macmillan, 2008), p. ix.
145. G. H. Landsman, *Reconstructing Motherhood and Disability in the Age of 'Perfect' Babies* (New York: Routledge, 2009), p. 142.
146. Oakley, *From Here*, pp. 67–8.
147. E. Shorter, 'The History of the Doctor-Patient Relationship', in W. F. Bynum and R. Porter (eds), *Companion Encyclopaedia of the History of Medicine*, Vol. 2 (London: Routledge, 1993), pp. 783–800, on pp. 787–92; M. Pugh, *Women and the Women's Movement in Britain, 1914–1999*, 2nd edn (Basingstoke: Macmillan, 2000), pp. 44–50, and pp. 83–90.
148. D. Elbourne, *Is the Baby All Right? Current Trends in British Perinatal Health* (London: Junction Books, 1981) pp. 16–25, and pp. 93–121.
149. Shorter, 'History', pp. 792–7; Bruley, *Women*, pp. 119–28, pp. 140–6, and pp. 158–74.
150. Good Housekeeping Family Centre, *Good Housekeeping's Mothercraft*, p. 240.
151. Jolly, *Book of Child Care*, p. 523.
152. Bayley, *Mental Handicap*, pp. 186–93; Glendinning, *Unshared Care*, pp. 31–40.
153. M. Hogg, 'A Mother's Story', in L. Medus, *No Hand to Hold and No Legs to Dance On: A Thalidomide Survivor's Story* (Bedlinog, Mid-Glamorgan: Accent Press, 2009), pp. 169–84, on p. 173.
154. S. Rolph and D. Atkinson, 'Emotion in Narrating the History of Learning Disability', *Oral History*, 38:2 (2010), pp. 53–63, on p. 57.
155. A. Turner, 'The History of Learning Disability in Glasgow, 1945 to the Present' (PhD dissertation, Strathclyde University, 2009), p. 134. See also pp. 122–4.
156. Turner, 'History', p. 175.
157. B. Spock and M. O. Lerrigo, *Caring for Your Disabled Child* (New York: Macmillan, 1965), p. 1, and p. 26.
158. P. Russell, *The Wheelchair Child* (London: Souvenir Press, 1978), p. 9.
159. J. Stone and F. Taylor, *A Handbook for Parents with a Handicapped Child* (London: Arrow, 1977), p. 7.
160. J. W. Scott, 'The Evidence of Experience', *Critical Inquiry*, 17:4 (1991), p. 778.
161. S. E. Kelly, '"A Different Light" – Examining Impairment through Parent Narratives of Childhood Disability', *Journal of Contemporary Ethnography*, 34:2 (2005), pp. 180–205, on p. 182.
162. Spock and Lerrigo, *Caring*, p. 7.

7 Förhammar and Nelson, 'Treating Children with Non-Pulmonary Tuberculosis in Sweden'

1. A. Winka, *Kyrkogården berättar: Minnesskrift om Apelvikens kyrkogård* (Varberg: Göranssons bokhandel, 1993), pp. 5–6.
2. A. Noymer and B. Jarosz, 'Causes of Death in Nineteenth-Century New England: The Dominance of Infectious Disease', *Social History of Medicine*, 21:3 (2008), pp. 573–8; J. Rogers, 'Reporting Causes of Death in Sweden', *Journal of the History of Medicine and Allied Sciences*, 54:2 (1999), pp. 190–209.
3. B. I. Puranen, *Tuberkulos: En sjukdoms förekomst och dess orsaker 1750–1980*. Umeå Studies in Economic History 7 (Umeå: Umeå University, 1984), pp. 99–126.
4. H. Bergstrand, *Svenska läkaresällskapet 150 år. Dess tillkomst och utveckling. En återblick* (Lund: Svenska läkaresällskapet, 1958), p. 253.
5. *Handlingar rörande Konung Oscar II's: Jubileumsfond utgivna av Komitén för utredning af frågan om Jubileumsfondens användning* (Stockholm, 1899).
6. W. Johnston, 'Tuberculosis', in K. F. Kiple (ed.), *The Cambridge World History of Human Disease* (Cambridge: Cambridge University Press, 1993), pp. 1061–2.
7. Puranen, *Tuberkulos*, p. 15.
8. L. Bryder, *Below the Magic Mountain: A Social History of Tuberculosis in Twentieth-Century Britain* (Oxford: Clarendon Press, 1988); F. B. Smith, *The Retreat of Tuberculosis 1850–1950* (London: Croom Helm, 1988).
9. K. Ott, *Fevered Lives: Tuberculosis in American Culture since 1870* (Cambridge, MA: Harvard University Press, 1996).
10. John Welshman highlights these points in his discussion of classic texts by Susan Sontag and David Armstrong. J. Welshman, *Municipal Medicine: Public Health in Twentieth-Century Britain* (Oxford: Peter Lang, 2000), pp. 125–6; S. Sontag, *Illness as Metaphor* (London: Allen Lane, 1979); D. Armstrong, *Political Anatomy of the Body: Medical Knowledge in Britain in the Twentieth Century* (Cambridge: Cambridge University Press, 1983).
11. C. A. Connolly, *Saving Sickly Children: The Tuberculosis Preventorium in American Life, 1909–1970* (New Brunswick, NJ: Rutgers University Press, 2008). For recent research on tuberculosis provision in northern Norway see, T. S. Ryymin, *Smitte, språk og kultur: Tuberkulosearbeidet i Finnmark* (Oslo: Scandinavian Academic Press, 2009).
12. See *Journal of the History of Childhood and Youth*, 2:2 (2009).
13. P. Burke, *What is Cultural History?* (Cambridge: Polity Press, 2005), pp. 70–2.
14. B. Ingsted and S. Reynolds Whyte (eds), *Disability and Culture* (Los Angeles, CA: University of California Press, 1995), pp. 6–7 and pp. 24–5; and R. Jenkins, 'Culture, Classification and (in) Competence', in R. Jenkins (ed.), *Questions of Competence: Culture, Classification and Intellectual Disability* (Cambridge: Cambridge University Press, 1998), p. 16.
15. For recent review of literature addressing the creation of welfare states, see B. Harris, *The Origins of the British Welfare State: Social Welfare in England and Wales 1800–1945* (Basingstoke: Palgrave Macmillan, 2004), pp. 15–27. It is, however, important to note that Scandinavian scholars draw an important distinction between the beguiling similarity of approaches noticed by outsiders and the country-specific policies and practices which often remained significant. J. Tøssebro, 'The Development of Community Services for People with Learning Disabilities in Norway and Sweden', in J. Welshman and J. Walmsley (eds), *Community Care in Perspective: Care, Control and Citizenship* (Basing-

stoke: Palgrave Macmillan, 2006), pp. 122–34, on p. 122. Thorough discussions of these issues are found in E. S. Einhorn and J. Logue, *Modern Welfare States: Scandinavian Politics and Policy in the Global Age*, 2nd edn (London: Praeger, 2003); N. F. Christiansen, K. Petersen, N. Edling and P. Haave (eds), *The Nordic Model of Welfare: A Historical Reappraisal* (Copenhagen: Museum Tusculanum Press, 2006).

16. G. Broberg and M. Tydén, 'Eugenics in Sweden: Efficient Care', in G. Broberg and N. Roll-Hansen (eds), *Eugenics and the Welfare State* (East Lansing: Michigan State University Press, 1996), pp. 77–149; M. Tydén, *Från politik till praktik: de svenska steriliseringslagarna 1935–1975*. Stockholm Studies in History 63 (Stockholm: Almqvist and Wiksell International, 2002).

17. M. Niemi, *Public Health and Municipal Policy Making: Britain and Sweden, 1900–1940* (Aldershot: Ashgate, 2007).

18. S. Sturdy, 'Introduction: Medicine, Health and the Public Sphere', in S. Sturdy (ed.) *Medicine, Health and the Public Sphere in Britain, 1600–2000* (London: Routledge, 2002), pp. 1–24.

19. S. Kilander, *Den nya staten och den gamla. En studie i ideologisk förvandling*. Acta Universitatis Upsaliensia, Studia Historica Upsaliensia 103 (Stockholm: Almqvist and Wiksell International, 1991), pp. 58–9, pp. 118–21 and pp. 213–17.

20. A-L. Seip, *Sosialhjelpstaten blir til. Norsk sosialpolitikk 1740–1920* (Oslo: Gyldendahl, 1984).

21. Kilander, *Den nya staten*.

22. N. F. Christiansen and P. Markkola, 'Introduction', in Christiansen et al. (eds), *The Nordic Model of Welfare*, pp. 9–29.

23. S. Förhammar, *Med känsla eller förnuft? Svensk debatt om filantropi 1870–1914*. Stockholm Studies in History, 59 (Stockholm: Almqvist and Wiksell International, 2000).

24. R. K. French, 'Scrofula (Scrophula)', in K. F. Kiple (ed.), *The Cambridge World History of Human Disease*, pp. 998–1000; S. Grzybowski and E. A. Allen, 'History and Importance of Scrofula', *Lancet*, 346: 8988 (1995), pp. 1472–4.

25. The printed annual reports for the sanatorium are found in a number of repositories. The authors used the reports found in the archives of Länsmuseet Varberg (The County Museum, Varberg, hereafter LMV) up until 1920 and reports stored in the Halland läns Landstingsarkiv (the archives of the Halland County), Halmstad (hereafter HLL), for 1921–30. The names of the annual reports vary slightly. *Redogörelse för kustsanatoriet Apelviken* (hereafter RKA) *1905–1906*, p. 3; B. Källgård and A. Peterson, *Apelviken – från kustsanatorium till kurort* (Varberg: Hembygdsföreningen Gamla Varberg, 2004), p. 9, pp. 13–14, and pp. 17–19.

26. J. S. Almer, *Kustsanatoriet Apelviken: Dess utveckling och nuvarande ståndpunkt.* (Varberg: Boktryckeribolaget, 1926), pp. 5–6.

27. The parliamentary papers of this era are printed and found in major Swedish libraries. *Riksdagshandlingar* (Parliamentary Papers). *Motioner i andra kammaren* (public bills in the second chamber) (hereafter MAK). MAK, 1909:59, p. 7.

28. RKA, 1906.

29. MAK, 1909:59, pp. 7–8.

30. The lists of members were included in the annual reports from 1905 to 1918.

31. RKA, 1905–1906, pp. 12–20.

32. RKA, 1905–1906, p. 4; O. Bjurling, *Halland läns landsting*. Vol. 1. 1863–1937 (Halmstad: Hallands läns landsting, 1937), pp. 84–85.

33. *Svensk Författningssamling* 1908:88, s. 1 f. The by-laws were modified in 1910 at the request of the national government, so that no changes could be made without governmental sanction. *Föreningen för kustvård åt skrofulösa barn: Styrelseberättelse*, 1911, p. 2.
34. RKA, 1905–1906, p. 8.
35. *Föreningen för kustvård åt skrofulösa barn,* 1930, pp. 19–21.
36. HLL, Kustsanatoriet Apelviken arkiv (the archives of the Coastal Sanatorium Apelviken); FIIA:1, Handlingar rörande landstingsbidrag 1914–1937, Sanatoriet landstingsbidrag 1914, Landstingsbidrag jämte bestämmelser 1915.
37. HLL, Kustsanatoriet Apelviken arkiv: FIIA:1, Landstingsarkivet Halmstad. Landstinget Hallands arkiv: Landstingens bestämmelser med samorganisationen 1924, Handlingar rörande landstingsbidrag 1914–1937, Utdrag av protokoll, hållet vid Hallands läns landstings sammanträde 1925, § 55; 1927 § 47; 1928 § 96; 1929, § 64.
38. RKA, 1905–1906, p. 5; Almer, *Kustsanatoriet Apelviken,* p. 4.
39. See, for example, *Meddelande från Kustsanatoriet Apelviken* 1907–1908, p. 6; *Föreningen för kustvård åt skrofulösa barn* 1915, p. 5; 1920, p. 9; 1925, p. 13; 1930, p. 19.
40. A. Harrington, *Reenchanted Science: Holism in German Culture from Wilhelm II to Hitler* (Princeton, NJ: Princeton University Press, 1996).
41. J.S. Almer, R. Hansson, E. Tengvall och H. Waldenström, 'Om vården av kirurgisk tuberkulos och skrofulos', Kap. 3 i *Svenska nationalförening mot tuberkulos utredning angående fortsatta åtgärder till tuberkulosens bekämpande i Sverige avlämnad till statsrådet och chefen för kungl. Socialdepartementet den 12 april 1929* (Stockholm: Socialdepartementet, 1929).
42. S. Johansson, *Bidrag till kännedom om och behandling av ben- och ledtuberkulosen under barnaåldern.* Avhandling (Stockholm: Karolinska institutet, 1924).
43. Almer, *Kustsanatoriet Apelviken,* pp. 49–52.
44. E. Lindahl, 'Om kustsanatorier', *Hygiea* (1901), pp. 291–6, pp. 424–43 and pp. 607–11; E. Lindahl, 'Kliniska studier på kustsanatorier och några andra sjukvårdsinrättningar utomlands', *Hygiea* (1903), pp. 74–88; E. Lindahl, 'Friluftsbehandling af sjuka i England', *Hälsovännen,* 16:8 (1901), pp. 127–9.
45. Johansson, *Bidrag till kännedom,* pp. 55–9 and pp. 62–5. This study showed positive results for this type of treatment.
46. S. Lomholt, *Niels R. Finsen* (Uppsala: A. Lindblads förlag, 1944).
47. Almer, *Kustsanatoriet Apelviken,* pp. 53–9.
48. Ibid., p. 60.
49. Almer et al., 'Om vården av kirurgisk tuberkulos och skrofulos'.
50. P. Silfverskiöld, 'Kustsjukhuset på Styrsö', *Hälsovännen,* 25:19 (2010), pp. 289–93, and 25:20 (2010), pp. 305–8.
51. S. Kilander, *'En nationalrikedom av hälsoskatt': om Jämtland och industrisamhället 1882–1910 (Hedamora:* Gidlunds, 2008). Kilander's book deals with the development of health resorts/ resorts in the mountains of Jämtland (close to the Norwegian border).
52. E. Mansén, *Ett paradis på jorden: Om den svenska kurortskulturen 1680–1880* (Stockholm: Atlantis, 2001), pp. 99–124.
53. K. Vik, *Varbergs Kurort-Apelviken* (Varberg: Kurortens samfällighetsförening, 1995), pp. 5–9.
54. See the photographs of Mathilda Ranch taken in 1904. LMV, Photo Collection, E6137, F2504.
55. Källgård and Peterson, *Apelviken,* p. 77.

56. H. Waldenström, 'Några ord om ljusbehandling särskilt bågljusbehandling, av ben-, led- och körteltuberkulos'. *Kvartalsskriften. Svensk nationalförening mot tuberkulos*, 20 (1925), pp. 11–20.
57. Almer, *Kustsanatoriet Apelviken.*
58. Johansson, *Bidrag till kännedom*, ch. 13.
59. J. Hallström, *Constructing a Pipe-Bound City: A History of Water Supply, Sewerage, and Excreta Removal in Norrköping and Linköping, Sweden, 1860–1910*. Linköping Studies in Arts and Sciences, 267 (Linköping: Department of Water and Environmental Studies, Linköping University, 2002).
60. M. C. Nelson and J. Rogers, 'Cleaning up the Cities: Application of the First Comprehensive Public Health Law in Sweden', *Scandinavian Journal of History*, 19:1 (1994), pp. 17–39; M. C. Nelson, 'Water, Health and Legislation in Sweden: An Historical Foundation', in T. Katko, O. Seppäla and J. Kaivo-Oja (eds) *Management of Water, Wastewater and Solid Waste Services in Comparative Historical and Future Perspective. A Nordic Research Workshop supported by NorFa*. Environmental Engineering and Biotechnology Report 13 (Tampere: Tampere University of Technology, 2001).
61. Welshman, *Municipal Medicine*, pp. 124–5.
62. Lindahl, 'Om kustsanatorier', p. 440.
63. Källgård and Peterson, *Apelviken*, p. 34.
64. Almer, *Kustsanatoriet Apelviken*, p. 60.
65. Almer, *Kustsanatoriet Apelviken*, pp. 49–52. An American example of this type of immobilizing treatment at home is described in the reprint of the autobiography by Katherine Butler Hathaway. K. B. Hathaway, *The Little Locksmith: A Memoir* (New York: The Feminist Press of the City University of New York, 2000).
66. Robert Hanson had worked at Styrsö before becoming Almer's assistant. He later succeeded Almer as head of the hospital and filled his place on the national committee. *Föreningen för kustvård åt skrofulösa barn*. Årsberättelse,1927, p. 5.
67. *Föreningen för kustvård åt skrofulösa barn*. Årsberättelse, 1927.
68. Almer et al., 'Om vården av kirurgisk tuberkulos och skrofulos', p. 109.
69. Ibid., pp. 130–6. Apparently this group had completed their study early in the 1920s.
70. Almer et al., 'Om vården av kirurgisk tuberkulos och skrofulos', p. 132.
71. *Föreningen för kustvård åt skrofulösa barn*. Årsberättelse, 1927.
72. Such facilities included St Göran Hospital's unit for surgical tuberculosis (Stockholm) and Borås Hospital for Children's Tuberculosis that opened in 1930. A substantial number of children were also cared for in orthopaedic clinics in Gothenburg's Children's Hospital, Sahlgrenska Hospital in Gothenburg, The Orthopaedic Clinic in Lund, the orthopaedic unit of the General Hospital in Malmö and The Institute for the Crippled in Helsingborg. See, Almer et al., 'Om vården av kirurgisk tuberkulos och skrofulos', pp.104–40.
73. Almer, *Kustsanatoriet Apelviken* , pp. 48–61.
74. There were a few from abroad, the first being from Finland.
75. From 1924 this was arranged through the cooperative organization of the west coast sanatoria.
76. *Föreningen för kustvård åt skrofulösa barn*. Årsberättelse, 1908–9; 1911–30.
77. Ibid., 1908–9; 1911–30; Almer, *Kustsanatoriet Apelviken*, pp. 62–73.
78. French, 'Scrofula (Scrophula)'; Grzybowski and Allen, 'History and Importance of Scrofula'.
79. Almer, *Kustsanatoriet Apelviken*, pp. 62–73.

80. The appeal, and dangers, of long distance travel for tuberculosis patients in search of restored health is captured in L. Bryder, '"A Health Resort for Consumptives": Tuberculosis and Immigration to New Zealand, 1880–1914', *Medical History*, 40:4, pp. 453–71. Other migration issues are discussed in E. K. Abel, *Tuberculosis and the Politics of Exclusion: A History of Public Health and Migration to Los Angeles* (New Brunswick, NJ: Rutgers University Press, 2007).

81. In 1914 the wages of a labourer were about 2–4 crowns/day, depending on where in the country the labourer lived. L. Jörberg, *A History of Prices in Sweden*, part 2 (Lund: Gleerup, 1972), p. 588.

82. Winka, *Kyrkogården berättar*, p. 33.

83. The testimony mostly covered the period after 1930. Källgård and Peterson, *Apelviken*, pp. 69–97.

84. Until the practice was outlawed in the 1918 Poor Law, indigent children were commonly 'auctioned off' within their municipalities; that is their care was entrusted to the lowest bidder.

85. Källgård and Peterson, *Apelviken*, pp. 69–97. Savela's interview, pp. 88–92.

86. Almer, *Kustsanatoriet Apelviken*, p. 75. It should be noted that there was growing European interest in holistic medicine, see, Harrington, *Reenchanted Science*.

87. Almer, *Kustsanatoriet Apelviken*, p. 75.

88. Bergstrand, *Svenska läkaresällskapet*, pp. 245–6 and pp. 249–51.

89. Ibid., pp. 264–5.

90. Riksdagshandlingar (Parliamentary Papers). Propositioner (Government Bills), P 1908:166, p. 4. Betänkande och förslag (Committee Report) af den 1905 tillsatta kommitté för verkställande af utredning angående åtgärder för människotuberkulosens bekämpande (Stockholm, 1907), p. IV; See also, M. C. Nelson and S. Förhammar, 'Swedish Seaside Sanatoria in the Beginning of the Twentieth Century', Journal of the History of Childhood and Youth, 2:2 (2009), pp. 249–66, on p. 254.

8 Dale, 'Health Visiting and Disability Issues in England before 1948'

1. B. Harris, *The Health of the Schoolchild: A History of the School Medical Service in England and Wales* (Buckingham: Open University Press, 1995); D. Hirst, 'The Early School Medical Service in Wales: Public Care or Private Responsibility?', in A. Borsay (ed.), *Medicine in Wales c. 1800–2000: Public Service or Private Commodity?* (Cardiff: University of Wales Press, 2003), pp. 65–85.

2. P. Dale, 'The Bridgwater Infant Welfare Centre, 1922–1939: From an Authoritarian Concern with "Welfare Mothers" to a More Inclusive Community Health Project?', *Family and Community History*, 11:2 (2008), pp. 69–83.

3. G. Owen (ed.), *Health Visiting* (London: Bailliere Tindall, 1977).

4. M. Jefferys, *An Anatomy of Social Welfare Services: A Survey of Social Welfare Staff and their Clients in the County of Buckinghamshire* (London: Michael Joseph, 1965), p. 64.

5. There is a tendency to confuse routine work with well babies with targeted interventions.

6. R. Dingwall, *The Social Organization of Health Visitor Training* (London: Croom Helm, 1977).

7. J. Ballantyne, *Deafness*, 3rd edn (Edinburgh: Churchill Livingstone, 1977), pp. 127–81. Also R. M. Powell, 'Medical Screening and Surveillance'; K. Jennings, 'The Role of the Health Visitor'; and A. MacCarthy and J. Connell, 'Audiological Screening and Assess-

ment', all in G. Lindsay (ed.), *Screening for Children with Special Needs: Multi-disciplinary Approaches* (London: Croom Helm, 1984), pp. 12–42, pp. 43–62 and pp. 63–85.

8. Department of Health and Social Security, *Child Abuse: A Study of Inquiry Reports 1973–81* (London: HMSO, 1982).

9. E. Ross, *Love and Toil: Motherhood in Outcast London, 1870–1918* (Oxford: Oxford University Press, 1993), pp. 204–9.

10. A. Symonds, '"It's a Funny Job Really": The Contradictions of Health Visiting', in A. Borsay (ed.), *Medicine in Wales*, pp. 171–94.

11. C. Moore, *George and Sam* (London: Viking Books, 2004).

12. P. Dale, 'Tension in the Voluntary-Statutory Alliance: "Lay Professionals" and the Planning and Delivery of Mental Deficiency Services, 1917–45', in P. Dale and J. Melling (eds), *Mental Illness and Learning Disability Since 1850: Finding a Place for Mental Disorder in the United Kingdom* (London: Routledge, 2006), pp. 154–178.

13. R. Viner and J. Golden, 'Children's Experiences of Illness', in R. Cooter and J. Pickstone (eds), *Medicine in the Twentieth Century* (Amsterdam: Harwood Academic Publishers, 2000), pp. 575–87.

14. J. Lewis, *The Politics of Motherhood: Child and Maternal Welfare in England, 1900–1939* (London: Croom Helm, 1980), p. 105.

15. Health visitors were influenced by changing ideas about the causes and treatment of disease. M. Worboys, *Spreading Germs: Disease Theories and Medical Practice in Britain, 1865–1900* (Cambridge: Cambridge University Press, 2000).

16. P. Hollis, *Ladies Elect: Women in English Local Government 1865–1914* (Oxford: Clarendon Press, 1987), p. 24.

17. H. Hendrick, *Child Welfare: England 1872–1989* (London: Routledge, 1994), pp. 1–15.

18. M. Thomson, *The Problem of Mental Deficiency: Eugenics, Democracy and Social Policy in Britain c. 1870–1959* (Oxford: Clarendon Press, 1998), pp. 1–35.

19. C. Davies, 'The Health Visitor as Mother's Friend: A Woman's Place in Public Health, 1900–1914', *Social History of Medicine*, 1:1 (1988), pp. 39–59.

20. Report of the Work of the Female Sanitary Inspectors (hereafter FSI Report), 20 September 1904, p. 4, in bound volume marked 1902–1911, Bradford Local Studies Centre, Bradford Central Library, B614 FEM.

21. P. Dale and C. Mills, 'Revealing and Concealing Personal and Social Problems: Family Coping Strategies and a New Engagement with Officials and Welfare Agencies c. 1900–12', *Family and Community History*, 10:2 (2007), pp. 111–25.

22. B. Thompson, 'Infant Mortality in Nineteenth-Century Bradford', in R. Woods and J. Woodward (eds), *Urban Disease and Mortality in Nineteenth-Century England* (London: Batsford, 1984), pp. 120–47.

23. C. Steedman, *Childhood, Culture and Class in Britain. Margaret McMillan, 1860–1931* (London: Virago, 1990).

24. Education Services Committee, Bradford Corporation, *Education in Bradford since 1870* (Bradford: Bradford Corporation, 1970).

25. FSI Report, 24 June 1905, p. 7.

26. This process would probably exclude the conditions that a modern practitioner would expect to encounter.

27. FSI Report, 25 March 1906, pp. 8–9.

28. Ibid., 31 March 1907, p. 8.

29. Ibid., 1 October 1909 to 30 September 1910, p. 17.

30. Ibid., 24 June 1905, p. 7.
31. It was unusual for the FSIs to recommend hospital treatment of rickets, but one such case involving several children from a 'respectable' home was discussed. FSI Report, 24 June 1905, p. 6.
32. D. Dwork, 'The Milk Option. An Aspect of the Infant Welfare Movement in England 1898–1908', *Medical History*, 31:1 (1987), pp. 51–69.
33. FSI Report, 30 December 1904, p. 5.
34. It was a Ministry of Health inspection that drew attention to these issues. Dr D. J. Williamson, Halifax County Borough: Survey Report, 1932 (hereafter Halifax PH Survey), National Archives, Kew, Surrey, Ministry of Health papers (hereafter NA MH), 66/1071.
35. H. Marland, 'A Pioneer in Infant Welfare: The Huddersfield Scheme 1903–1920', *Social History of Medicine*, 6:1 (1993), pp. 25–50.
36. R. Millward and F. Bell, 'Infant Mortality in Victorian Britain: The Mother as Medium', *Economic History Review*, 54:4 (2001), pp. 699–733.
37. Report of the Medical Officer of Health for Halifax (hereafter Halifax MOH Report) for 1908, p. 29, Halifax Library, Halifax, 614HAL; and Halifax MOH Report for 1928, p. 59.
38. Halifax PH Survey, paragraph 311.
39. The committee changed its name and remit several times, but a key phase was *c.* 1906–10 when responsibility for school meals and medical inspections was combined with control of admissions to special and industrial schools. See Halifax County Borough Council Minutes, Halifax Library, 352HAL.
40. The health visitors were occasionally used to investigate cases of unusual sensitivity, for example those involving concern about the moral welfare of girls under the care and control of the mental deficiency committee.
41. The Ministry of Health was very critical about the public health arrangements in Exeter. Dr A. C. Parsons, Exeter County Borough, Public Health Survey, 1930, NA MH 66/608.
42. A. Knox and C. Gardner-Thorpe, *The Royal Devon and Exeter Hospital 1741–2006* (Exeter: A. Knox and C. Gardner-Thorpe, 2008), p. 161.
43. The Halifax MOH Reports mention fifteen ON cases in 1914 and twelve in 1915. Warnings about ON continued, for example Halifax MOH Report, 1928, p. 45.
44. Halifax MOH Report, 1922, p. 16 and p. 23.
45. Halifax PH Survey, paragraph 564.
46. Ibid, paragraphs 529–32 and 540.
47. L. Bryder, '"Wonderlands of Buttercup, Clover and Daisies": Tuberculosis and the Open-Air School Movement in Britain, 1907–1939', in R. Cooter (ed.), *In the Name of the Child: Health and Welfare,1880–1940* (London: Routledge, 1992), pp. 72–95.
48. Halifax MOH Report, 1928, pp. 61–2.
49. For discussion about social and medical aspects of disability designed for a practitioner audience see M. Oliver, 'Flexible Services', *Nursing Times*, 84:16 (1988), pp. 25–9.
50. For summary of the medical model and its limitations see A. Borsay, *Disability and Social Policy in Britain since 1750: A History of Exclusion* (Basingstoke: Palgrave Macmillan, 2005), p. 186 and p. 194.

9 Martínez-Pérez, Porras, Báguena and Ballester, 'Spanish Health Services and Polio Epidemics in the Twentieth Century'

1. E. Rodríguez-Ocaña (ed.), 'Child Health, A Paradigmatic Issue in Modern History', *Dynamis,* 23 (2003), pp. 17–166.
2. P. K. Longmore and L. Umansky, 'Introduction: Disability History: From Margins to the Mainstream', in P. K. Longmore and L. Umansky (eds), *The New Disability History. American Perspectives* (New York: New York University Press, 2001), pp. 1–29, on p. 20. See also, A. Borsay, 'History, Power and Identity', in C. Barnes, M. Oliver, and L. Barton (eds), *Disability Studies Today* (Cambridge: Polity Press, 2002), pp. 98–119; A. L. Aguado-Díaz, *Historia de las Deficiencias* (Madrid: Escuela Libre Editorial, 1995).
3. E. Sass (ed.), *Polio's Legacy: An Oral History* (London: University Press of America, 1996); D. J. Wilson, *Living with Polio. The Epidemic and its Survivors* (Chicago, IL: University of Chicago Press, 2005); M. Shell, *Polio and its Aftermaths. The Paralysis of Culture* (Cambridge, MA: Harvard University Press, 2005).
4. R. Cooter (ed.), *In the Name of the Child: Health and Welfare, 1880–1940* (London: Routledge, 1992); For Spanish policies, see, R. Ballester and E. Balaguer, 'La Infancia Como Valor y Como Problema en las Luchas Sanitarias de Principios de Siglo en España', *Dynamis,* 15 (1995), pp. 177–92; E. Rodríguez-Ocaña, 'La Construcción de la Salud Infantil. Ciencia, Medicina y Educación en la Transición Sanitaria en España', *Historia Contemporánea,* 18 (1999), pp. 19–52; E. Perdiguero (ed.), *Salvad al Niño. Estudios Sobre la Protección a la Infancia en la Europa Mediterránea a Comienzos del Siglo XX* (Valencia: Seminari d´Estudis Sobre la Ciència, 2004).
5. M. del Cura, 'La Infancia Anormal, en España' (PhD dissertation, Castilla-La Mancha University, 2010).
6. J. Martínez-Pérez, 'Consolidando el Modelo Médico de Discapacidad: Sobre la Poliomielitis y la Constitución de la Traumatología y Ortopedia Como Especialidad en España (1930–1950)', in J. Martínez-Pérez (ed.), 'Dossier: The poliomyelitis and its Contexts: Collectives and Individual Experiences in the Face of the Disease in the Twentieth Century', *Asclepio,* 61:1 (2009), pp. 117–42.
7. M. I. Porras, M. J. Báguena and R. Ballester, 'Methodological Approaches to the Study of Sanitary Conditions of the Cities. The Case of Poliomyelitis in Spain (1913–1929)', in *Seminario Sobre Salud y Ciudades en España, 1880–1940* (Barcelona, 2010).
8. R. Gómez Ferrer, 'Parálisis Espinal Infantil. Etiología y Patogenia', in *Actas III Congreso Español de Obstetricia, Ginecología y Pediatría* (Valencia, 1913), pp. 210–93.
9. M. I. Porras-Gallo, 'La Lucha Contra las Enfermedades "Evitables" en España y la Pandemia de Gripe de 1918–1919', *Dynamis,* 14 (1994), pp. 159–83.
10. E. Fernández Sanz, 'Campaña Sanitaria Contra la Poliomielitis Aguda (Parálisis Infantil)', in *Campaña Sanitaria Contra la Parálisis Infantil (Poliomielitis Aguda)* (Madrid: V. Tordesillas, 1916), pp. 20–40; M. Martín Salazar, 'Prólogo', in *Campaña Sanitaria,* pp. 3–19; M. Martín Salazar, *Epidemiología y Régimen Sanitario de la Parálisis Infantil* (Madrid: V. Tordesillas, 1916), p. 11. The act including polio as an avoidable disease, appeared in *Gaceta de Madrid,* 28 August 1916.
11. Porras-Gallo, 'La Lucha Contra las Enfermedades'. It is important to emphasize the role played by the Rockefeller Foundation in the reform of the healthcare system. E. Rodríguez-Ocaña, J. Bernabeu and J. L. Barona, 'La Fundación Rockefeller y España, 1914–1936', in J. L. García, J. M. Moreno and G. Ruiz (eds), *Estudios de Historia de las*

Técnicas, la Arqueología Industrial y las Ciencias (Salamanca: Junta de Castilla y León, 1998), vol. 2, pp. 531–9.

12. J. Fernández Pérez, *Epidemiología de la Parálisis Infantil* (Madrid: Impr. J. Cosano, 1932); M. J. Báguena, 'Saberes y Prácticas en Torno a la Polio en la Medicina Valenciana (1900–1950)', in J. Martínez-Pérez et al. (eds), *La Medicina en el Nuevo Milenio. Una Perspectiva Histórica* (Cuenca: Ed. UCLM, 2004), pp. 949–62; F. Martínez-Navarro et al., 'Estudio de la Epidemia de Poliomielitis Infantil Presentada en Madrid Durante el Año 1929 por el Dr. Laureano Alvadalejo. Primera Memoria Anual de los Trabajos Llevados a Cabo por el Servicio Epidemiológico Central (1929)', in Martínez-Pérez et al. (eds), *La Medicina en el Nuevo Milenio*, pp. 963–87.

13. A. M. Payne, 'Poliomyelitis as a World Problem', in *Poliomyelitis. Papers and Discussions Presented at the Third International Poliomyelitis Conference* (Philadelphia, PA: Lippincoat, 1955), pp. 391–400.

14. Here it is useful to contrast the large number of US publications with the more modest, and later, work on Europe. N. Rogers, *Dirt and Disease. Polio before FDR* (New Brunswick, NJ: Rutgers University Press, 1992); Shell, *Polio and its Aftermaths*; Wilson, *Living with Polio*; D. M. Oshinsky, *Polio. An American Story* (Oxford: Oxford University Press, 2005); D. J. Wilson, *Silent Voices: An Oral History from the American Polio Epidemics and Worldwide Eradication Efforts* (Westport: Praeger Publishers, 2007); N. Rogers '"Silence has its own Stories": Elizabeth Kenny, Polio and the Culture of Medicine', *Social History of Medicine,* 21:1 (2008), pp. 145–61; U. Lindner, and S. Blume 'Vaccine Innovation and Adoption: Polio Vaccines in the UK, the Netherlands and West Germany, 1955–1965', *Medical History*, 50:4 (2006), pp. 425–46; P. Axelsson, *Hostens spöke. De svenska polioepidermias historia.* (Stockholm: Carlssons, 2004), an English summary of this Swedish text appears on pp. 230–8. The most recent and comprehensive study, with an updated bibliography, is Martínez-Pérez (ed.), 'Dossier', pp. 7–192.

15. R. Cooter, 'The Disabled Body', in R. Cooter and J. Pickstone (eds), *Companion to Medicine in the Twentieth Century* (London: Routledge, 2002), pp. 367–83.

16. J. Palacios-Sánchez, 'Evolución Histórica', in J. Palacios-Sánchez (ed.), *Historia del C.P.E.E. de Reeducación de Inválidos. Antiguo INRI* (Madrid: M.E.C.-C.P.E.E, 1990), pp. 50–90.

17. J. Martínez-Pérez, 'La Organización Científica del Trabajo y las Estrategias Médicas de Seguridad Laboral en España (1922–1936)', *Dynamis,* 14 (1994), pp. 131–58; J. Martínez-Pérez, 'Medicina del Trabajo y Prevención de la Siniestralidad Laboral en España (1922–1936)', in J. Atenza and J. Martínez-Pérez, *El Centro Secundario de Higiene Rural de Talavera de la Reina y la Sanidad Española de su Tiempo* (Toledo: Junta de Comunidades de Castilla-La Mancha, 2001), pp. 235–57.

18. J. Martínez-Pérez, 'The Recovered Worker: Occupational Medicine, Orthopaedics, and the Impact of Medical Technology on the Social Image of Persons with Disabilities (Spain, 1922–1936)', *História, Ciencias, Saúde-Manguinhos, 13* (2006), pp. 349–73; J. Martínez-Pérez and M. I. Porras-Gallo, 'Hacia una Nueva Percepción de las Personas con Discapacidades: Legislación, Medicina y los Inválidos del Trabajo en España (1900–1936)', *Dynamis*, 26 (2006), pp. 195–219. Anne Borsay has examined the way in which orthopaedics also helped in Britain to establish a model to treat disabilities. A. Borsay, 'Disciplining Disabled Bodies. The Development of Orthopaedic Medicine in Britain *c.* 1800–1939', in D. M. Turner and K. Stagg (eds), *Social Histories of Disability and Deformity* (London: Routledge, 2006), pp. 97–116.

19. *Gaceta de Madrid*, 14 December 1933, p. 1821.

20. Ibid.
21. M. J. Báguena, M. I. Porras, and R. Ballester, 'Poliomyelitis in Urban and Rural Spain (1890–1970). Epidemiological Trends, Social and Medical Responses', in A. Andresen, J. L. Barona, and S. Cherry (eds), *Making a New Countryside: Health Policies and Practices in European History ca. 1860–1950* (Peter Lang: Frankfurt am Main, 2010), pp. 115–34.
22. M. J. Báguena, 'Estudios Epidemiológicos y Virológicos Sobre la Poliomielitis en Valencia', *Asclepio,* 61:1 (2009), pp. 39–54.
23. E. Rodríguez-Ocaña, 'Foreign Expertise, Political Pragmatism and Professional Elite: The Rockefeller Foundation in Spain, 1919–39', *Studies in History and Philosophy of Biology and Biomedical Science,* 31:3 (2000), pp. 447–61.
24. M. I. Porras, M. J. Báguena and R. Ballester, 'Spain and the International Scientific Conferences on Polio, 1940s–1960s', *Dynamis,* 30 (2010), pp. 91–118. A wider overview of international influences is provided by J. L. Barona and J. Bernabeu, *La Salud y el Estado. El Movimiento Sanitario Internacional y la Administración Española* (Valencia: Universidad de Valencia, 2008).
25. The first report was F. K. Safford, *Rapport sur une Mission en Espagne,* WHO Records and Archives, Geneva, Switzerland, Centralized files, Third Generation, R4/418/2 SPA.
26. J. Bosch Marín and E. Bravo, 'Aportación de España a la Lucha Contra la Poliomielitis', in *Aportación Española al V Symposium Europeo Sobre Poliomielitis. Madrid, 28–30 de Septiembre 1958* (Madrid: Publicaciones 'Al servicio del niño español', Mº de la Gobernación, 1958), p. 45.
27. In the context of the Cold War, prophylactic vaccines were used as defensive weapons on both sides. J. Smith, *Patenting the Sun: Polio and the Salk Vaccine* (New York: W. Morrow, 1990).
28. J. Tuells, 'Los Testimonios de los Expertos y su Participación en las Primeras Campañas de Vacunación Antipoliomielitica en España', in T. Ortiz-Gómez et al. (eds), *La Experiencia de Enfermar en Perspectiva Histórica* (Granada, Universidad de Granada, 2008), pp. 321–4.
29. R. Ballester and M. I. Porras, 'El Significado Histórico de las Encuestas de Seroprevalencia Como Tecnología de Laboratorio Aplicada a las Campañas de Vacunación: el Caso de la Poliomielitis en España', *Asclepio,* 61:1 (2009), pp. 55–80.
30. One of the national newspapers in which this approach is to be found is the *ABC,* for example *ABC,* 14 May 1960, p. 62; 5 June 1960, p. 101; 21 December 1960, p. 89; 2 April 1961, p. 73. The most comprehensive study of mass immunization campaigns in Spain is J. A. Rodríguez-Sánchez and J. Seco-Calvo, 'Las Campañas de Vacunación Contra la Poliomielitis en España en 1963', *Asclepio,* 61:1 (2009), pp. 81–116.
31. M. Mezquita, *Evaluación de los Resultados de la Primera Campaña de Vacunación Contra la Poliomielitis por via Oral en España* (Madrid: Dirección General de Sanidad, 1965), p. 21.
32. See M. I. Porras and M. J. Báguena, 'La Poliomielitis en la España Franquista a Través de la Prensa General', in Ortiz-Gómez et al. (eds), *La Experiencia de Enfermar,* pp. 325–9.
33. Ballester offers a systematic review of documentaries and other kinds of contemporary films on polio. R. Ballester, 'Imágenes de la Vulnerabilidad. Las Fuentes Fílmicas de la Poliomielitis en España', in Ortiz-Gómez et al. (eds), *La Experiencia de Enfermar,* pp. 335–9.
34. These interviews are part of the national project mentioned in the acknowledgements at the end of the chapter and further described in J. A Rodríguez-Sánchez, J. Seco-Calvo

and I. Guerra, 'La Fuentes Orales en la Construcción de una Historia de la Polio', in J. R. Pita, J. A. Rodríguez-Sánchez et al., *A poliomielite na Península Iberica. Reflexoes Para a sua Comprensao Histórica* (Coimbra: Universidade de Coimbra, in press).

35. H. Castells and V. Carulla, *La Fisioterapia de la Parálisis Infantil. Resultados de la Roentgenoterapia Profunda* (Barcelona: Hijos de Nicolás Moyá, 1926). p. 1.
36. C. Elordi, S. Falcón García, 'Tratamiento de la Parálisis Espinal Infantil con Prostigmina', *Rev. San. Hig. Pub.*, 20 (1946), pp. 1313–33.
37. Our findings are consistent with those obtained by the research group from the Universities of Salamanca and Leon, headed by J. A. Rodríguez-Sánchez.
38. V. Cohn, *Sister Kenny: The Woman who Challenged the Doctors* (Mineapolis, MN: University of Minnesota Press, 1975).
39. D. J. Wilson, 'And They Shall Walk: Ideal Versus Reality in Polio Rehabilitation in the United States', *Asclepio*, 61:1 (2009), pp. 175–92.
40. J. A. Rodríguez-Sánchez, 'Los Primeros Movimientos Asociativos: de ALPE a FRATER', in J. A. Rodríguez-Sánchez (ed.) *La Memoria Paralizada. Identidades y Vivencias de la Poliomielitis y el Síndrome Postpolio* (Salamanca, Universidad de Salamanca, in press).
41. M. J. Gámez Fuentes, 'Representing Disability in 90's Spain: The case of ONCE', *Journal of Spanish and Cultural Studies*, 6 (2005), pp. 305–28.
42. R. Sales-Vázquez and C. Ballús-Pascual, 'Los Problemas Psicosociales en la Poliomielitis y su Orientación Asistencial', *Acta Pediátrica Española*, 201 (1959), pp. 493–507.
43. R. Ballester, 'Himno a la Esperanza de Javier Aguirre: un Documental Insólito', in Rodríguez-Sánchez (ed.), *La Memoria Paralizada*.

10 Wheatcroft, 'Cured by Kindness? Child Guidance Services during the Second World War'

1. R. Means, S. Richards and R. Smith (eds), *Community Care: Policy and Practice*, 3rd edn (Basingstoke: Palgrave, 2003), pp. 16–42.
2. S. Wheatcroft, 'Children's Experiences of War: Handicapped Children in England during the Second World War', *Twentieth Century British History*, 19:4 (2008), pp. 480–501.
3. J. Cassidy and P. R. Shaver (eds), *Handbook of Attachment: Theory, Research and Clinical Applications* (London: Guilford Press, 1999).
4. C. Rayner, *How did I get here from there?* (London: Virago, 2003), pp. 277–8 and p. 219.
5. M. Oswin, *The Empty Hours: A Study in the Weekend Life of Handicapped Children in Institutions* (Harmondsworth: Penguin, 1973).
6. For a wider survey of psychological influences and practices see M. Thomson, *Psychological Subjects: Identity, Culture and Health in Twentieth-Century Britain* (Oxford: Oxford University Press, 2006).
7. D. Thom, 'Wishes, Anxieties, Play and Gestures: Child Guidance in Interwar England', in R. Cooter (ed.), *In the Name of the Child: Health and Welfare 1880–1940* (London: Routledge, 1992), pp. 200–19; J. Stewart, 'The Scientific Claims of British Child Guidance, 1918–45', *British Journal for the History of Science*, 42:3 (2009), pp. 407–32.
8. H. Hendrick, *Child Welfare: Historical Dimensions, Contemporary Debate* (Bristol: Policy Press, 2003), pp. 21–3.

9. G. Donaldson, 'Between Practice and Theory: Melanie Klein, Anna Freud and the Development of Child Analysis', *Journal of the History of Behavioural Sciences*, 32 (1996), pp. 160–176.

10. O. C. Samson, *Child Guidance: Its History, Provenance and Future* (London: British Psychological Society, 1980).

11. Report of the Child Guidance Council,1935, National Archives (hereafter NA), Kew, ED 50/273, p. 4.

12. Thom, 'Wishes, Anxieties', p. 215.

13. Department of Education and Science, *The School Health Service* (London: HMSO, 1975), p. 24.

14. 'Cured by Kindness', *Times Educational Supplement*, 22 July 1939.

15. As 'emotional disturbance' was not recognized under Part V of the Education Act 1921, those sent by the LEAs (the home was run by a charitable trust) were paid for under section 80 of the same act, which provided for the treatment of elementary schoolchildren and was interpreted as covering the residential treatment of 'behavioural problems'. Letter from Maudslay (Ministry of Health) to Wrigley (Board of Education), 22 December 1939, NA, ED 50/273.

16. It is not clear when this school opened but there was discussion about its inspection from early 1934 and a Kent team inspected it in September 1935, NA, ED 32/384.

17. The other members were the Central Association for Mental Welfare (CAMW), the National Council for Mental Hygiene (NCMH), the Association of Mental Health Workers (AMHW) and the Association of Psychiatric Social Workers (APSW).

18. Letter from Mental Health Emergency Committee (MHEC) to the Board of Education, 19 April 1939, NA, ED 50/273.

19. Concern was also raised about psychological problems amongst adults during the war. Thomson, *Psychological Subjects*, pp. 225–31.

20. Letter from Evelyn Fox to the Director of Education, 16 May 1939, NA, ED 50/273.

21. 'Billeting Misfits', *Times Educational Supplement*, 28 October 1939.

22. Hostels for 'difficult' children should be distinguished from those for the elderly, homeless, and children with infectious diseases. John Welshman suggests that after the war the hostel system contributed to the wider development of community care. J. Welshman, 'Inside the Walls of the Hostel, 1940–1974', in P. Dale and J. Melling (eds), *Mental Illness and Learning Disability since 1850: Finding a Place for Mental Disorder in the United Kingdom* (London: Routledge, 2006), pp. 200–23.

23. Board of Education, Interview Memorandum, 30 September 1939, NA, ED 50/273.

24. Ministry of Health, *Memorandum EV8: Government Evacuation Scheme* (London, HMSO, 1940).

25. In September 1939 eighteen CGCs closed and it took time to relocate the LSE course to Cambridge. Report of the APSW, 26 October 1939, Modern Records Centre (hereafter MRC), University of Warwick, MSS.378.APSW/P/20/5/7.

26. Child Guidance Council, Note on Present Activities, August 1940, MRC, MSS.378/APSW/P/20/5/19.

27. The Standing Joint Committee of Industrial (later Working) Women's Organizations was set up in 1916 and became an integral part of the Labour Party's organization, many members had social work experience and/or links to children's courts. Letter of the Joint Committee of Working Women's Organizations to R. A. Butler, 2 December 1941; and the minutes of a meeting with the President of the Board of Education and the Parliamentary Secretary, 7 May 1942, NA, ED 50/274.

28. Board of Education, Circular 866: Reserved Occupations – Supplementary List, issued by the Ministry of Labour, 31 March 1939, NA, ED 50/273.
29. M. Opie, 'A Child Guidance Experiment under Emergency Conditions', *Labour Woman*, September 1942.
30. Mr Wills, 'The Delinquents Abroad', *Times Educational Supplement*, 13 April 1940. Mr Wills was superintendent of a hostel for difficult children.
31. S. Isaacs (ed.), *Cambridge Evacuation Survey: A Wartime Study in Social Welfare and Education* (London: Methuen, 1941), p.118.
32. Report of the Child Guidance Council, 1935, NA, ED 50/273.
33. William Healy, Institute for Juvenile Research, 1934, MRC, MSS.16C/5/0/60.
34. Opie, 'A Child Guidance Experiment'.
35. R. Padley and M. Cole (eds), *Evacuation Survey, A Report to the Fabian Society* (London: Routledge, 1940), p. 189.
36. Ibid., p. 193.
37. Ministry of Health, *Hostels for 'Difficult' Children: A Survey of Experience under the Evacuation Scheme* (London: HMSO, 1944).
38. Ibid., p. 4.
39. Ibid., p. 6.
40. Letter of the Secretary of Friends Education Council to Bosworth-Smith, Board of Education, 1941, NA, ED 32/247.
41. Reports of Visits, 22 January 1943 and 5 February 1943, NA, ED 122/21.
42. A. G. Salaman to the Board of Education, 12 February 1943 and Reports of Visits, NA, ED 122/21.
43. Board of Education, *Report on a Five Year Experiment in the Combination of Open-Air Medical and Psycho-Therapeutic Treatment in a Midland Town* (1945), p. 2.
44. The play therapist employed at Brambling house was Phyllis Traill, who in 1945 wrote a paper on her experiences of the Lowenfeld technique at the Birmingham CGC in 1937. See: P. M. Traill, 'An Account of Lowenfeld Technique in a Child Guidance Clinic, with a Survey of Therapeutic Play Technique in Great Britain and U.S.A.', *Journal of Mental Science*, 91:382 (1945), pp. 43–78.
45. J. Stewart, 'I Thought You Would Want to Come and See His Home: Child Guidance and Psychiatric Social Work in Interwar Britain', in M. Jackson (ed.), *Health and the Modern Home* (London: Routledge, 2007), pp. 111–27, on p. 123.
46. K. M. Wolf, 'Evacuation of Children in Wartime: A Survey of the Literature, with Bibliography', *Psychoanalytic Study of the Child*, 1 (1945), pp. 389–404, on p. 389.
47. B. Wicks, *No Time to Wave Goodbye* (London: Bloomsbury, 1988).
48. For a further study of Bowlby's work in this area see, J. Bowlby, *Forty-Four Juvenile Thieves: Their Characters and Home Life* (London: Bailliere, Tindall & Cox, 1946).
49. The Caldecott Nursery was founded in 1911 for children whose families, through poverty or neglect, could not care for them, and became known as the Caldecott Community when evacuated during the First World War.
50. Report of the Provisional National Council for Mental Health, 1943–4, p. 22.
51. Letter from Lowndes (Board of Education) to Evelyn Fox (MHEC), 9 February 1942, NA, HLG 97/296.
52. A. Freud and D. Burlingham, *Young Children in Wartime in a Residential Nursery* (London: Allen & Unwin, 1942). The Hampstead nursery accommodated 138 children (of which thirty-five were non-resident).
53. Freud and Burlingham, *Young Children in Wartime*, p. 42.

54. Ibid., pp. 75–6.
55. Ibid., p. 42.
56. J. Kanter, 'Residential Care with Evacuated Children: Lessons from Clare Winnicott', *Cyc-online*, 80 (September 2005), at http://www.cyc-net.org/cyc-online/cycol-0905-kanter.html [Accessed 1 November 2008].
57. P. H. J. H. Gosden, *Education in the Second World War: A Study in Policy and Administration* (London: Methuen, 1976), p. 176.
58. Today parents are actively involved in child guidance services. J. Hodgson, S. Mattison, E. Phillips and G. Pollack, 'Consulting Parents to Improve a Child Guidance Service', *Educational Psychology in Practice*, 17:3 (2001), pp. 263–72.
59. Stewart, 'I Thought You Would Want to Come and See His Home', p. 215.
60. J. Bowlby, 'Psychological Aspects', in Padley and Cole (eds), *Evacation Survey*, pp. 186–96.
61. Notes of an informal discussion between members of the Board of Education and the Inspectorate, 17 June 1943, NA, ED 10/216.
62. The 1944 Education Act changed and extended the official categories of children's handicap. However, it did not define the new categories, it merely empowered the Ministry of Education to do so, and this was done in 'The Handicapped Pupils and School Health Service Regulations', 1945.
63. Ministry of Education, *Pamphlet 30: Education of the Handicapped Pupil 1945–55* (London: HMSO, 1956).
64. H. Hendrick, 'Children and Social Policies', in H. Hendrick (ed.), *Child Welfare and Social Policy* (Bristol: Policy Press, 2005), p. 44.
65. Hendrick, *Child Welfare: Historical Dimensions*, pp. 125–40; Hendrick, 'Children and Social Policies', pp. 43–5.

11 Turner, 'Education, Training and Social Competence'

1. W. B. Dockrell, W. R. Dunn and A. Milne (eds), *Special Education in Scotland* (Edinburgh: Scottish Council for Research in Education, 1978), p. 2.
2. A. Borsay, *Disability and Social Policy in Britain since 1750: A History of Exclusion* (Basingstoke: Palgrave Macmillan, 2005), pp. 94–116.
3. P. Bartlett and D. Wright (eds), *Outside the Walls of the Asylum: The History of Care in the Community 1750–2000* (London: Athlone Press, 1999).
4. S. French (ed.), *An Oral History of the Education of Visually Impaired People: Telling Stories for Inclusive Futures* (New York: Edwin Mellen Press, 2006).
5. J. S. Hurt, *Outside the Mainstream: A History of Special Education* (London: Batsford, 1988); T. Cole, *Apart or A Part: Integration and the Growth of British Special Education* (Milton Keynes: Open University Press, 1989); D. Armstrong, *Experiences of Special Education: Re-evaluating Policy and Practice through Life Stories* (London: Routledge-Falmer, 2003).
6. P. Conrad, 'Medicalization and Social Control', *Annual Review of Sociology*, 18 (1992), pp. 209–32, on p. 210.
7. A. Carey, 'Beyond the Medical Model: A Reconsideration of "Feeblemindedness", Citizenship and Eugenic Restrictions', *Disability and Society*, 18:4 (2003), pp. 411–30, on p. 413.
8. House of Commons Commissioners Reports (1946–47), XI, Primary Education: Report of the Advisory Council of Education in Scotland, p. 107.

9. M. Choiko, 'The Teacher and the Child', paper given at Annual Conference of the Guild of Teachers of Backward Children, Leicester, 1963 (London: National Society for Mentally Handicapped Children, 1963).
10. Transcript of interview with Betty Dowling conducted and transcribed by Angela Turner, 2 March 2007, Scottish Oral History Centre Archive (hereafter SOHCA), University of Strathclyde, SOHCA/024/6 (hereafter BD interview).
11. Education Act (1944).
12. J. R. Mercer, 'Sociological Perspectives on Mild Mental Retardation', in W. Swann (ed.) *The Practice of Special Education* (Oxford: Blackwell, 1981), p. 14; See also, document titled 'The Handicapped', undated, Glasgow University Archives, Thomas Ferguson Collection (hereafter GUA TFC), DC57/20.
13. Report of the Medical Officer of Health (hereafter MOH), City of Glasgow, Corporation of Glasgow (hereafter CG), 1961, p. 15–16. These MOH reports are available from the University of Strathclyde library.
14. Scottish Society for Mentally Handicapped Children (hereafter SSMHC, and after 1973 SSMH), Newsletter (June 1963), p. 3, ENABLE Collection, 9 Lynedoch Street, Glasgow; Also SSMHC, Newsletter (September 1968), p. 2.
15. R. K. McKnight, 'The Development of Child Guidance Services', in Dockrell, Dunn and Milne (eds) *Special Education in Scotland* , pp. 97–109, on pp. 100–4.
16. J. Stewart, 'Child Guidance in Interwar Scotland: International Influences and Domestic Concerns', *Bulletin of the History of Medicine*, 80:3 (2006), pp. 513–39, on p. 513.
17. F. J. Schonell, *Backwardness in the Basic Subjects* (Edinburgh: Oliver and Boyd, 1945), p. vi.
18. N. Munn, *Psychology: The Fundamentals of Human Adjustment* (London: George G. Harrap, 1946), pp. 11–15.
19. The Corporation of Glasgow, *Report of the Working Party on the Provision Made for Slow Learning Children in the First Two Years of Secondary School*, June, 1972, p. 18
20. McKnight, 'The Development of Child Guidance Services', p. 97.
21. Munn, *Psychology*, p. 424.
22. Ibid., p. 423.
23. 'Handicapped Children', 1945, GUA TFC, DC 57/104.
24. Ministry of Education, *Special Educational Treatment*, Pamphlet No. 5 (HMSO, London, 1946), Cmnd. 6922, pp. 18–19.
25. D. M. McIntish, 'Discussion of Mental Survey', Association of Directors of Education Conference Reports, 1 November 1946; G. Thomson, 'Scottish Mental Survey', Association of Directors of Scottish Education, Conference Reports, 13 May 1949; W. McLelland, 'Selection for Secondary Education', all in *Publications for the Scottish Council for Research in Education XIX* (London: University of London Press, 1949).
26. McLelland, 'Selection for Secondary Education'.
27. 'Average Intelligence Lower Each Generation', *Glasgow Herald*, 4 January 1952, p. 3.
28. The Association for the Directors of Education in Scotland (hereafter ADES) Conference Reports, 26 May 1944, Jordanhill Archives (hereafter JA), University of Strathclyde, Archives of the ADES.
29. Hansard: *Orders of the Day, Education Bill* (355), XXVII, 1944, cols 208–16.
30. 'Handicapped Children', *Glasgow Herald*, 4 December 1950, p. 3.
31. Ministry of Education, *Special Educational Treatment*, p. 36.
32. Munn, *Psychology*, p. 423.
33. 'Handicapped Children', 1950, GUA TFC, DC57/20.

34. ADES Conference Reports, 3 November 1946, JA, Archives of the ADES, ADESC5.
35. E. A. Broadly and B. Rogerson, 'A School Leavers Programme', in Scottish Council for Educational Technology (hereafter SCET), Occasional Working Paper 1 (hereafter OWP1), *Resources in Special Education* (1975), pp. 11–12.
36. BD Interview.
37. Scottish Education Department (SED), *The Education of Mildly Mentally Handicapped Pupils of Secondary School Age* (Edinburgh: HMSO, 1981), p. 30.
38. G. F. Mackay, 'The Named Person in Context', in *The Named Person*, A Set of Papers based on a series of meetings held in November and December, Jordanhill College of Education 1984, p. 4. These papers are archived in JA.
39. SED, *The Education of Mildly Mentally Handicapped Pupils*, p. 30.
40. BD Interview.
41. Corporation of the City of Glasgow (hereafter CG), *Backward Pupils in Secondary Schools*, 1947, p. 6.
42. Ibid., p. 7.
43. F. McKee (Psychologist, Glasgow Child Guidance Service), 'Social Education for the Mentally Handicapped', in SCET, OWP1, *Resources in Special Education* (1975), pp. 37–8.
44. P. Feely, '"The Kerr Family" in St Aidens School, Glasgow', SCET, OWP1, *Resources in Special Education* (1975), p. 40.
45. SED, *The Education of Pupils with Learning Difficulties in Primary and Secondary Schools in Scotland: A Progress Report by H. M. Inspectors of Schools, Scottish Education Department* (HMSO, Edinburgh, 1978), p. 5
46. BD Interview.
47. Ibid.
48. Ibid.
49. Ibid.
50. SSMH, Newsletter (February 1977), p. 6.
51. M. Egan, 'The "Manufacture" of Mental Defectives: Why the Number of Mental Defectives Increased in Scotland, 1857–1939', in P. Dale and J. Melling (eds), *Mental Illness and Learning Disability Since 1850: Finding a Place for Mental Disorder in the United Kingdom* (London: Routledge, 2006), pp. 131–53.
52. For history of this organization see document created by M. Benathan, A. Rimmer and T. Cole at http://www.sebda.org/information/SEBDA_history.pdf [accessed 5 November 2010].
53. Cole, *Apart*, p. 104.
54. Ibid., p. 104.
55. Ibid., p. 169.
56. Armstrong, *Experiences*, p. 78 and p. 80.
57. Cole, *Apart*, p. 154.
58. Pupils in Glasgow accounted for about a third of the children (estimated in 1974 to be 8,000–10,000) diagnosed as mentally handicapped and attending special schools in Scotland. See M. M. Clark, 'A Study of Ascertainment for Special Education in Scotland 1973–75', and A. Milne, 'Current Provision in Special Education in Scotland', both in Dockrell, Dunn and Milne (eds), *Special Education in Scotland*, pp. 76–92, and pp. 117–25, on p. 120.
59. Report of the MOH, CG, 1962, p. 107.
60. Ibid., (1963), p. 105.

61. Ibid., (1970), p. 82.
62. Cole, *Apart*, p. 131.
63. Ibid., p. 136.
64. Ibid.
65. SED, *The Education of Mildly Mentally Handicapped Pupils*, p. 7.
66. Cole, *Apart*, p. 154.
67. Ibid., p. 158.
68. Ibid.
69. SED, *The Education of Mildly Mentally Handicapped Pupils*, p. 15
70. Report of the MOH, CG, 1962, p. 207.
71. Scottish Health Service Planning Council, *A Better Life: Report on Services for the Mentally Handicapped in Scotland,* A report by a programme planning group of the Scottish Health Service Planning Council and the Advisory Council on Social Work (HMSO, Edinburgh, 1971), p. 37.
72. Letter from European Social Fund, Association of Directors of Social Work Archive (hereafter ADSWA), Glasgow Caledonian University Library, Association of Directors of Social Work Executive Committee Minutes (hereafter ADSW ECM), ADSWA1/1.1.62.
73. ADSW ECM, 2 May 1979, ADSWA1/1.1.66.
74. SCET, OWP1, *Resources in Special Education*, 1975, Introduction.
75. Secretary of State for Scotland, *Special Education: An Extract of the Report of the Secretary of State for Scotland on Education in Scotland in 1966* (HMSO; Edinburgh, 1967), p. 3.
76. BD Interview.
77. H. Jones, C. Kemp and F. McIlhenny, *Still at School: A Report of a Research Project into School Provision for Young People Over 16 Years of Age Recorded as Having Moderate Learning Difficulties*, Division of Special Educational Needs, Jordanhill College, 1989, p. 22. This report is archived in JA.
78. S. Tomlinson, 'Professionals and ESN (M) Education', in Swann (ed.), *The Practice of Special Education*, pp. 260–79, on p. 265.
79. M. Blythman, 'The Education of Pupils with Learning Difficulties in Mainstream Schools in Scotland', in The Joint Committee of Colleges of Education in Scotland, *Ten Years On, A Review of Developments since the Publication of the HMI Report 'The Education of Pupils with Learning Difficulties in Primary and Secondary Schools in Scotland'* (October 1988), p. 4.
80. SSMH, Newsletter (February 1977), p. 26.
81. J. Reid, 'Description of a Urban Special School-The Mary Russell School in Glasgow', in Dockrell, Dunn and Milne (eds), *Special Education in Scotland*, pp. 24–9, on pp. 26–7.
82. Interview with Marilyn Goodson carried out by Angela Turner, 13 February 2006, SOCHA/024/4 (hereafter MG interview).
83. Interview with David Colston carried out by Angela Turner, 24 February 2006, SOHCA/024/3.
84. BD Interview.
85. MG Interview.
86. Ibid.
87. 'Keith', quoted in Armstrong, *Experiences*, p. 52.
88. 'Trevor', quoted in Armstrong, *Experiences*, p. 58.
89. National Prospectus: Diplomas in Special Educational Needs, JA, JCE/12/18/13x.

90. A. Peacock and K. Denvir, *Scottish Postgraduate Research into Maladjustment 1974–1983* (Edinburgh: Scottish Council for Research into Education, 1985).
91. Strathclyde Department of Education, Glasgow Council for Remedial Education in Secondary Schools, *Report of a Working Party on Remedial Education* (1984), p. 10.
92. SCET, OWP1, *Resources in Special Education*, p. 4.
93. M. Warnock, 'The Way Forward', from the *Times Educational Supplement*, reprinted in SSMH, Newsletter (January 1979), pp. 8–11.
94. BD Interview.
95. Cole, *Apart*, p. 132.
96. Milne, 'Current Provision in Special Education in Scotland', p. 121.
97. H. M. Inspectors of Schools (in collaboration with colleagues from Scottish Home and Health Department and Social Work Services Group), *Provision for Profoundly Mentally Handicapped Children, Three Years On* (June 1980), p. 10
98. Jones, Kemp, and McIlhenny, *Still at School,* p. 30
99. *SDSA News*, Magazine of the Scottish Down's Syndrome Association, 24 (Summer 1990).
100. Strathclyde Regional Council, Department of Education, *Every Child is Special: A Policy for All* (1992), p. 6.
101. Borsay, *Disability and Social Policy*, p. 137.

12 Smith, 'Hyperactivity and American History'

1. I use the term hyperactivity because it has been the term most commonly employed, recognized and understood by patients, parents and physicians during the last fifty years. Hyperactivity has also been called minimal brain damage, minimal brain dysfunction, hyperkinesis and Attention Deficit Disorder (ADD). ADHD was not readily employed until the 1990s. Centers for Disease Control and Prevention (hereafter CDC), 'Summary Health Statistics for U.S. Children: National Health Interview Survey, 2006', *Vital and Health Statistics*, 10:234 (2007), p. 5, at http://www.cdc.gov/nchs/data/series/sr_10/sr10_234.pdf [accessed 9 June 2010]; CDC, 'Diagnosed Attention Deficit Hyperactivity Disorder and Learning Disability: United States, 2004–2006', *Vital and Health Statistics*, 10:237 (2007), at http://www.cdc.gov/nchs/data/series/sr_10/Sr10_237.pdf [accessed 9 June 2010].
2. Cincinnati Children's Hospital Medical Center, 'Study Shows ADHD Underdiagnosed and Undertreated', at http://www.cincinnatichildrens.org/health/subscribe/ped-insights/01-08/adhd-study.htm [accessed 9 June 2010]; P. Conrad, *Identifying Hyperactive Children: The Medicalization of Deviant Behavior* (Toronto: Lexington Books, 1976); P. Schrag and D. Divoky, *The Myth of the Hyperactive Child: And Other Means of Child Control* (1975; New York: Penguin, 1982).
3. For more on the debates about adult hyperactivity, see: M. Smith, 'A History Lesson', *BMJ*, 340:4 (2010), p. 2241; J. Moncrieff and S. Timimi, 'Is ADHD a Valid Diagnosis in Adults? No', *BMJ*, 340:3 (2010), p. 547; P. Asherson and colleagues, 'Is ADHD a Valid Diagnosis in Adults? Yes', *BMJ*, 340:3 (2010), p. 549.
4. P. S. Latham and P. H. Latham, 'Attention Deficit Hyperactivity Disorder ADHD, Education, and the Law', *NYU Child Study Center*, 3 (1998), pp. 1–4.
5. D. M. Hamner, 'Pathologizing Behaviors: The Case of Attention-Deficit/Hyperactivity Disorder' (PhD dissertation, Boston University, 1998); C. Malacrida, 'Alternative Therapies and Attention Deficit Disorder: Discourses of Maternal Responsibility and Risk',

Gender and Society, 16:3 (2002), pp. 366–85; A. Rafalovich, *Framing ADHD Children: A Critical Examination of the History, Discourse, and Everyday Experience of Attention Deficit/Hyperactivity Disorder* (Lanham, Md.: Lexington Books, 2004); I. Singh, 'Bad Boys, Good Mothers, and the Miracle of Ritalin', *Science in Context*, 15:4 (2002), pp. 577–602; I. Singh, 'Biology in Context: Social and Cultural Perspectives on ADHD', *Children and Society*, 16:5 (2002), pp. 360–7; I. Singh, 'Boys Will Be Boys: Fathers' Perspectives on ADHD Symptoms, Diagnosis, and Drug Treatment', *Harvard Review of Psychiatry*, 11:6 (2003), pp. 308–16; I. Singh, 'Doing Their Jobs: Mothering with Ritalin in a Culture of Mother Blame', *Social Science and Medicine*, 59:6 (2004), pp. 1193–1205.

6.   M. T. Brancaccio, 'Education Hyperactivity: The Historical Emergence of a Concept', *Intercultural Education*, 11:2 (2000), pp. 165–77; A. Lakoff, 'Adaptive Will: The Evolution of Attention Deficit Disorder', *Journal of the History of the Behavioral Sciences*, 36:2 (2000), pp. 149–69; R. Mayes and A. Rafalovich, 'Suffer the Restless Children: The Evolution of ADHD and Paediatric Stimulant Use, 1900–1980', *History of Psychiatry*, 18:4 (2007), pp. 435–57; N. Moon, 'The Amphetamine Years: A Study of the Medical Applications and Extramedical Consumption of Psychostimulant Drugs in the Postwar United States, 1945–1980' (PhD dissertation, Georgia Institute of Technology, 2009); A. Rafalovich, 'The Conceptual History of Attention Deficit/Hyperactivity Disorder: Idiocy, Imbecility, Encephalitis, and the Child Deviant', *Deviant Behavior*, 22:2 (2001), pp. 93–115.

7.   H. Hoffman, *Struwwelpeter: Merry Stories and Funny Pictures* (1844; New York: Frederick Warne and Co., Inc., 1848), http:www.gutenberg.org/files/12116/12116-h/12116-h.htm [accessed 10 January 2011].

8.   For more on the prehistory of hyperactivity, see M. Smith, 'The Uses and Abuses of the History of Hyperactivity', in L. Graham (ed.), *(De)constructing ADHD: Critical Guidance for Teachers and Teacher Educators* (New York: Peter Lang, 2010), pp. 21–39.

9.   For a recent take on the broader history of intellectual disability, see A. C. Carey, *On the Margins of Citizenship: Intellectual Disability and Civil Rights in Twentieth Century America* (Philadelphia, PA: Temple University Press, 2009).

10.   M. W. Laufer, E. Denhoff and G. Solomons, 'Hyperkinetic Impulse Disorder in Children's Behavior Problems', *Psychosomatic Medicine*, 19:1 (1957), pp. 38–49, on p. 48.

11.   Ibid., p. 39.

12.   H. Fischer, '50 Years Ago in the *Journal of Pediatrics*: Hyperkinetic Behavior Syndrome in Children', *Journal of Pediatrics*, 150:5 (2007), p. 520.

13.   For example, G. F. Still, 'The Goulstonian Lectures on Some Abnormal Psychical Conditions in Children. Lecture I', *Lancet*, 159:4102 (1902), pp. 1008–12, on p. 1008.

14.   Laufer, Denhoff and Solomons, 'Hyperkinetic Impulse Disorder', p. 45.

15.   J. J. Brumberg, *Fasting Girls: The History of Anorexia Nervosa* (Cambridge, MA: Harvard University Press, 1989); A. Young, *The Harmony of Illusions: Inventing Posttraumatic Stress Disorder* (Princeton, NJ: Princeton University Press, 1995).

16.   M. Smith, 'Putting Hyperactivity in its Place: Cold War Politics, the Brain Race and the Origins of Hyperactivity in the United States, 1957–1968', in E. Dyck and C. Fletcher (eds), *Locating Health* (London: Pickering and Chatto, 2011), pp. 57–69.

17.   I. Bernstein, *Promises Kept: John F. Kennedy's New Frontier* (New York: Oxford University Press, 1991), p. 219; E. T. May, *Homeward Bound: American Families in the Cold War Era* (1988; New York: Basic Books, 1999), p. 76, and pp. 120–1; D. Owram, *Born at the Right Time: A History of the Baby-Boom Generation* (Toronto: University of Toronto Press, 1996), p. 6, and p. 116.

18. P. L. Gardner, 'Guidance: An Orientation for the Classroom Teacher', *Clearing House*, 36 (1961–2), pp. 36–8, on p. 38.
19. Laufer, Denhoff and Solomons, 'Hyperkinetic Impulse Disorder', p. 46.
20. J. B. Conant, *The American High School Today: A First Report to Interested Citizens* (New York: McGraw-Hill, 1959), pp. 44–5.
21. A. S. Knowles, 'For the Space Age: Education as an Instrument of National Policy', *Phi Delta Kappa*, 39 (1958), pp. 305–10; Conant, *The American High School Today*; H. G. Rickover, *American Education – A National Failure: The Problem of Our Schools and What We Can Learn from England* (New York: E. P. Dutton, 1963); M. Rafferty, *Suffer Little Children* (New York: Devin-Adair, 1963); M. Rafferty, *What They Are Doing to Your Children* (New York: New American Library, 1964); M. Rafferty, *Max Rafferty on Education* (New York: Devin-Adair, 1968).
22. D. Ravitch, *The Troubled Crusade: American Education, 1945–1980* (New York: Basic Books, 1983), pp. 43–6.
23. H. Ozmon, 'Progressive Education and Some of its Critics', *Peabody Journal of Education*, 43:3 (1965), pp. 169–74.
24. K. Reeves, 'Each in His Own Good Time', *Grade Teacher*, 74 (1956–7), p. 8 and p. 117, on p. 8.
25. A. Davids and J. Sidman, 'A Pilot Study – Impulsivity, Time Orientation, and Delayed Gratification in Future Scientists and Underachieving High School Students', *Exceptional Children*, 29:4 (1962–3), pp. 170–4, on p. 170.
26. Ibid., p. 174.
27. For more discussion about how children have been similarly perceived in New Labour Britain see, H. Hendrick, 'The Child as Social Actor in Historical Sources: Problems of Identification and Interpretation', in P. Christensen and A. James (eds) *Research with Children: Perspectives and Practices* (London: Falmer Press, 2000), pp. 36–62; H. Hendrick, *Child Welfare: Historical Dimensions, Contemporary Debate* (Bristol: The Policy Press, 2003).
28. D. Barclay, 'A Turn for the Wiser', *Pediatrics*, 23:4 (1959), pp. 759–60, on p. 760.
29. Anon., 'Millions of Children Need Psychiatric Aid', *JAMA*, 209:3 (1969), p. 356.
30. D. Healy, *The Antidepressant Era* (Cambridge, MA: Harvard University Press, 1997), pp. 43–77.
31. Ibid., pp. 180–1; D. Healy, *Let Them Eat Prozac: The Unhealthy Relationship Between the Pharmaceutical Industry and Depression* (New York: New York University Press, 2004), p. xii, and pp. 1–5; D. Herzberg, *Happy Pills in America: From Miltown to Prozac* (Baltimore, MD: Johns Hopkins University Press, 2009), p. 4.
32. C. Bradley, 'The Behavior of Children Receiving Benzedrine', *American Journal of* Psychiatry, 94:3 (1937), pp. 577–85; Anon., 'New Drug Rouses Mental Patients', *Science News-Letter*, 68 (1955), p. 184; N. Rasmussen, *On Speed: The Many Lives of Amphetamine* (New York: New York University Press, 2008), p. 136, and p. 156; N. Moon, 'The Amphetamine Years', pp. 74–7.
33. D. Mahler, 'Review of the Film: The Hyperactive Child', *Exceptional Children*, 38 (1971–1972), p. 161; Schrag and Divoky, *Myth of the Hyperactive Child*, pp. 80–4.
34. D. M. Ross and S. A. Ross, *Hyperactivity: Research, Theory, and Action* (New York: John Wiley & Sons, 1976), p. 99.
35. R. L. Jenkins, 'Classification of Behavior Problems of Children', *American Journal of Psychiatry*, 125:8 (1969), pp. 1032–9, on pp. 1032–3; M. Smith, 'Psychiatry Limited:

Hyperactivity and the Evolution of American Psychiatry, 1957–1980', *Social History of Medicine*, 21:3 (2008), pp. 541–59.

36. P. F. Kernberg, 'The Problem of Organicity in the Child: Notes on Some Diagnostic Techniques in the Evaluation of Children', *Journal of the American Academy of Child Psychiatry*, 8:3 (1969), p. 8, and pp. 517–41, on p. 537; L. Eisenberg, A. Gilbert, L. Cyrtyn and P. A. Molling, 'The Effectiveness of Psychotherapy Alone and in Conjunction with Perphenazine or Placebo in the Treatment of Neurotic and Hyperkinetic Children', *American Journal of Psychiatry*, 116:12 (1961), pp. 1088–93.

37. Maurice Laufer, quoted in R. Reinhold, 'Drugs that Help Control the Unruly Child', *New York Times*, 5 July 1970, p. 96.

38. Eric Denhoff quoted in Reinhold, 'Drugs that Help', p. 96.

39. C. K. Conners and L. Eisenberg, 'The Effects of Methylphenidate on Symptomology and Learning in Disturbed Children', *American Journal of Psychiatry*, 120:5 (1963), pp. 454–64.

40. B. Ehrenreich and D. English, *For Her Own Good: 150 Years of the Experts' Advice to Women* (Garden City, NY: Anchor Books, 1979); R. Apple, *Perfect Motherhood: Science and Childrearing in America* (New Brunswick, NJ: Rutgers University Press, 2006).

41. Singh, 'Bad Boys', p. 593.

42. Telephone Interview with L. Freeman, conducted by Matthew Smith, 28 January 2008.

43. Ibid.

44. Ibid.

45. R. Reinhold, 'Learning Parley Divided on Drugs', *New York Times*, 6 February 1968, p. 40.

46. R. Schnackenberg, 'Caffeine as a Substitute for Schedule II Stimulants in Hyperkinetic Children', *American Journal of Psychiatry*, 130:7 (1973), pp. 796–8.

47. M. Smith, 'Into the Mouths of Babes: Hyperactivity, Food Additives and the Reception of the Feingold Diet', in M. Jackson (ed.) *Health and the Modern Home* (New York: Routledge, 2007), pp. 304–21; M. Smith, *An Alternative History of Hyperactivity: Food Additives and the Feingold Diet* (New Brunswick, NJ: Rutgers University Press, 2011).

48. J. S. Werry, 'Food Additives and Hyperactivity', *Medical Journal of Australia*, 2:8 (1976), pp. 281–2, on p. 282.

49. D. McCann et al., 'Food Additives and Hyperactive Behaviour in 3-Year-Old and 8/9-Year-Old Children in the Community: A Randomised, Double-Blinded, Placebo-Controlled Trial', *Lancet,* 370:9598 (2007), pp. 1560–7.

50. A. Schonwald, 'ADHD and Food Additives Revisited', *AAP Grand Rounds,* 19 (2008), p. 17.

51. T. Hartman, *The Edison Gene: ADHD and the Gift of the Hunter Child* (Rochester, VT: Park Street Press, 2003).

52. For an early British take on hyperactivity, see Anon., 'Hyperactivity', *Lancet*, 312: 8089 (1978), p. 561.

INDEX

0 1341 1571774 3

DATE DUE	RETURNED